PCCN® EXAM PREP
STUDY GUIDE

PCCN® EXAM PREP
STUDY GUIDE

No part of this publication may be reproduced, stored in a retrieval system, or transmitted in any form or by any means, electronic, mechanical, photo-copying, recording, or otherwise, without the prior permission of Springer Publishing Company, LLC, or authorization through payment of the appropriate fees to the Copyright Clearance Center, Inc., 222 Rosewood Drive, Danvers, MA 01923, 978-750-8400, fax 978-646-8600, info@copyright.com or at www.copyright.com.

Springer Publishing Company, LLC
11 West 42nd Street, New York, NY 10036
www.springerpub.com

Acquisitions Editor: Jaclyn Koshofer
Compositor: Exeter Premedia Services Private Ltd.

ISBN: 978-0-8261-6402-5
ebook ISBN: 978-0-8261-6407-0
DOI: 10.1891/ 9780826164070

23 24 25 26 / 5 4 3 2 1

The author and the publisher of this Work have made every effort to use sources believed to be reliable to provide information that is accurate and com-patible with the standards generally accepted at the time of publication. The author and publisher shall not be liable for any special, consequential, or exemplary damages resulting, in whole or in part, from the readers' use of, or reliance on, the information contained in this book. The publisher has no responsibility for the persistence or accuracy of URLs for external or third-party Internet websites referred to in this publication and does not guarantee that any content on such websites is, or will remain, accurate or appropriate.

PCCN® is a registered trademark of the American Association of Critical-Care Nurses (AACN). AACN does not endorse this resource, nor does it have a proprietary relationship with Springer Publishing Company.

Library of Congress Control Number: 2023930029

Contact sales@springerpub.com to receive discount rates on bulk purchases.

Publisher's Note: **New and used products purchased from third-party sellers are not guaranteed for quality, authenticity, or access to any included digital components.**

Printed in the United States of America by Gasch Printing.

CONTENTS

PREFACE

This *Exam Prep Study Guide* was designed to be a high-speed review—a last-minute gut check before your exam day. We created this review to supplement your certification preparation studies. We encourage you to use it in conjunction with other study aids to ensure you are as prepared as possible for the exam.

This book follows the American Association of Critical-Care Nurses' most recent exam content outlines and uses a succinct, bulleted format to highlight what you need to know. The aim of this book is to help you solidify your retention of information in the month or so leading up to your exam. It is written by certified progressive care nurses who are familiar with the exam and the content you need to know. Special features appear throughout the book to call out important information, including:

- **Complications**: Problems that can arise with certain disease states or procedures
- **Nursing Pearls**: Additional patient care insights and strategies for knowledge retention
- **Alerts**: Need-to-know details on how to handle emergency situations or when to transfer care
- **Pop Quizzes**: Critical-thinking questions to test your ability to synthesize what you learned (answers in the back of the book)
- **Two Full-Length Practice Tests:** One printed in the book, one online
- **Free One-Month Access to ExamPrepConnect:** The digital study platform that guides you confidently through your exam prep journey

We know life is busy. Being able to prepare for your exam efficiently and effectively is paramount, which is why we created this *Exam Prep Study Guide*. You have come to the right place as you continue on your path of professional growth and development. The stakes are high, and we want to help you succeed. Best of luck to you on your certification journey. You've got this!

PASS GUARANTEE

1 ABOUT THE EXAMINATION

OVERVIEW

Congratulations on taking one step closer to becoming a progressive care certified nurse (PCCN). The PCCN® examination is written and administered by the American Association of Critical-Care Nurses (AACN) and accredited by the National Commission for Certifying Agencies (NCCA). This exam is designed for RNs and APRNs who practice in progressive care units or provide direct care for acutely ill patients.

PCCN CERTIFICATION REQUIREMENTS

To be eligible to sit for the PCCN® exam, test takers must meet the following requirements:

- Have a current, unencumbered nursing license as either an RN or APRN in the United States.
- Meet the requirements of either of the following: Minimum of 2 years of direct care of acutely ill patients, totaling 1,750 clinical hr, with 875 of those hr obtained in the year before application; or have 5 years and at least 2,000 clinical hr of direct care of acutely ill patients, with 144 of those hr in the most recent year before application.
- Be prepared to provide the name and contact information for a direct supervisor or coworker who can verify clinical hr fulfillment.

ABOUT THE EXAMINATION

- The PCCN® examination is a 2.5-hr exam with 125 multiple choice questions.
- Of the 125 multiple choice questions, 100 are scored, and 25 are sample test questions to be used on future exams.
- Passing point/cutoff score: A passing point/cutoff score is predetermined by the exam development committee who carefully reviews each examination question to determine the basic level of knowledge or skill that is expected. The passing point/cutoff score is based on the panel's established difficulty ratings for each examination question. Test takers who meet or exceed this passing point/cutoff score will become PCCN certified.
- Test plan: The test covers two main topics: Clinical Judgment and Professional Caring/Ethical Practice. Clinical Judgment accounts for 80% of the questions and covers each body system, as well as its related diagnostic tests and nursing interventions. Questions are further broken down by body system and include the following topics: Cardiovascular (27%), Pulmonary (17%), Endocrine/Hematology/Neurology/Gastrointestinal/Renal (20%), and Musculoskeletal/Multisystem/Psychosocial (16%). Professional Caring/Ethical Practice accounts for 20% of the questions and includes the following topics: Advocacy/Moral Agency, Caring Practices, Response to Diversity, Facilitation of Learning, Collaboration, Systems Thinking, and Clinical Inquiry.

HOW TO APPLY

- To apply to take the PCCN® examination or for additional information, visit the AACN website at www .aacn.org/certification/get-certified or download the PCCN® Exam Handbook from the AACN's website.
- The examination cost for AACN members is $195, and the cost for nonmembers is $300.
- After applying, there is a 90-day window for scheduling and taking the exam at a PSI testing center.

HOW TO RECERTIFY

- After successfully passing the PCCN® examination, certification is active for 3 years.
- Online renewal is available to active PCCN certifications 4 months before the scheduled renewal date.
- Nurses who want to recertify must have completed at least 432 hr actively working clinically in acute or critical care. At least 144 of those hr need to be in the year leading up to recertification.
- Certification holders may renew through the following: *Continuing Education Recognition Program (CERP)*: Complete 100 CERP points in the following: *Category A:* Clinical Judgment/Clinical Inquiry (60 to 80 points), *Category B:* Advocacy and Moral Agency, Caring Practices, Response to Diversity, and Facilitation of Learning (10 to 30 points), and *Category C:* Collaboration, and Systems Thinking (10 to 30 points). *Examination*: Take the PCCN certification exam. *Inactive status*: Nurses can change their status to inactive if they do not meet the criteria for renewal. Inactive status extends the time frame by 3 years to meet the eligibility requirements for recertification. Nurses may not use the PCCN credential while inactive.
- For more information on certification renewal, visit www.aacn.org/certhandbooks.

AACN CONTACT INFORMATION

For more information, visit the AACN website at www.aacn.org/certification/get-certified/pccn-adult. The AACN can also be reached as follows:

- Main Office: (800) 809-2273 available Monday to Friday 7:30 a.m. to 5:30 p.m. PT
- Customer Care: (800) 899-2226 available Monday to Friday 7:30 a.m. to 4:30 p.m. PT
- Mailing Address:
  American Association of Critical-Care Nurses
  27071 Aliso Creek Road
  Aliso Viejo, CA 92656-3399

RESOURCES

American Association of Critical-Care Nurses. (2022, October). *PCCN exam handbook: Acute/critical care nursing certification adult*. https://www.aacn.org/~/media/aacn-website/certification/get-certified/handbooks/ pccnexamhandbook.pdf

American Association of Critical-Care Nurses. (n.d.-a). *PCCN (adult): Initial eligibility requirements & fees*. https:// www.aacn.org/certification/get-certified/pccn-adult

American Association of Critical-Care Nurses. (n.d.-b). *PCCN (adult): Renewal eligibility requirements & fees*. https:// www.aacn.org/certification/certification-renewal/pccn-adult?tab=Renewal%20by%20Synergy%20CERPs

ACUTE CORONARY SYNDROME

Overview

- Acute coronary syndrome (ACS) describes a group of conditions resulting from a sudden obstruction of the coronary arteries.
- ACS can manifest in three ways: non-ST-elevation myocardial infarction (NSTEMI), ST-elevation myocardial infarction (STEMI), and unstable angina.
- Treatments range from medical management to invasive procedures inducing cardiac catheterization or coronary artery bypass grafting (CABG).
- With timely recognition, ACS can be effectively treated and managed.

Signs and Symptoms

- Patients experiencing ACS may present with any of the following symptoms, with some symptoms varying depending on the manifestation of ACS (Table 2.1): anxiety, fear, or feelings of imminent demise; decreased pallor; diaphoresis; dyspnea; extra heart sounds (S3, S4, and/or holosystolic murmurs); fatigue and weakness; initial hypertension and tachycardia, which progresses to hypotension; jugular vein distention (JVD); mental status changes; nausea and vomiting; severe chest pain, heaviness or pressure unrelieved by rest, position changes, and/or medication; palpitations; presyncope or syncope; and radiating pain to the chest, neck, jaw, arms, back, and/or epigastrium.

Diagnosis

Labs

- B-type natriuretic peptide (BNP) may be used.
- Cardiac enzymes: Creatine kinase (CK) may be elevated >308 U/L for men and >192 U/L for women. Creatine kinase-myocardial band (CK-MB) may be elevated >25 IU/L. Troponin may be elevated >0.4 ng/mL. ▶

 COMPLICATIONS

A sudden coronary artery obstruction, if unrecognized and/or untreated, can cause decreased blood flow to the heart and, subsequently, decreased oxygenation of the heart. This can lead to cell injury, dysrhythmia, infarction, left ventricular failure, pericarditis, thromboembolism, and tissue injury, and can cause sudden death of the person. Immediate recognition and intervention of obstructions are necessary to prevent deteriorating conditions that can progress to cardiac arrest and death.

 NURSING PEARL

The difference between stable and unstable angina can be identified by symptom presentation. Stable angina involves chest pain that is precipitated by activity and relieved by rest and nitroglycerin. In contrast, unstable angina occurs at rest with no precipitating physical activity.

 ALERT!

Risk factors associated with ACS include age, diabetes, dyslipidemia, gender, genetics/family history, high fat diet, hypertension, obesity, sedentary lifestyle, and tobacco use. Nurses should recognize the potential development of ACS in high-risk patients.

 ALERT!

Symptoms and presentation of ACS can vary between gender and in those with diabetes mellitus and/or prior surgical history of CABG or cardiac transplantation. Women are more likely to present with atypical symptoms, such as jaw, neck, or upper back pain with dyspnea and/or fatigue. Patients with a history of diabetes mellitus, CABG, or cardiac transplant may present with silent ischemia, complaining of dyspnea and fatigue without angina.

TABLE 2.1 Acute Coronary Syndrome Categories

UNSTABLE ANGINA	NSTEMI	STEMI	SYMPTOMS
✓			Chest pain may be relieved by nitroglycerin
✓	✓	✓	Chest pain may occur at rest
✓	✓	✓	Chest pain has increased frequency and severity
✓	✓	✓	Chest pain lasts >20 minutes
		✓	Unrelenting chest pain
		✓	Patient has dyspnea, pallor, diaphoresis, or cool clammy skin
		✓	Patient has vagal symptoms (bradycardia, nausea, and vomiting)

NSTEMI, non-ST-elevation myocardial infarction; STEMI, ST-elevation myocardial infarction.

Labs (continued)
- C-reactive protein (CRP) may be elevated >10 mg/L.
- Comprehensive metabolic panel (CMP) may show elevated or low potassium or calcium, which may worsen kidney or liver functions.
- Complete blood count (CBC) can be utilized.
- Lipid panel may be normal or elevated.

Diagnostic Testing
- 12-lead EKG may show ST elevation (Table 2.2)
- Cardiac catheterization: coronary angiogram and percutaneous coronary intervention (PCI)
- Chest x-ray
- Continuous EKG monitoring
- Stress test
- Transthoracic echocardiogram (TTE)

[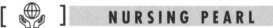]   **NURSING PEARL**

One popular mnemonic, MONA-B, can be used to recall the common medications used when treating ACS patients (morphine, oxygen, nitroglycerin, aspirin, and beta blockers).

TABLE 2.2 EKG Changes in ACS

EKG LEAD CHANGES	ANATOMICAL LOCATION	VESSEL(S) INVOLVED
V1–V2	Septal wall	LAD
V2–V4	Anterior LV	LAD
I, aVL	High lateral wall	Left circumflex
V5–V6	Low lateral LV	LAD
II, III, aVF	Inferior LV	RCA, left circumflex
V8–V9	Posterior wall	Posterior descending, RCA or left circumflex
V3R, V4R	Right ventricular	RCA

ACS, acute coronary syndrome; LAD, left anterior descending; LV, left ventricular; RCA, right coronary artery.

Treatment

- Requires timely diagnosis and intervention
- Immediate for suspected ACS: 12-lead EKG and continuous EKG monitoring; intravenous (IV) access, oxygen if indicated to maintain an oxygen saturation >90%
- Medications (Table 2.3): angiotensin-converting enzyme inhibitors (ACEI), antiplatelet inhibitors, anticoagulation, aspirin, beta-adrenergic blockers, fibrinolytic therapy (Table 5.1), morphine (Table A.2), nitroglycerin, and oxygen
- Possible cardiac catheterization or CABG (see Cardiac Catheterization section)

TABLE 2.3 Cardiovascular Medications

INDICATIONS	MECHANISM OF ACTION	CONTRAINDICATIONS, PRECAUTIONS, AND ADVERSE EFFECTS
ACEIs (e.g., lisinopril, enalapril, and captopril)		
• Left-sided HF • HTN	• Inhibit the conversion of angiotensin I to angiotensin II • Reduce vascular resistance to improve function of the left ventricle • Dilate veins, which decreases venous return	• Use with caution in patients experiencing hemodynamic instability and AKI. • Medication may need to be discontinued if patient develops new onset cough. • Monitor for signs of hyperkalemia and hypotension. • Avoid the use of two renin–aldosterone system inhibitors, especially in patients with renal failure. • Use with insulin or other antidiabetic agents may enhance hypoglycemic effect.
Alpha adrenergic blockers (e.g., prazosin and doxazosin)		
• BP control and management	• Vasodilate by blocking alpha 1 and 2 receptors	• Medication is contraindicated in hypotension. • Use with caution in patients with cataracts and older adults. • Adverse effects include hypotension, tachycardia, weakness, and tremors.
Antiarrhythmics, class 1-A (procainamide, disopyramide, and quinidine)		
• A-fib • V-tach • CPR	• Inhibit sodium transport through myocardial cells, prolonging the recovery period after repolarization thereby slowing the impulse and allowing for conversion	• Use with caution when administering in cardiogenic, hemorrhagic shock, hypotension, renal, or hepatic dysfunction. • Do not administer in patients with second- or third-degree AV block or SLE.
Antiarrhythmics, class 1-B (lidocaine)		
• Treatment of V-tach or V-fib	• Inhibit an influx of sodium in myocardial tissue, increasing recovery period after repolarization and allowing for conversion out of dysrhythmia	• Use with caution in geriatric patients, HF, hepatic disease, and hypotension.

(continued)

TABLE 2.3 Cardiovascular Medications (*continued*)

INDICATIONS	MECHANISM OF ACTION	CONTRAINDICATIONS, PRECAUTIONS, AND ADVERSE EFFECTS
Antiarrhythmics, class 1-C (flecainide, propafenone)		
• Prevention of ventricular dysrhythmias • Prevention or conversion of A-fib, atrial flutter, or SVT	• Inhibit sodium channels and shorten action potential of Purkinje fibers without impacting other myocardial tissues, thus preventing or converting dysrhythmias	• Hepatic and renal disease can alter excretion of flecainide. • Do not administer in patients with cardiogenic shock. • Use with caution with prolonged QRS or PR interval.
Antiarrhythmics, class II, beta blockers (e.g., atenolol and metoprolol)		
• Left- and right-sided HF • BP and HR control and management	• Block the effects of epinephrine and norepinephrine in the body to decrease HR, contractility, and vascular resistance • Reduce BP via vasodilation, thereby decreasing afterload	• Use with caution in patients with asthma, as it may cause bronchospasm. • Do not use in patients with heart blocks, sick sinus syndrome, or other bradycardias. • Use with other HR reducers can cause bradycardia.
Antiarrhythmics, class II and class III (sotalol)		
• Maintenance of NSR with symptomatic A-fib or atrial flutter	• Beta-blocking effects and class III antiarrhythmic activity to lengthen refractory period in cardiac tissue, allowing for maintenance of an NSR	• Do not abruptly discontinue. • Use with caution in hypotensive patients or patients with renal impairment.
Antiarrhythmics, class III (e.g., amiodarone and ibutilide)		
• Rate control with multiple tachydysrhythmias	• Delay of repolarization • Depress SA and AV node automaticity • Vasolytic effects resulting in slowed HR	• Amiodarone is not recommended in the context of HF cardiogenic shock due to negative inotropic effects. • Use with caution in patients with underlying heart block or hepatic impairment.
Antiarrhythimcs, class IV, calcium channel blockers (e.g., diltiazem)		
• Rate control with supraventricular tachydysrhythmias • Antihypertensive	• Inhibit calcium influx across myocardial and smooth muscle • Slow AV conduction	• Use with caution in patients with hypotension or HF.
Antiarrhythmics, miscellaneous (e.g., adenosine)		
• Narrow complex, monomorphic tachycardia • Wide complex tachycardia	• Stimulate adenosine-sensitive potassium channels in the atrial and sinoatrial node, causing outflow of potassium, resulting in sinus bradycardia	• Adenosine is contraindicated in patients with sinus node disease. • Use with caution in patients with Wolff–Parkinson–White syndrome. • This medication is not effective for A-fib, atrial flutter, or V-tach.

(*continued*)

TABLE 2.3 Cardiovascular Medications (*continued*)

INDICATIONS	MECHANISM OF ACTION	CONTRAINDICATIONS, PRECAUTIONS, AND ADVERSE EFFECTS
Antiarrhythmic, unclassified-cardiac glycosides (e.g., digoxin)		
• Left-sided symptomatic HF • Irregular heartbeat (such as atrial fibrillation)	• Slow conduction through the AV node to improve cardiac contractility in left-sided HF by eliciting a positive inotropic effect	• Hold for patients with digoxin toxicity, tachy/brady dysrhythmias, bradycardia, and AV block. • Hypokalemia, hypomagnesemia, and hypercalcemia exacerbate digoxin toxicity. • Do not administer to patients with Wolff–Parkinson–White syndrome or hypertrophic subaortic stenosis. • Use with caution in patients with impaired renal function, thyroid disease, and MI. • Medication may increase risk of digitalis toxicity when used with potassium-depleting diuretics. Use with digoxin and sympathomimetics or succinylcholine increases risk of cardiac dysythmias.
Anticholinergics (e.g., atropine and glycopyrrolate)		
• Bradycardia • Decrease oral secretions preoperatively or at end of life	• Competitively inhibit autonomic cholinergic receptors • Block parasympathetic actions on the heart, resulting in increased SA node rate	• Flushing of the face may occur, which does not indicate anaphylaxis. • Risk of tachycardia if dose above 2 to 3 mg.
Antidiuretic hormones (e.g., vasopressin)		
• Hypotension • Cardiogenic or septic shock • During cardiac arrest and after resuscitation • Central diabetes insipidus • GI bleeding	• Initiates antidiuretic effect by increasing water absorption at the renal collecting ducts • Stimulate contraction of smooth muscle and capillaries, small arterioles, and venules, resulting in increased BP	• Use with caution in patients with heart and renal failure, seizure disorders, migraines, asthma, CHF, CAD, and in older adults. • Adverse reactions include water intoxication, myocardial/mesenteric ischemia, hyponatremia, hypertension, headache, nausea, diarrhea, tremor, and abdominal pain.
Antiplatelets (e.g., aspirin and clopidogrel)		
• A-fib/A-flutter • CAD • PVD • Acute coronary syndrome • Postoperative antithrombotic prophylaxis	• Inhibit platelet aggregation	• Use with caution in patients with underlying conditions which may cause bleeding, including hepatic impairment and trauma. • Monitor for signs of bleeding. • Adverse effects include generalized bleeding, GI bleeding, and Stevens-Johnson syndrome (aspirin).

(*continued*)

TABLE 2.3 Cardiovascular Medications (*continued*)

INDICATIONS	MECHANISM OF ACTION	CONTRAINDICATIONS, PRECAUTIONS, AND ADVERSE EFFECTS
ARBs (e.g., valsartan and losartan)		
• Left-sided HF • HTN • Patients who cannot tolerate ACEIs due to renal function or other side effects	• Block the binding of angiotensin I to angiotensin II receptors	• Use with caution in patients experiencing hemodynamic instability and AKI. • Avoid use of two renin–aldosterone system inhibitors, especially in patients with renal failure. • Use with insulin or other antidiabetic agents may enhance hypoglycemic effect.
Beta blocker with alpha blockade (e.g., labetalol)		
• HTN, rate control	• Block beta 1 receptors in the heart • Block beta 2 receptors in the bronchial and vascular smooth muscle • Block alpha 1 receptors in vascular smooth muscle • Vasodilation and decreased PVR to decrease BP	• Medication is contraindicated in patients with severe bradycardia, AV block, cardiogenic shock, or prolonged hypotension or asthma. • Use with caution in pheochromocytoma, cerebrovascular disease, diabetes, hepatic disease, or while operating machinery. • Do not abruptly discontinue.
Calcium supplements (calcium chloride)		
• Treatment for hypocalcemia	• Supplement low-circulating calcium • Assist with maintaining homeostasis	• Calcium supplements are contraindicated in hypercalcemia and V-fib. • Do not give intramuscularly or subcutaneously. • Use with caution in hyperparathyroidism, nephrolithiasis, and sarcoidosis.
Corticosteroids (e.g., prednisone and dexamethasone)		
• Cardiac inflammation of autoimmune etiology	• Suppress inflammation and normal immune response	• Medication is contraindicated in patients who are pregnant or have active, untreated infections. It also should not be used together with live virus vaccines. • Use with caution in hypothyroidism and liver disease. • Adverse effects include thromboembolism, peptic ulcers, anorexia, nausea and vomiting, decreased wound healing, bruising, hyperglycemia, osteoporosis, and increased susceptibility to infection.

(continued)

TABLE 2.3 Cardiovascular Medications (*continued*)

INDICATIONS	MECHANISM OF ACTION	CONTRAINDICATIONS, PRECAUTIONS, AND ADVERSE EFFECTS
Diuretics: Aldosterone antagonists (e.g., spironolactone)		
• Left- and right-sided HF • For patients with fluid overload	• Block the effects of aldosterone in the body, thereby blocking sodium reabsorption, causing diuresis without loss of potassium	• Use with caution in patients who have renal failure, as medication is potassium sparing; hyperkalemia may occur. • Monitor magnesium levels as long-term use may cause increase in renal tubular reabsorption of magnesium, causing hypermagnesemia, especially in patients taking magnesium supplements. • Use with angiotensin II receptor antagonists, ACEIs, or ARBs may cause increased serum potassium levels and increased creatinine in patients with HF.
Diuretics: Loop diuretics (e.g., furosemide)		
• Left-sided HF with fluid overload • Right-sided HF for symptom management but in lower doses • Hypertension • Edema associated with liver cirrhosis and renal disease	• Inhibit sodium and chloride reabsorption at proximal and distal tubules and loop of Henle, causing excretion of sodium, potassium, magnesium, calcium, bicarbonate, and water	• Monitor for dehydration, AKI, GFR <30, and hypotension. • Monitor for pancreatitis, ototoxicity, and aplastic anemia. • Monitor for hypokalemia, hyponatremia, hypochloremia alkalosis, hyperglycemia, hyperuricemia, and hypocalcemia. • Monitor for digitalis toxicity when administering digoxin with loop diuretics. • Monitor and correct potassium levels when used with medications that potentiate hypokalemia: Corticosteroids, insulin, and beta antagonists.
Diuretics: Thiazide (hydrochlorothiazide)		
• Fluid overload • Pulmonary hypertension • HF • Hypertension	• Increase water excretion by inhibiting reabsorption of sodium and chloride at the distal tubules	• Diuretics are contraindicated in anuria and renal failure. • Use with caution in hepatic disease, hypotension, hypovolemia, and diabetes. • Adverse effects include photosensitivity, hypokalemia, and hyperglycemia.
Immunosuppressants (azathioprine)		
• Autoimmune-induced cardiac inflammation	• Suppress cell-mediated immunity and altered antibody function	• Medication is contradicted in concurrent use with mycophenolate. • Use caution in infection, cancer, radiation therapy, and severe renal impairment. • Adverse effects include chills, fever, nausea and vomiting, anorexia, hepatotoxicity, and pulmonary edema.

(continued)

TABLE 2.3 Cardiovascular Medications (*continued*)

INDICATIONS	MECHANISM OF ACTION	CONTRAINDICATIONS, PRECAUTIONS, AND ADVERSE EFFECTS
Inotropic agents (dobutamine, dopamine)		
• Left-sided HF • Patients who require positive inotropic support	• Improve stroke volume and cardiac output by beta adrenergic agonist action • Increases myocardial contractility (positive inotropic effects), chronotropy, and systemic vascular resistance	• Monitor electrolytes and renal function, as it may cause hypokalemia. • Monitor due to increased risk for ventricular dysrhythmias, especially in patients with atrial fibrillation. • Use with alpha blockers, vasodilators, and other adrenergic sympathomimetics may antagonize CV effects. • Do not use with beta blockers, as they will negate each other's effects.
IVIG		
• Autoimmune induced cardiac inflammation	• Inactivate autoreactive T-cells	• There are no contraindications. • Use with caution in critical illness. • Adverse effects include headache, fever, chills, fatigue, nausea, vomiting, tachycardia, pleural effusion, and acute renal failure.
Nitrates (e.g., nitroglycerin and isosorbide nitrates)		
• Stable or unstable angina • Adjunct therapy in MI • HTN (IV)	• Increase oxygenation to the coronary arteries, resulting in decreased preload and afterload, thus decreasing workload of the heart • Decrease cardiac workload to alleviate chest pain and lower BP	• Nitrates are contraindicated in patients with cardiac tamponade, constrictive pericarditis, or in patients taking PDE-5 inhibitors. • Use with caution in patients with hypovolemia, head trauma, cardiomyopathy, or cardioversion (transdermal patch). • Adverse effects include hypotension, tachycardia, headache, and dizziness.
Sympathomimetic agents (e.g., epinephrine, norepinephrine, phenylephrine)		
• Acute hypotension • Cardiogenic shock • Sepsis or septic shock • During cardiac arrest and after resuscitation	• Epinephrine: Nonselective adrenergic agonist and acts on both alpha and beta receptors, resulting in cardiac stimulation and arteriolar vasoconstriction • Norepinephrine: Acts on alpha-adrenergic receptors to increase systemic BP and coronary artery blood flow • Phenylephrine: Alpha-1 adrenergic agonist results in potent vasoconstriction	• Use with caution in hypovolemic, HTN, hyperthyroid, and closed angle glaucoma. • Caution should be observed to avoid extravasation. • Adverse effects include peripheral vasoconstriction or ischemia, tissue necrosis, PVCs, ST-T wave changes, and bradycardia.

(*continued*)

TABLE 2.3 Cardiovascular Medications (*continued*)

INDICATIONS	MECHANISM OF ACTION	CONTRAINDICATIONS, PRECAUTIONS, AND ADVERSE EFFECTS
Vasodilators (e.g., nitroglycerin and nitroprusside)		
• Hypertensive emergency • Stable or unstable angina • Adjunct therapy in MI • Hypertension • Acute HF • Mitral regurgitation	• Acts directly on arterial and venous smooth muscle, resulting in peripheral vasodilation and decreased left ventricular afterload, which lowers BP • Decreases myocardial oxygen demand	• Do not administer in aortic coarctation, AV shunt, or high output acute HF. • Nitroprusside can cause cyanide toxicity. Monitor plasma thiocyanate concentrations. • Nitrates are contraindicated in patients with cardiac tamponade, constrictive pericarditis, or in patients taking PDE-5 inhibitors. • Use with caution in patients with hypovolemia, head trauma, cardiomyopathy, or cardioversion (transdermal patch). • Adverse effects include hypotension, tachycardia, headache, and dizziness.

ACEI, angiotensin-converting enzyme inhibitors; A-fib, atrial fibrillation; AKI, acute kidney injury; ARB, angiotensin receptor blockers; AV, atrioventricular; BP, blood pressure; CAD, coronary artery disease; CHF, congestive heart failure; CV, cardiovascular; GFR, glomerular filtration rate; GI, gastrointestinal; HF, heart failure; HTN, hypertension; IVIG, intravenous immunoglobulin; MI, myocardial infarction; NSR, normal sinus rhythm; PVC, premature ventricular contraction; PVD, peripheral vascular disease; PVR, pulmonary vascular resistance; SA, sinoatrial; SLE, systemic lupus erythematosus; SVT, supraventricular tachycardia; V-fib, ventricular fibrillation; V-tach, ventricular tachycardia.

Nursing Interventions

- Assess and manage anxiety as needed.
- Draw serial laboratory tests as ordered and monitor results.
- Update patient and/or family on current clinical status, plan of care, and upcoming tests or procedures.
- Perform continuous physiologic monitoring through frequent physical assessment of cardiac, pulmonary, and neurologic systems for signs of worsening condition or complications.
- Monitor vital signs (VS): Maintain oxygenation and perfusion. Position patient with head of bed (HOB) >30°. Titrate appropriate oxygen delivery system to achieve oxygen saturation >90%. Use continuous SpO$_2$ monitoring. Prepare for transfer to higher level of care if hemodynamically unstable or unable to maintain adequate oxygenation and ventilation. Assess EKG monitoring system for presence of dysrhythmias. Assess for both hypertension and/or hypotension.
- See the Cardiac Catheterization section for information relating to cardiac catheterization treatment and management.

[ ]   **NURSING PEARL**

When monitoring vital signs for a patient experiencing ACS, blood pressure (BP) and heart rate (HR) may initially be elevated. As cardiac output decreases, the patient may develop acute hypotension. This decreased perfusion can result in acute kidney injury (AKI) and decreased urine output.

Patient Education

- Adhere to dietary recommendations as ordered for lipid and sodium control (Dietary Approaches to Stop Hypertension [DASH] diet).
- See the Cardiac Catheterization section for information on care of the femoral access site post cardiac catheterization. Increase physical activity as recommended. If referred by the provider, participate in a cardiac rehab program.
- Follow up as appropriate with outpatient appointments.
- Follow exercise and weight management recommendations.
- Pursue smoking cessation as advised.
- Take medication as prescribed.

ACUTE INFLAMMATORY DISEASE

Overview

- Acute inflammatory disease of the heart consists of endocarditis, myocarditis, and pericarditis. It can manifest with a wide range of signs and symptoms depending on etiology and type. *Endocarditis:* inflammation of the inner lining of the heart (endocardium). *Myocarditis:* inflammation of the middle layer of the heart (myocardium). *Pericarditis:* inflammation of the outermost layer of the heart (pericardium).
- Treatments include lifestyle modifications, medications, and invasive procedures.

Signs and Symptoms

- Endocarditis may have vague or nonspecific symptoms involving multiple organ systems: abdominal pain, chills, clubbing of fingers, fatigue, fever, headache, malaise, myalgia, new or changing heart murmur, and weakness.
- Pericarditis symptoms may include dyspnea, pericardial friction rub, and severe chest pain.
- Myocarditis may present with a range of symptoms: angina, crackles, dyspnea, fatigue, fever, heart failure (HF), JVD, lymphadenopathy, myalgia, nausea and vomiting, peripheral edema, S3 heart sounds, and syncopal episodes.

Diagnosis

Labs

- Blood cultures to identify organisms responsible for infection
- CBC to show elevated white blood cells (WBCs)
- Cardiac enzymes: possible troponin elevation in cardiac inflammation ▶

[ ]   **ALERT!**

The DASH diet is a nutrition and lifestyle modification approach to moderate BP. The DASH diet includes restricting daily sodium intake to 1,500 mg in addition to increasing fruit and vegetable intake, decreasing meat intake to one 6 oz. portion or less of lean meat a day, and limiting sweets, fats, and alcohol intake.

[ ]   **POP QUIZ 2.1**

A 48-year-old female is admitted to the progressive care unit (PCU) with ACS. Her EKG in the emergency department showed no ST elevation; however, after completing her admission EKG in the PCU, there are ST elevations in leads II, III, and AVF. She complains of worsening shortness of breath and anxiety. HR is 136, BP is 98/62, oxygen saturation is 89% on 2 L nasal cannula, and oral temperature is 99°F (37.2°C). What should the nurse's next action be?

[ ]   **COMPLICATIONS**

- A severe complication of inflammatory cardiac disease, specifically infective endocarditis, is the development of a septic pulmonary embolism (PE). Bacterial vegetations, which develop on or near the heart valves, become dislodged, travel through the vasculature, and disrupt circulation and perfusion like native clots, ruptured plaques, or emboli. These septic emboli can affect any organ system and can result in sudden death.
- Risk factors for developing an acute inflammatory disease of the heart include age; alcohol and/or IV drug use; family history; gender; poor dentition; medical conditions including cancer, diabetes, renal disease, and/or conditions that alter the body's immune system such as HIV/AIDs; severe burns, or trauma.

Labs (continued)
- Possible inflammatory marker elevation in infection or inflammatory process: erythrocyte sedimentation rate (ESR) and CRP
- Viral titers: possible elevation if viral infection present

Diagnostic Testing
- 12-lead EKG
- Cardiac biopsy
- Cardiac catherization
- Chest x-ray
- CT or MRI
- Echocardiogram
- Pericardiocentesis

ALERT!

Prior to performing invasive procedures, coagulation values should be drawn and treated if elevated to decrease the risk for additional bleeding in the pericardial space. Excessive bleeding can worsen the patient's condition, leading to pericardial effusion and/or tamponade.

Treatment

- Medications (Table 2.3): antiarrhythmics, antibiotic and/or antifungal IV therapy (Table A.1), autoimmune/immunosuppressive therapy
- Intraaortic balloon pump (IABP) (requires transfer to higher level of care)
- Valve replacement

Nursing Interventions

- Administer antibiotic, antifungal, or immunosuppressant therapy as ordered.
- Follow institutional policy for accessing and administering IV medications through peripherally inserted central catheter (PICC) line to prevent central line-associated bloodstream infections (CLABSIs).
- Monitor VS and physical assessment for any changes. Notify provider immediately if condition worsens.
- Position patient to decrease cardiac workload.
- Perform or have patient perform daily oral hygiene.
- Refer patients with history of IV drug use to treatment as appropriate.

ALERT!

Patients with a suspected or confirmed history of IV drug use are at high risk for developing infective endocarditis. Most commonly, these patients present with methicillin-susceptible *Staphylococcus aureus* (MSSA) or methicillin-resistant *Staphylococcus aureus* (MRSA) infections. Both methicillin-susceptible Staphylococcus aureus (MSSA) and MRSA are treated with long-term antibiotics. This may require a PICC line or other long-term IV injection devices. Patients with IV drug use history are often reluctant to comply with this course of treatment, which worsens the infection and results in valvular disease and/or HF.

Patient Education

- Avoid lifestyle actions that create a risk for recurrence of IV drug use.
- Avoid others who are ill, especially with upper respiratory infections.
- Consider participating in a drug or alcohol rehabilitation program.
- Determine the cause of inflammatory disease (if identifiable).
- Educate on PICC line maintenance and care if receiving IV antibiotic therapy in outpatient or home health setting.
- Perform daily oral hygiene practices and regularly visit the dentist.
- Use antibiotic prophylaxis for dental or other procedures.

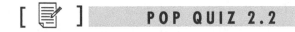

POP QUIZ 2.2

A 67-year-old female is admitted to the PCU after a motor vehicle accident. She was restrained (as evidenced by a positive seatbelt sign), and the airbags were deployed. In the emergency department, she complains of frequent sharp chest pain. She says the pain is worse when she takes a deep breath or lies down. The pain radiates to her shoulders and upper back. EKG shows no ST elevation, and cardiac enzymes are negative. VS are as follows: HR 122, BP 130/81 mmHg, SpO$_2$ 98% on 2 L nasal cannula, T 98.4°F (36.9°C). What should the nurse's next action be?

ANEURYSM
Overview

- An aneurysm is an abnormal outpouching or dilation of a vessel wall that can occur in the abdominal aorta, thoracic aorta, or as a cerebral aneurysm.
- While abdominal and thoracic aortic aneurysms often present with no symptoms, dissection or rupture of the aneurysm presents with sudden and severe excruciating pain in the chest and/or back with hypotension.
- Cerebral aneurysms are also asymptomatic, usually only presenting with symptoms after rupture.
- The mortality rate of ruptured or dissecting aneurysms (regardless of location) is high.
- Treatment requires strict BP management and surgical repair.

Signs and Symptoms

- Aortic and thoracic aneurysm: Most commonly asymptomatic and found on routine, unrelated examinations, or imaging; symptoms, if any, include the following: Epigastric pain, dull generalized back or chest pain, pulsatile mass in the periumbilical area, and bruits may be present on abdominal auscultation.
- Aortic or thoracic aneurysm dissection presents with dyspnea; mental status changes; sudden severe pain radiating to the back, shoulders, chest, and/or neck often described as tearing, ripping, or sharp; hypotension; and signs and symptoms of hemorrhagic or cardiovascular shock.
- Cerebral aneurysms: Often asymptomatic and usually found in unrelated imaging studies. Rupture symptoms include severe headache that may be accompanied with a brief loss of consciousness, nausea and vomiting, and a sudden onset headache (described as a thunderclap headache or as "the worst headache of my life"). Cerebral aneurysms leading to subarachnoid hemorrhage may have a sentinel leak, also known as a warning leak, presenting 6 to 20 days before the event.

Diagnosis

Labs

There are no labs specific to diagnose aneurysm. However, the following may be helpful when determining severity and treatment:

- CBC
- Coagulopathies and clotting: D-dimer, fibrinogen, international normalized ratio (INR), interleukin-6, prothrombin time (PT)/partial thromboplastin time (PTT)

Diagnostic Testing

- 12-lead EKG
- Angiography
- Chest x-ray
- Chest, abdomen, or head CT scan
- Echocardiogram
- MRI
- Ultrasound

[🧠]   **COMPLICATIONS**

A life-threatening complication of aortic aneurysm and dissection includes rupture and hemorrhage that can lead to exsanguination, hypovolemia, and death. Rupture of cerebral aneurysm can result in a devastating hemorrhagic stroke, resulting in total loss of voluntary function and cognitive ability and may result in herniation or death. Preventing these complications requires rapid identification, monitoring, and BP management.

[⚙]   **ALERT!**

For patients with abdominal aortic aneurysm with or without suspected dissection, strict BP control is essential to prevent dissection growth or rupture. BP control is managed with pain medication, antihypertensives, and continuous bedside monitoring. Instruct patients to immediately report any change in pain or status.

Treatment

- Medications; BP control (Table 2.3) and opioid analgesics (Table A.2)
- Surgical repair: endovascular cerebral aneurysm repair (EVAR), open aortic surgical repair, and open cerebral aneurysm surgical repair.

Nursing Interventions

- In patients with known aortic aneurysm: Monitor BP to maintain a goal of systolic blood pressure (SBP) of 110 mmHg. Encourage bedrest and a quiet, calm environment. See the Cardiac Catheterization section for post procedure care and management. Gather a complete history and detailed physical assessment. If the patient presents with symptoms of a retroperitoneal bleed post cardiac catheterization, immediate surgical consult should be made as retroperitoneal bleed is a surgical emergency. Manage pain and anxiety. Monitor for new onset of sudden pain in the back, chest, or abdomen; diaphoresis; weakness, and VS changes (hypotension and/or tachycardia). Monitor vital signs.

Patient Education

- Adhere to dietary recommendations as ordered for lipid and sodium control (e.g., DASH diet).
- During suspected or confirmed aortic dissection, patients must be educated on the importance of remaining in bed and minimizing exertion.
- Explain the purpose of any medication therapy.
- Follow up as appropriate with outpatient appointments.
- Follow exercise and weight management recommendations.
- Increase physical activity as recommended and, if referred by provider, participate in a cardiac rehab program.

ALERT!

If decompensating, alert the provider and call for the rapid response team to ensure all available resources are available for intubation and transfer to a higher level of care.

NURSING PEARL

Patients experiencing aortic dissection are at risk to develop cardiac tamponade. Remember, the hallmark signs for cardiac tamponade include Beck's triad: hypotension, distended neck veins, and muffled heart sounds.

POP QUIZ 2.3

A 65-year-old male is admitted to the PCU after a witnessed syncopal episode in the yard while gardening with his wife. The patient fell forward and hit a large rock during the syncopal episode. While in the emergency department, a chest x-ray revealed a right-sided hairline fracture in rib 5, but most notably a dilation in the aorta, which is concerning for an abdominal aortic aneurysm. The physician has ordered a STAT CT and BP goals of SBP 110 mmHg. What additional orders should the nurse request at this time?

CARDIAC CATHETERIZATION

Overview

- Cardiac catheterizations are performed to provide visualization of the vascular system and/or coronary arteries using contrast media and x-rays.
- There are two types of cardiac catheterization: left heart catheterizations and right heart catheterizations.
- Left heart catheterization angiography can help identify areas and lesions of concern in the coronary arteries. If a concerning lesion is identified, it may be treated with balloon angioplasty or stent placement.
- Not all lesions can be treated with a balloon angioplasty or stent placement. If revascularization is not possible with stenting or balloon angioplasty, then a CABG is indicated.

COMPLICATIONS

Complications of cardiac catheterization and/or stent placement include reocclusion of the stent/vessel, dysrhythmia, arterial dissection, pseudoaneurysm, hematoma, retroperitoneal bleed, myocardial infarction, and death.

Signs and Symptoms

A cardiac catheterization is indicated if a patient presents with the following signs, symptoms, or past medical history:

- Dysrhythmia
- Congenital heart disease
- New or worsening symptoms of HF including dyspnea, increasing oxygen requirements, fluid overload, pulmonary edema, or cardiogenic shock
- Sudden onset of chest pain with or without anxiety, fear, or feelings of imminent demise; decreased pallor; diaphoresis; dyspnea; extra heart sounds (S3, S4, and/or holosystolic murmurs); fatigue and weakness; initial hypertension and tachycardia, which progresses to hypotension; JVD; mental status changes; nausea and vomiting; palpitations; presyncope or syncope; radiating pain to the chest, neck, jaw, arms, back, and/or epigastrium; ST changes; and severe chest pain, heaviness, or pressure unrelieved by rest, position changes, and/or medication

Diagnosis

Labs

- Lab drawn prior to beginning a cardiac catheterization procedure
- Basic metabolic panel (BMP): creatinine, magnesium, and potassium
- Coagulopathies: INR will be evaluated for patients taking Coumadin; PT; PTT is a baseline evaluation as heparin is given intraoperatively and will increase coagulation times
- CBC, hematocrit, and hemoglobin; platelets indicate potential clotting issues, whereas WBCs indicate whether infection is present
- Type and screen

ALERT!

Patients receiving iodine contrast are at risk for developing an AKI due to the nephrotoxic properties of contrast. Patients receiving iodine contrast for a catheterization procedure should be well hydrated pre and post procedure. Additionally, baseline renal function should be assessed to monitor for the development of AKI post procedure.

Diagnostic Testing

- 12-lead EKG
- Continuous EKG monitoring
- Positive Allen test for radial approach
- TTE

Treatment

- Before the procedure, patients should receive the following: aspirin as ordered pre procedure, IV access, IV fluid replacement as ordered, potassium or magnesium supplementation if needed based on potassium or magnesium labs, and vitamin K as needed based on INR (Table 5.4).
- If coronary angiogram demonstrates evidence of blockage of the coronary arteries, patients may receive the following: Balloon angioplasty, bare metal stent, and drug-eluting stent.
- Post procedure, patients should receive the following: clopidogrel or prasugrel if PCI performed (Table 2.3); strict bedrest procedures until femoral sheath is removed and hemostasis is achieved; complications of stent placements include coronary artery perforation, device embolization, and longitudinal stent deformity; post-procedure, 12-lead EKG. ▶

Treatment (*continued*)

■ Assess for bleeding or hematoma around cardiac catheterization insertion site (usually the femoral or radial arteries).

Nursing Interventions

■ Assess and manage anxiety.

■ Assess vital signs for hemodynamic and oxygenation changes. Assess for evidence of reperfusion dysrhythmias or HR change. Assess for both hypertension and/or hypotension. Maintain oxygenation and perfusion.

■ Draw serial laboratory tests as ordered and monitor results.

■ Describe what to expect during the procedure.

■ Prep the patient pre procedure, including clipping hair and cleaning the site.

■ Discuss bedrest orders post procedure.

■ Explain sedation. Typically, patients receive a combination of versed and fentanyl.

■ Perform continuous physiologic monitoring through frequent physical assessment of the cardiac, pulmonary, and neurologic systems.

■ Monitor for symptoms of internal and external manifestations of bleeding or hemorrhage. These may present as bleeding or oozing around the puncture or catheter insertion site, hematoma and/or ecchymosis around the catheter insertion site, or retroperitoneal bleeding.

[🌐]   NURSING PEARL

During catheter removal and pressure application to the site to achieve hemostasis, patients may experience a vasovagal response. During this vasovagal response, the patient may complain of feeling nauseous and hot. They may also become diaphoretic, hypotensive, and bradycardic. Atropine and fluid bolus may be indicated for this symptomatic bradycardia.

Patient Education

■ Adhere to dietary recommendations as ordered for lipid and sodium control. Follow the DASH diet.

■ Maintain care of the femoral access site. Post procedure: Notify the nurse or proceed to the ED if the patient experiences cold, numbness, tingling pain, or burning in the extremity distal to the femoral insertion site; change in color to the extremity; intense pain at the femoral access site; or increased bruising or swelling at the femoral access site. For frank bleeding from femoral access site: Lay down flat, hold pressure, and immediately call for help.

■ Follow up as appropriate with outpatient appointments.

■ Follow exercise and weight management recommendations.

[📝]   POP QUIZ 2.4

A 52-year-old female returns to the PCU post cardiac catheterization. She was found to have a 99% blockage in the left circumflex, an 85% blockage in the right anterior descending artery, and 85% blockage in the left anterior descending artery. Vital signs are as follows: HR 109, BP 110/85 mmHg, respiratory rate (RR) 16, SpO$_2$ 96% on 2 L of oxygen via nasal cannula, and T 97.2°F (36.2°C). She received 100 mcg of fentanyl and 2 mg of midazolam for sedation. She did not receive any stenting or balloon angioplasty during the procedure. What should the nurse expect as the next step for the patient in treating her blockages?

■ Increase physical activity as recommended. If referred by a provider, participate in a cardiac rehab program.

■ Perform self-assessments of the femoral access site for any new swelling, changes in bruising, bleeding, or oozing.

■ Pursue smoking cessation as advised.

■ Take medication as prescribed.

CARDIAC TAMPONADE

Overview

- Cardiac tamponade develops when there is fluid or blood accumulation in the pericardial sac surrounding the heart. As fluid and/or blood accumulation increases in the pericardial sac, the heart's pumping ability is constricted. This constriction decreases the cardiac output of the heart and sends patients into shock.
- The most common causes of cardiac tamponade are pericarditis, surgical complications, and trauma.

Signs and Symptoms

- Beck's triad: muffled heart sounds, bulging neck veins, and hypotension
- Chest pain
- Dizziness
- Dyspnea
- Mental status changes
- Narrowed pulse pressures
- Palpitations
- Pulsus paradoxus (SBP drop of >10 mmHg on inspiration)
- Syncopal episodes
- Tachycardia

Diagnosis

Labs

Labs are not specifically diagnostic for detecting cardiac tamponade; rather, labs provide more information to guide the treatment plan.

- BMP
- CBC
- Coagulation labs: PT/PTT; INR

Diagnostic Testing

- Chest x-ray
- Chest CT scan
- MRI
- Pressure monitoring during cardiac catheterization
- TTE

Treatment

- Needle pericardiocentesis
- Surgical intervention through the pericardial window or an open thoracotomy, which is done as a surgical procedure in the operator room
- Vasopressors (Table 2.3)
- Volume replacement

[🧠] **COMPLICATIONS**

Cardiac tamponade is a medical emergency that requires immediate intervention to prevent shock and death. As cardiac tamponade progresses, patients rapidly develop hypotension and shock. If surgical intervention is not urgently performed, the patient will experience a cardiac arrest and death.

[⚙] **ALERT!**

Coagulation time values (PT, PTT, INR, etc.) alone do not help diagnose cardiac tamponade; however, this information is valuable pre- and postoperatively. Reversal agents may be ordered as needed. Elevated coagulation times place patients at a higher risk for bleeding, making drainage of the pericardium or performing a pericardial window difficult.

Nursing Interventions

- Continuously monitor VS: HR, BP, and oxygen saturation.
- If condition deteriorates, prepare for arterial line insertion and/or transfer to a higher level of care.
- If patient undergoes a surgical procedure, monitor for signs and symptoms of infection post procedure: chills, fever, foul-smelling drainage, pus or purulent drainage, redness around the surgical site, and warmth or pain to touch around the incision site.
- Maintain continuous physiologic monitoring and assessment: heart and lung sounds, mental status changes, peripheral pulses, and skin color and temperature. Assess for worsening chest pain, dizziness, dyspnea, palpitations.
- Maintain oxygenation and perfusion. Administer oxygen therapy as ordered, increasing oxygen as needed.
- Prepare for possible bedside pericardiocentesis.

Patient Education

- Educate on the severity and time-sensitive nature of treating cardiac tamponade.
- Discuss the possibility of transfer to the ICU and/or OR.
- Discuss surgical treatment options.
- Discuss the full plan for course of recovery.
- Educate on what to expect during and after invasive procedure.
- Notify the nurse of new or worsening chest pain, dizziness, dyspnea, and palpitations.
- Review the purpose of bedside EKG monitoring.
- Once cardiac tamponade is resolved, follow up with cardiologist after discharge home.
- Take all prescribed medications.

CARDIOGENIC SHOCK

Overview

- Cardiogenic shock is a type of systemic shock defined as decreasing cardiac output and evidence of tissue hypoxia and end-organ hypoperfusion in the presence of adequate intravascular volume.
- Cardiogenic shock can develop following myocardial infarctions, HF, dysrhythmias, acute valvular dysfunction, ventricular or septal rupture, myocardial or pericardial infections, massive pulmonary embolism, cardiac tamponade, or drug toxicity.
- Cardiogenic shock results in decreased ventricular filling which then causes decreased stroke volume, ultimately decreasing cardiac output despite adequate filling pressures.

Signs and Symptoms

- Abnormal heart sounds: diastolic murmur with aortic insufficiency, muffled heart tones with cardiac tamponade, murmurs if aortic stenosis or mitral regurgitation, and S3 or S4
- Abnormal lung sounds: rales or crackles associated with pulmonary vascular congestion and/or fluid overload ▶

NURSING PEARL

Patients with cardiac tamponade can quickly decompensate. Ensure that emergency supplies are readily available and discuss plan of care with a responsible provider.

POP QUIZ 2.5

A patient is admitted to the progressive care unit 24 hr after CABG. The patient begins to exhibit sudden shortness of breath, palpitations, and chest pain. The nurse notices that he has JVD, is hypotensive, and has muffled heart sounds. Given his recent cardiac surgery and clinical presentation, the nurse suspects he may be developing cardiac tamponade. What is the nurse's next action?

COMPLICATIONS

Complications associated with cardiogenic shock include dysrhythmia, cardiac arrest, renal failure, ventricular aneurysm, stroke, pulmonary embolism, and death. Prompt recognition and treatment is necessary to improve outcomes.

Signs and Symptoms (*continued*)

- Altered mental status
- Cool, clammy, or mottled extremities
- Cyanosis
- Decreased peripheral pulses
- JVD
- Peripheral edema

Diagnosis

Labs

- Blood gases: arterial blood gas (ABG) to show hypoxia; venous blood gas (VBG) to show hypoxia
- BMP with magnesium
- BNP
- Cardiac enzymes may be elevated: CK, CK-MB, troponin
- CBC
- Coagulation studies may be either high or low: INR, PT, PTT
- Lactate may be elevated in shock

Diagnostic Testing

- 12-lead EKG
- Cardiac catheterization/angiogram with PCI if indicated
- Cardiac pressure assessment in the cardiac catheterization lab
- Continuous EKG monitoring
- Chest x-ray
- Cardiac CT

ALERT!

Serial ABGs and lactate values can help determine if interventions are improving the patient's condition. Increasing lactate levels indicate the status of myocardial and other organ and tissue ischemia or hypoperfusion. This can be treated with fluid, as permitted by cardiac function. Other values in the ABG, such as PCO_2, PaO_2, and HCO_3 can be best treated with mechanical ventilation IABP deployment.

Treatment

- CABG
- Hemodialysis if kidney damage is extensive
- Coronary angiography/PCI
- Medications: anticoagulation/antiplatelets, antiplatelet drugs, antiarrhythmics, diuretics if pulmonary edema is present, fluids, fibrinolytic therapy (transfer to higher level of care), and vasopressors and inotropes
- Ventricular assistive devices
- Ventilator/oxygen support

Nursing Interventions

- Assess airway, breathing, and circulation.
- Assess vital signs and telemetry monitor.
- Maintain continuous physiologic monitoring through physical assessment and VS.
- Manage anxiety through nonpharmacologic methods (e.g., guided imaging and deep breathing) and/or pharmacologic methods as ordered by provider. ▶

NURSING PEARL

Patients with cardiac tamponade can quickly decompensate. Ensure that emergency supplies are readily available and discuss plan of care with responsible provider.

Nursing Interventions (*continued*)

- Position patient as appropriate: flat with HOB elevated if prepping for extracorporeal membrane oxygenation (ECMO)/IABP deployment and transfer to higher level of care, Trendelenburg if severe drop in BP, and semi-Fowler's to decrease the work of breathing.
- Reduce activity to decrease cardiac workload.

Patient Education

- Adhere to full plan for course of recovery.
- Ask questions about clinical condition.
- Discuss what to expect during/after invasive procedures.
- Notify the nurse (if possible) of new or worsening chest pain, dizziness, dyspnea, and/or palpitations.
- Once cardiac tamponade is resolved, follow up with the cardiologist after discharge home.
- Recognize the severity and time-sensitive nature of treating cardiac tamponade.
- Review surgical treatment options.
- Review the purpose of bedside EKG monitoring.
- Take all prescribed medications.

CARDIOMYOPATHY

Overview

- *Cardiomyopathy* classifies a group of disorders that affect the myocardium.
- Cardiomyopathy can be further classified as dilated, hypertrophic, or restrictive based on clinical presentation and diagnostic testing.

Signs and Symptoms

Signs and symptoms of cardiomyopathies are outlined in Table 2.4.

Diagnosis

Labs

- ABG is used to determine acid–base balance and compensation.
- BNP may be elevated >100 pg/mL.
- BMP with magnesium is used to determine electrolyte balance, as well as renal and liver function.
- Cardiac enzyme (CK, CK-MB, and troponin) elevation is evaluated.
- HIV viral loads: HIV can result in direct myocardial damage, autoimmune reactions, and cardiac inflammation, which may result in left ventricular dysfunction. Antiretroviral therapy is also known to contribute to additional myocardial damage.
- Iron studies are used to rule out hemochromatosis.
- Thyroid function elevation: Long-term untreated hyperthyroidism can cause dilated cardiomyopathy.
- Toxicology screening for cocaine and methamphetamines: Illicit drug use can cause cardiomyopathy.

POP QUIZ 2.6

A patient is admitted in suspected cardiogenic shock. Vital signs are as follows: HR 138, BP 100/64, RR 24, SpO$_2$ 94% on 4 L of oxygen via nasal cannula, and T 99°F (37.2°C). He has IV fluids running through a 20-gauge peripheral IV in his right hand. He also has an 18-gauge peripheral intravenous line (PIV) in the left antecubital. The provider places an order for a dobutamine drip. What should the nurse's next action be?

COMPLICATIONS

Complications of cardiomyopathy include HF, renal or hepatic damage, dysrhythmia, valvular dysfunction, pulmonary hypertension, thromboembolism, cardiac arrest, and/or sudden death. Patients with progressive HF and cardiomyopathy can receive a ventricular assistive device as a bridge to cardiac transplant. Otherwise, patient outcomes are poor and may result in death.

TABLE 2.4 Signs and Symptoms of Cardiomyopathies

Dilated cardiomyopathy	• Anorexia
	• Cough
	• Crackles
	• Decreased peripheral pulses
	• Dysrhythmia
	• Edema
	• Hepatomegaly
	• JVD
	• Nausea and vomiting
	• Narrow pulse pressure
	• Palpitations
	• PMI and apical pulse lateral displacement
	• S3 and S4 heart sounds
	• Tricuspid insufficiency
	• Vital sign changes
Hypertrophic cardiomyopathy	• Angina
	• Dysrhythmias (A-fib, SVT, V-tach, V-fib)
	• Lateral displacement of apical pulse
	• Paroxysmal nocturnal dyspnea
	• S4 and systolic murmur
Restrictive cardiomyopathy	• Ascites
	• Cardiac enlargement
	• Edema
	• Hepatojugular reflex
	• JVD
	• Mitral and tricuspid insufficiency
	• Pulmonary congestion
	• S3 and S4 heart sounds
Findings common to all types	• Dyspnea on exertion
	• Fatigue
	• Orthopnea

A-fib, atrial fibrillation; JVD, jugular vein distention; PMI, point of maximum impulse; V-fib, ventricular fibrillation; V-tach, ventricular tachycardia.

Diagnostic Testing

- 12-lead EKG
- Cardiac biopsy
- Continuous EKG monitoring
- Coronary angiogram (right- and left-sided)
- Cardiac catheterization
- CT scan
- Chest x-ray
- Genetic testing
- Nuclear stress test
- Transesophageal echocardiography (TEE) and/or TTE

[⚙]   ALERT!

Early identification and treatment of cardiomyopathy is essential to enhance and improve patient outcomes. There is currently no cure to cardiomyopathy. Patients are managed with lifestyle modifications, medication management, and bridge to cardiac transplantation. Nearly 50% of patients diagnosed with dilated cardiomyopathy, progress to HF and a life expectancy of no greater than 5 years. To improve outcomes, diet, exercise, and medication compliance is essential.

Treatment

- Cardiac transplantation (if severe)
- Identification of underlying causes of cardiomyopathy and reverse if possible (e.g., infection)
- Implantable cardioverter-defibrillator (ICD)
- Left ventricular assist device (LVAD)
- Medication to optimize afterload and preload using ACEIs, beta blockers, and antiarrhythmics (Table 2.3)
- Pacing if indicated (transfer to higher level of care)
- Sodium restriction

Nursing Interventions

- Assess for signs of decreased cardiac output as evidenced by worsening chest pain, dyspnea, edema, fatigue, JVD, lung crackles, orthopnea, palpitations, skin color changes, skin temperature changes (cool/clammy), and weight gain (assess weight daily).
- Closely monitor vital signs: BP, HR, heart rhythm, dysrhythmia presence, and SpO$_2$.
- Maintain oxygen saturation >90%. Titrate oxygen and switch oxygen delivery system as ordered.
- Position patient in semi-Fowler's position to decrease cardiac workload.

Patient Education

- Adhere to a sodium and fluid restriction.
- Continuously update and educate on status and situation.
- Discuss the plan of care and what to expect.
- Discuss the importance of interventions and diagnostic testing.
- Exercise as advised.
- Follow BP control guidelines.
- Follow antibiotic prophylaxis prior to dental procedures to reduce risk of infective endocarditis as prescribed.
- Take medications as prescribed.

NURSING PEARL

Dietary education and modification are essential for appropriate management of cardiomyopathy and associated HF. Consultation with a dietician may be warranted to improve patient and family understanding of necessary dietary changes.

POP QUIZ 2.7

A 35-year-old patient is admitted to the progressive care unit with a diagnosis of idiopathic dilated cardiomyopathy. The nurse notices that he has a pending HIV antibody test. How could the HIV antibody test result impact the patient's diagnosis?

DYSRHYTHMIAS

Overview

- To understand and identify dysrhythmias, a basic understanding of normal sinus rhythm (NSR) is essential.
- NSR includes the presence of an upright P wave (indicating depolarization of the atria), a QRS complex (indicating ventricular depolarization and atrial repolarization), and an upright T wave (indicating ventricular repolarization). PR intervals should be between 0.12 and 0.2 seconds. QRS intervals should be <0.1 seconds. QT intervals should be <0.38 seconds. There should be one P wave for every QRS complex (Figure 2.1). ▶

COMPLICATIONS

Dysrhythmias can cause complications including stroke, HF, cognitive impairments, and cardiac arrest. Rhythm identification is essential to providing appropriate intervention to prevent complications.

FIGURE 2.1 Normal sinus rhythm.

NSR, normal sinus rhythm.

Source: From Thaler, M. S. (2019). *The only EKG book you'll ever need* (9th ed.). Wolters Kluwer.

Overview (*continued*)

- A dysrhythmia is a disturbance of the NSR that can have a wide variety of presentations.
- Recognition of dysrhythmias is key to delivering appropriate intervention and care.
- Often, the cause of dysrhythmias results from accessory pathways, cardiomyopathy, conduction, defects, HF, myocardial infarction, infection, trauma, shock, or valvular disease.
- In the progressive care setting, patients are particularly vulnerable and may develop dysrhythmias due to medications, fluid and electrolyte imbalances, and blood loss, as well as other causes.
- Some dysrhythmias can be lethal, so adequate understanding of the advanced cardiac life support (ACLS) protocol is essential and should be reviewed.
- Dysrhythmias can be classified as atrial dysrhythmias, sinus dysrhythmias, ventricular dysrhythmias, and myocardial conduction system abnormalities.

Atrial Dysrhythmias

- *Atrial fibrillation*, or A-fib, is an abnormal electrical conduction in the atria that causes quivering of the upper chambers and results in ineffective pumping of the heart (Figure 2.2). Rapid ventricular response (RVR), a potential sequela of A-fib, is common during critical illness and can lead to hemodynamic instability. A-fib with RVR can be treated with medications (e.g., metoprolol, amiodarone, and diltiazem) or cardioversion. P waves will not be seen on the EKG because the atrial rate is so fast and the action potentials produced are of such low amplitude. The QRS rate is variable, and the rhythm is irregular. In patients with A-fib with RVR, the ventricles may beat >100 times per minute, resulting in elevated HR. The irregularity of the atrial contraction causes decreased filling time of the atria. This results in a smaller volume of oxygenated blood being circulated. A-fib may be caused by any of the following: advanced age, congenital heart disease, underlying heart disease, alcohol consumption, hypertension (systemic or pulmonary), endocrine abnormalities, genetic predisposition, cerebral hemorrhage or stroke, mitral or tricuspid valve disease, left ventricular dysfunction, pulmonary embolism, obstructive sleep apnea (OSA), myocarditis, or pericarditis.
- *Atrial flutter* occurs when the atria beat more rapidly than the ventricles (Figure 2.3). The hallmark sign of this arrythmia is a "saw tooth"-like EKG tracing. EKG shows a P rate between 251 and 300 and a PR interval is usually not observable. Irregularity and rate of atrial contraction causes decreased filling time of the atria. This results in a smaller volume of oxygenated blood being circulated. The cause begins with an ectopic beat which depolarizes one segment of the normal conduction pathway. ▶

FIGURE 2.2   Atrial fibrillation.

Source: From Knechtel, M. A. (2021). *EKGs for the nurse practitioner and physician assistant* (3rd ed.). Springer Publishing Company.

Atrial Dysrhythmias (continued)

- *Premature atrial contractions* are contractions of the atria that are triggered by the atrial myocardium but have not originated from the sinoatrial node (Figure 2.4). Early P waves are often caused by hypercalcemia, altered action potentials, hypoxia, or elevated preload. EKG shows early P waves with normal PR interval and one QRS complex for each P wave. Irregularity of rhythm can sometimes decrease filling times and BP. The cause is commonly idiopathic; however, higher incidence of pulmonary artery catherizations (PACs) occurs in patients with myocardial infarction (MI), congestive heart failure (CHF), hypertension (HTN), diabetes mellitus (DM), chronic obstructive pulmonary disease (COPD), community acquired pneumonia (CAP) hypertrophic cardiomyopathy, left ventricular hypertrophy, valvular heart disease, septal defects, or congenital heart disease. Medications like beta-agonists, digoxin, chemotherapy, tricyclic antidepressants, and monoamine oxidase inhibitors (MAOIs) can also induce PACs.
- *Sinus dysrhythmia* is a variation of a NSR with an R–R interval >0.12 seconds (Figure 2.5). This is a normal finding in children and young adults which requires no treatment. Incidence decreases with age.

FIGURE 2.3   Atrial flutter.

Source: From Knechtel, M. A. (2021). *EKGs for the nurse practitioner and physician assistant* (3rd ed.). Springer Publishing Company.

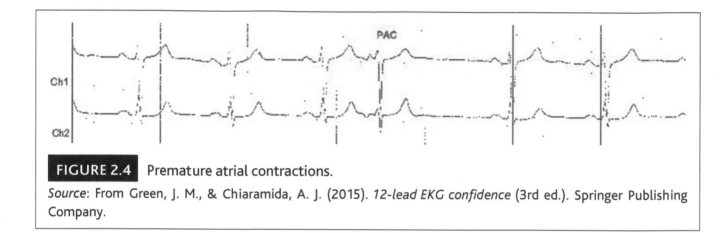

FIGURE 2.4 Premature atrial contractions.

Source: From Green, J. M., & Chiaramida, A. J. (2015). *12-lead EKG confidence* (3rd ed.). Springer Publishing Company.

Ventricular Dysrhythmias

- *Supraventricular tachycardia* is a rapid heartbeat that develops when the electrical impulses in the atrioventricular (AV) node affect the atria (Figure 2.6). The patient's HR can be anywhere from 150 to 220 beats per minute. EKG shows a narrow QRS complex and rhythm between 150 and 220 beats per minute. Supraventricular tachycardia (SVT) results in decreased cardiac output from loss of atrial contribution to ventricular preload for the beat.
- *Ventricular tachycardia* (VT) has a wide QRS complex and ventricular beat >100 beats per minute (Figure 2.7). VT can be further classified as monomorphic or polymorphic based on characteristics of the QRS complex. Torsades de Pointes is an example of polymorphic VT. EKG has an absent or independent P wave with a QRS >0.11 and rate >100 beats per minute. VT results in decreased cardiac output and increased myocardial demand. It can occur commonly in patients with underlying ischemic heart disease, structural heart disease, abnormal electrical conduction, infiltrative cardiomyopathy, electrolyte imbalances, cocaine or methamphetamine use, or digitalis toxicity. Common triggering events for VT include hypokalemia and hypomagnesemia. ▶

FIGURE 2.5 Sinus dysrhythmia.

Source: From Knechtel, M. A. (2021). *EKGs for the nurse practitioner and physician assistant* (3rd ed.). Springer Publishing Company.

FIGURE 2.6   Paroxysmal supraventricular tachycardia.

Source: From Roberts, D. (2020). *Mastering the 12-lead EKG* (2nd ed). Springer Publishing Company.

Ventricular Dysrhythmias (continued)

- *Ventricular fibrillation* (VF) is a quivering or shaking of the ventricles. This results in ventricular standstill and incomplete pumping (Figure 2.8). VF is a life-threatening dysrhythmia that requires prompt recognition and treatment to improve outcomes. VF has an absent P wave with a QRS rate >300 and is usually not observable. VF is a life-threatening dysrhythmia and often causes ventricular standstill. VF can occur commonly in patients with underlying structural heart disease, MI, A-fib, electrolyte abnormalities, hypothermia, hypoxia, cardiomyopathies, QT abnormalities, and alcohol use. Common triggering events for VF include hypo/hyperkalemia and hypomagnesemia. Myocardial conduction system abnormalities include first-degree AV block, second-degree AV block types 1 and 2, and third-degree AV block.
- *First-degree AV block* results when there is an abnormally slow conduction through the AV node, resulting in a prolonged PR interval (Figure 2.9). First-degree AV block has a PR interval >0.2 seconds. Patients with first-degree AV block may not have any symptoms and may only be detected with a routine EKG. First-degree AV block may result from hyperkalemia or hypokalemia, or with the formation of myocardial abscess in endocarditis. ▶

FIGURE 2.7   Ventricular tachycardia.

Source: From Knechtel, M. A. (2021). *EKGs for the nurse practitioner and physician assistant* (3rd ed.). Springer Publishing Company.

FIGURE 2.8   Ventricular fibrillation.

Source: From Knechtel, M. A. (2021). *EKGs for the nurse practitioner and physician assistant* (3rd ed.). Springer Publishing Company.

Ventricular Dysrhythmias (continued)

- *Second-degree AV block* (Mobitz type I, or Wenckebach) includes a progressively prolonged PR interval until one QRS is dropped (Figure 2.10). Second-degree AV block has progressive prolongation of the PR interval until one QRS complex is dropped. It may result from electrolyte abnormalities (hypokalemia), digoxin toxicity, or beta blockade. It may also result from preexisting CAD, MI, hypoxia, increased preload, valvular surgery or disease, and diabetes.
- *Second-degree AV block* (Mobitz type II) includes occasionally dropped P and QRS complexes (Figure 2.11). A second-degree AV block (Mobitz type II) has occasionally absent P waves with the loss of a QRS complex for that beat. Second-degree AV block (Mobitz type II) can cause an occasional decrease in cardiac output with increased preload for the following beat. It may result from hypokalemia, anti-dysrhythmics, or tricyclic antidepressant medications, or in patients with preexisting CAD, MI, hypoxia, increased preload, valvular surgery or disease, and diabetes mellitus. ▶

FIGURE 2.9   First-degree AV block.

AV, atrioventricular.

Source: From Knechtel, M. A. (2021). *EKGs for the nurse practitioner and physician assistant* (3rd ed.). Springer Publishing Company.

P Wave, No QRS

FIGURE 2.10   Second-degree AV block Mobitz type I.

AV, atrioventricular.

Source: From Knechtel, M. A. (2021). *EKGs for the nurse practitioner and physician assistant* (3rd ed.). Springer Publishing Company.

Ventricular Dysrhythmias (continued)

■ *Third-degree AV block* (complete heart block) includes P waves and QRS complexes that beat independently of one another (Figure 2.12). P waves and QRS complex are both present; however, there is no observable relationship between the P wave and QRS complex. Rate is usually <60 beats per minute. Third-degree AV block may result from hypokalemia, conduction abnormalities in the bundle of His, or MI (inferior wall). Third-degree AV block can cause decreased cardiac output.

Other Lethal Dysrhythmias

■ *Asystole* includes a complete absence of electrical activity as evidenced by no palpable pulse, paired with a flat waveform on EKG monitoring (Figure 2.13).

■ *Pulseless electrical activity* includes a complete absence of electrical activity with no palpable pulse; however, P waves and QRS complexes may be present on EKG.

Signs and Symptoms

Any disruption to regular HR and heart rhythm may result in the following symptoms:

■ Anxiety and/or feelings of impending doom
■ Dyspnea
■ Diaphoresis ▶

P RI   PRI

P Wave, No QRS

FIGURE 2.11   Second-degree AV block Mobitz type II.

AV, atrioventricular.

Source: From Knechtel, M. A. (2021). *EKGs for the nurse practitioner and physician assistant* (3rd ed.). Springer Publishing Company.

FIGURE 2.12 Third-degree AV block.

AV, atrioventricular.

Source: From Knechtel, M. A. (2021). *EKGs for the nurse practitioner and physician assistant* (3rd ed.). Springer Publishing Company.

Signs and Symptoms (*continued*)

- Dyspnea
- Mental status changes and/or syncope resulting from decreased cerebral perfusion
- Nausea and/or vomiting
- Pain in chest, back, or arms
- Pallor
- Palpitations
- Nausea and/or vomiting
- VS changes: decreasing oxygen saturation, hypotension or hypertension, and irregular HR and rhythm findings on continuous EKG monitoring
- Weak and/or irregular peripheral pulses

FIGURE 2.13 Asystole.

Source: From Knechtel, M. A. (2021). *EKGs for the nurse practitioner and physician assistant* (3rd ed.). Springer Publishing Company.

Diagnosis

Labs

There are no labs specific to detect dysrhythmias. However, the following labs may be indicated to treat potential causes of dysrhythmias:

- BMP with magnesium
- Cardiac enzymes: CK, CK-MB, and troponin

Diagnostic Testing

- 12-lead EKG
- Continuous EKG monitoring
- Coronary angiogram
- Echocardiogram
- Electrophysiology study
- Holter monitor for extended cardiac monitoring
- Stress test

Treatment

Treatment is highly dependent on the type of dysrhythmia (Table 2.5). Adhere to the ACLS protocol if patient is acutely decompensating or experiencing cardiac arrest.

[⚡]   **ALERT!**

Failure to capture may occur if the pacer voltage is too low. Notify provider and increase voltage as ordered or per institutional protocol until capture is achieved at desired rate (Table 2.7).

TABLE 2.5 Dysrhythmia Treatments		
DYSRHYTHMIA	**TREATMENT**	**OTHER INTERVENTIONS**
Atrial		
• Atrial fibrillation	• Amiodarone • Ibutilide • Disopyramide • Flecainide • Procainamide • Propafenone • Quinidine • Sotalol • Dofetilide • Anticoagulation • Calcium channel blockers (e.g., diltiazem) • Digoxin • Dronedarone • Metoprolol	• Ablation • Cardioversion • Pacemaker implantation
• Atrial flutter	• Ibutilide • Flecainide • Propafenone • Sotalol • Procainamide • Amiodarone • Beta blockers • Calcium channel blockers • Digoxin	• Ablation • Cardioversion • Pacemaker implantation

(continued)

TABLE 2.5 Dysrhythmia Treatments (*continued*)

DYSRHYTHMIA	TREATMENT	OTHER INTERVENTIONS
• PACs	• Electrolyte replacement (Table 8.3)	• Reverse hypoxia or other identifiable causes of elevated preload
Sinus		
• Sinus dysrhythmia	• No treatment required	• None
Ventricular		
• SVT	• Adenosine	• Vagal maneuvers
• Monomorphic V-tach	• Amiodarone • Epinephrine • Lidocaine	• Cardioversion if pulse present • High-quality CPR and defibrillation if pulse not present • ICD (if recurrent V-tach)
• Polymorphic ventricular tachycardia (also referred to as Torsades de Pointes)	• Magnesium	• Cardioversion if pulse present • High-quality CPR and defibrillation if pulse not present
• V-fib	• Amiodarone • Epinephrine • Lidocaine	• High-quality CPR • Defibrillation
Myocardial conduction abnormalities		
• First-degree AV block	• None	• Usually involves minimal treatment; identify/correct cause
• Second-degree AV block (Mobitz type I or Wenckebach)	• If hypotensive or experiencing altered LOC: Atropine	• Pacemaker
• Second-degree AV block (Mobitz type II)	• None	• Pacemaker
• Third-degree AV block (complete heart block)	• Atropine • Dopamine • Epinephrine	• Transcutaneous pacing • Permanent pacemaker
Other lethal dysrhythmias		
• Asystole	• Epinephrine	• High-quality CPR • Obtain advanced airway if not already in place
• Pulseless electrical activity	• Epinephrine	• High-quality CPR • Obtain advanced airway if not already in place

AV, atrioventricular; ICD, implantable cardioverter-defibrillator; LOC, loss of consciousness; PAC, pulmonary artery catherizations; SVT, supraventricular tachycardia; V-fib, ventricular fibrillation; V-tach, ventricular tachycardia.

TABLE 2.6 Pacemaker Characteristics

FIRST INITIAL—CHAMBER THAT IS PACED	SECOND INITIAL—CHAMBER THAT IS SENSED	THIRD INITIAL—RESPONSE OF PACER TO INTRINSIC ACTIVITY
• A—atria • V—ventricle • D—dual	• A—atria • V—ventricle • D—dual	• I—inhibits pacer • D—inhibits or triggers pacer • O—neither

Nursing Interventions

- Administer ordered medications and titrate drips to achieve ordered parameter goals.
- Assess airway, breathing, and circulation.
- Insert at least two large bore peripheral IVs and consider the need for central line placement.
- If a pacemaker is implanted, assess implantation site for bleeding; colored or foul-smelling drainage; capturing, sensing, and pacing within ordered parameters (Tables 2.6 and 2.7); icepack placement over pacemaker implantation site to reduce swelling; erythema; and warmth.
- Maintain continuous physiologic monitoring and observe for changes in diaphoresis, changes in pallor, changes in peripheral pulses, and mental status change.
- Monitor vital signs for hemodynamic instability.
- Monitor telemetry for rhythm changes or conversion to potentially unstable dysrhythmias.
- Perform 12-lead EKG if rhythm change is observed.
- Provide therapeutic support for patient and family. A chaplain can be called to the bedside to provide additional support if needed.

Patient Education

- Notify the nurse if the following symptoms are present: Difficulty in breathing, dizziness, nausea/vomiting, new onset or changes to chest pain, and palpitations.

[🌐]   **NURSING PEARL**

Electrolyte replacement in patients with cardiac dysfunction or dysrhythmia is essential. Electrolyte imbalance affects the electrical conduction of the heart and can predispose already at-risk patients for worsening dysrhythmias. Closely monitor these laboratory values and notify providers of abnormal results.

HEART FAILURE

Overview

- HF is a disorder in which the ventricles of the heart either do not fill or do not eject blood efficiently, resulting in decreased cardiac output. It develops when there is impaired cardiac pumping (contractility) or filling. ▶

TABLE 2.7 Types of Pacer Failure and Common Causes

FAILURE TO PACE	FAILURE TO CAPTURE	FAILURE TO SENSE
• Battery failure • Lead or wire dislodgement • Sensing threshold too low	• Battery failure • Lead or wire dislodgement • Pacer voltage too low • Ventricular perforation	• Battery failure • Lead or wire dislodgement • Sensitivity set too high

Overview (*continued*)

- HF can be classified as either chronic or acute right- or left-sided HF, each with distinguishable symptoms and varying treatment.
- Risk factors for HF include a past medical history of HTN, CAD, MI, diabetes, tobacco use, obesity, elevated cholesterol levels, and advanced age.

Signs and Symptoms

- CHF: abdominal distention, anorexia, dyspnea, fatigue, peripheral edema
- Acute HF: dyspnea at rest or on exertion, lightheadedness, orthopnea, palpitations, and paroxysmal nocturnal dyspnea
- Left-sided HF: altered mental status/confusion, anxiety, crackles on auscultation, dyspnea (with or without exertion), extra heart sounds (S3/S4), fatigue, orthopnea, pink frothy sputum, pleural effusion, pulmonary edema, tachycardia, tachypnea, and weakness
- Right-sided HF: anorexia, edema/anasarca, fatigue, heart murmur, hepatomegaly, JVD, nausea, tachycardia, and weight gain

Diagnosis

Labs

- ABG
- BMP with magnesium
- BNP
- CBC
- Cardiac enzymes
- Thyroid function

Diagnostic Testing

- 12-lead EKG
- Cardiac biopsy
- Chest x-ray
- Continuous EKG monitoring
- Coronary angiogram/catheterization (right and/or left sided)
- Stress test
- TTE

Treatment

- Cardiac catheterization
- Cardiac transplantation
- Cardiac rehab at time of discharge
- Diet: sodium and fluid restriction ▶

 POP QUIZ 2.8

A 38-year-old male is admitted to the PCU after having a syncopal episode at work. He reports feeling nauseous and dizzy. The patient is alert and oriented x4. Heart sounds are irregular and rapid with no S1 or S2 sound noted. Lungs are clear, diminished at the bases, and peripheral pulses in the lower extremities are diminished. A 12-lead EKG reveals atrial fibrillation with rapid ventricular rhythm, with an HR of 130. Other VS are BP 95/60 mmHg, SpO_2 95% on room air, RR 20, and T 98.4°F (36.9°C). After notifying the provider of new onset atrial fibrillation and assessment findings, what should the nurse's next action be?

 COMPLICATIONS

Complications of HF include dysrhythmia, pleural effusion, hepatomegaly, renal failure, thromboembolism, and sudden death. Medical management is possible with collaborative care of medication compliance and lifestyle modifications; however, HF resistant to medical intervention may require more invasive interventions, including IABP and/or cardiac transplantation.

 NURSING PEARL

New York Heart Association Heart Failure Classes
- Class 1: No limitations on physical activity
- Class 2: Slight limitation on physical activity
- Class 3: Marked limitation on physical activity
- Class 4: Discomfort with any physical activity, symptomatic even at rest

 ALERT!

Close monitoring of potassium levels is essential to protect electrical conduction of the heart. This is especially important if patients are taking thiazide or loop diuretics, as they can cause hypokalemia. Replacement electrolytes should be administered as ordered to maintain a potassium level >4 mmol/L.

Treatment (*continued*)

- ICD
- IABP or LVAD: Requires transfer to higher level of care for initial implantation/deployment; chronic LVADs managed in PCU.
- Medications: ACEIs, angiotensin receptor blockers (ARBs), beta blockers, aldosterone antagonists, diuretics, vasodilators, and digoxin (Table 2.3).
- Pacemaker (Tables 2.5 and 2.6)
- Supplemental oxygen

Nursing Interventions

- Administer prescribed medication as ordered.
- Assess airway, breathing, and circulation.
- Assess the need for noninvasive oxygen or intubation and transfer to higher level of care.
- Assess for elevated or low BP, fluid retention, or electrolyte imbalances.
- Assess for signs of decreased cardiac output as evidenced by worsening chest pain, dyspnea, edema, fatigue, JVD, lung crackles, mental status, orthopnea, palpitations, skin color changes, and/or skin temperature changes (cool/clammy).
- Elevate HOB to alleviate orthopnea and dyspnea and decrease cardiac workload.
- Monitor weight daily and report weight gain >2 to 3 lbs over 24 hr or over 5 lbs in 1 week. This may indicate high fluid retention.
- Monitor VS continuously for changes.
- Maintain oxygen saturation >90%. Titrate oxygen and upgrade oxygen delivery device as needed.
- Monitor strict intake and output (I/O) due to the potential for fluid retention.

Patient Education

- Adhere to a low-sodium, fluid-restricted diet if ordered by the provider.
- Follow physical restrictions and take breaks between activities as needed.
- Take medications as prescribed and follow up with any outpatient appointments after discharge.
- Once discharged, engage in a physical activity program as ordered and tolerated. Consider participating in a cardiac rehabilitation program if recommended by your provider.

HYPERTENSION AND HYPERTENSIVE CRISIS

Overview

- *HTN* is defined as an abnormal elevation in BP. See Table 2.8 for stages of HTN.
- HTN can be managed with lifestyle modifications and medications. ▶

NURSING PEARL

Daily weights are essential to monitor fluid retention and volume status. Weight gain of >3 lbs in a 24-hr period indicates fluid retention and volume overload. The provider should be notified if sudden weight gain occurs in a 24-hr period.

POP QUIZ 2.9

A 59-year-old male with CHF is admitted to the PCU. He complains of worsening fatigue, anorexia, nausea, and new onset of blurred vision. He also notices the presence of halos around objects in his vision. Past medical history is notable for HF, diabetes, and anxiety. Current medications include metformin 1,000 mg by mouth twice a day (PO BID), furosemide 80 mg PO daily, captopril 25 mg PO BID, and digoxin 0.125 mg PO daily. VS are as follows: HR 126, BP 96/70, RR 24, SpO$_2$ 94% on 4 L of oxygen via nasal cannula and T 98.1°F (36.7°C). Given the patient's medications and clinical presentation, what is happening with this patient?

TABLE 2.8 Stages of Hypertension	
Normal	Systolic <120
	Diastolic <80
Elevated	Systolic 120–129
	Diastolic <80
Stage 1: Hypertension	Systolic 130–139
	Diastolic 80–89
Stage 2: Hypertension	Systolic >140
	Diastolic ≥90
Stage 3: Hypertension (hypertensive crisis)	Systolic >180
	Diastolic ≥120

Source: Data from American Heart Association.

Overview (*continued*)

- A *hypertensive crisis* is a marked elevation in BP that is associated with end-organ damage as evidenced by pulmonary edema, myocardial ischemia, acute renal failure, aortic dissection, or neurologic deficits including mental status changes and/or stroke. Hypertensive crisis cannot be managed outside of the hospital and is considered a medical emergency. The increased SVR places additional pressure on vasculature and organ structures resulting in end-organ damage. While it is imperative to lower BP during a hypertensive crisis, it must be lowered gradually to prevent refractory ischemia. The goal is to lower mean arterial pressures (MAPs) by 20% to 25% in the first 1 to 2 hr.

Signs and Symptoms

- Often asymptomatic with symptom manifestation only if severe
- Severe HTN symptoms include activity intolerance, agitation, angina, anxiety, altered level of consciousness (if hypertensive encephalopathy), AV nicking (finding on ophthalmic examination), dizziness, headache, nausea and vomiting, pain (chest, back, or abdomen), palpitations, restlessness, retinopathy, papilledema, transient focal neurologic deficits, and vision changes

Diagnosis

Labs
- BMP
- Cardiac enzymes: CK, CK-MB, troponin
- CBC
- Lipid panel
- Thyroid-stimulating hormone (TSH)
- Uric acid
- Urinalysis

COMPLICATIONS

Complications of hypertension and a hypertensive crisis include renal failure, hemorrhagic stroke, arterial dissection, MI, visual disturbances and/or loss of vision, CAD, left ventricular hypertrophy, HF, and death. In patients with hypertensive crisis and no evidence of organ damage, BP must be gradually lowered over 48 hr as tolerated to maintain cerebral perfusion and prevent ischemia stroke. If organ damage or aortic dissection is present, BP should be lowered to <140 mmHg in the first hr of treatment.

ALERT!

Hyperthyroidism is a common secondary cause for hypertension. In patients with hyperthyroid-induced hypertension, first-line treatment should start with thyroid regulation before progressing to antihypertensive medications.

Diagnostic Testing

- 12-lead EKG
- Echocardiogram
- Head CT scan
- Brain MRI
- Ophthalmic examination: AV nicking
- Renal ultrasound

Treatment

- First 1 to 2 hr for hypertensive emergency: lower MAP by 20% to 25% or BP to 160/100 mmHg
- Lifestyle modifications: alcohol intake reduction, anxiety and stress reduction, diet, physical activity, smoking cessation, and weight loss
- Medication (Table 2.3); ACEIs, alpha adrenergic inhibitors, ARBs, beta adrenergic blockers, beta blockers, calcium channel blockers, diuretics, and vasodilators
- Transition from IV to oral medication within 12 to 24 hr (if possible)

Nursing Interventions

- Administer antihypertensive medications as ordered.
- Assess airway, breathing, and circulation.
- Assess neurologic status, including level of consciousness and for focal deficits.
- Assess for signs of stroke. See Chapter 10 for more information on stroke.
- Assess for tissue ischemia, coronary ischemia, T-wave inversion, and cerebral ischemia related to overly aggressive lowering of BP.
- Implement anxiety and stress reduction practices as needed.
- Limit caffeine intake for accurate BP readings.
- Monitor BP and VS as ordered.
- Monitor I/O to optimize fluid balance.
- Monitor sodium intake and fluid as ordered.
- Monitor weight daily.

Patient Education

- Adhere to dietary recommendations as ordered for lipid and sodium control.
- Continuously update (if alert and oriented) on current status, plan of care, and upcoming tests or procedures.
- Follow the DASH diet.
- Follow exercise and weight management recommendations.
- Follow up as appropriate with outpatient appointments.
- If referred by provider, participate in cardiac rehab program.
- Increase physical activity as recommended.
- Limit alcohol intake.
- Pursue smoking cessation as advised.
- Take medications as prescribed.

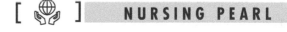

ALERT!

Nitroprusside is the gold standard treatment in the management of hypertensive crisis. Watch for signs of cyanide toxicity: Blurred vision, tinnitus, altered mental status, hyperreflexia, or seizure. Risk of toxicity is elevated with prolonged therapy >48 hr and in patients with renal failure.

NURSING PEARL

If IV beta blockers are administered rapidly, patient can become severely bradycardic. Though this resolves quickly, avoid rapid administration of IV beta blocker.

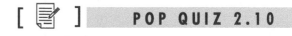

POP QUIZ 2.10

A patient with newly diagnosed hypertension was admitted to the PCU 3 days ago. His BP on admission was 189/102 mmHg. With medication therapy, his BP is now 141/84 mmHg, HR 102, RR 16, SpO$_2$ 96% on 4 L nasal cannula, and T 96.8°F (36°C). With the healthcare team's permission, the patient's wife brought food and snacks into the hospital from home. As the nurse enters the room around lunchtime, the patient and his wife have finished eating takeout Chinese food with multiple soy sauce packets on the bedside table. The wife asks if she can bring in a breakfast sandwich from the drive-thru the next morning. What should the nurse's first action be?

POST ICU CARE
Overview

- Patients in the ICU have likely undergone procedures or have been diagnosed with critical illnesses which required additional specialized monitoring.
- As such, patients transferred to the PCU from the ICU should be monitored closely for hemodynamic instability, post-procedure complications, or other changes in status.

Signs and Symptoms

- Complications associated with cardiac catheterization and angiography include bruising and/or hematoma noted around access site, loss of peripheral pulse distal to the insertion site, redness/swelling around the access site, skin cool to touch and pale distal to insertion site, and severe back pain.
- Hemodynamic instability: angina/chest pain, dysrhythmia development, diaphoresis, dyspnea, dizziness, mental status changes, nausea/vomiting, palpitations, and tachycardia/bradycardia.

Diagnosis
Labs
The following labs are typically assessed daily:

- CBC
- Coagulation: PT/PTT, INR
- CMP/BMP

Diagnostic Testing
- 12-lead EKG
- Chest x-ray
- Doppler ultrasound
- Echocardiogram

Treatment

- If the patient is experiencing hemodynamic instability, identify the cause and treat with appropriate therapy: ACLS protocol and ICU transfer, as indicated, antiarrhythmic drugs, antihypertensives (hypertension), fluid volume replacement, and vasodilators (HTN).
- Monitor for complications post procedure.
- Other common reasons for readmission to ICU: HF exacerbation, hemorrhage/surgical emergency, hyperkalemia unresponsive to treatment, loss of consciousness/unresponsiveness, new infection/sepsis, new MI or stroke, poor ventilation/inability to protect airway, and reemergence of hemodynamically unstable dysrhythmia (V-tach, A-fib with RVR, etc.) requiring cardioversion.

[🧠]   **COMPLICATIONS**

Patients newly admitted to the PCU must be closely watched for decompensation and worsening condition, requiring transfer back to the ICU. To prevent this, close hemodynamic monitoring and assessment of post-procedure complications are essential. Early detection and treatment of deteriorating conditions can prevent an unnecessary rebound to the ICU.

ALERT!

If the patient becomes hemodynamically unstable or may require a higher level of care, notify the provider immediately and consider calling a rapid response to assemble all necessary disciplines to address the rapid response situation and facilitate quick transfer to a higher level of care.

ALERT!

Stent thrombosis following PCI can occur early (as an acute event in the first 24 hr or as a subacute event between 24 hr and 1 month post procedure), late (between 1 and 12 months post procedure), and very late (after 12 months post procedure). Stent thrombosis at any stage is thought to occur due to ineffective anticoagulation. Be sure the patient receives the ordered anticoagulation before and after the procedure and educate the patient on the importance of continuing their anticoagulation for at least a year as directed by their provider.

Nursing Interventions

- Administer medications as ordered.
- Monitor vital signs as ordered.
- Perform a detailed head-to-toe physical assessment every shift. Access site status (increased bruising, swelling, hematoma, etc.); color, sensation, and movement of extremities distal to invasive access sites; edema and signs of fluid overload monitoring; and peripheral pulses.
- Closely monitor continuous telemetry.
- Continuous SpO_2 monitoring.

Patient Education

- Notify the nurse for any of the following symptoms: new onset or worsening chest pain; dizziness; confusion; palpitations; nausea/vomiting; diaphoresis or dyspnea; active bleeding from access site; increased swelling or pain in access site; and cold, numb, or tingly extremities.
- Work with PT to engage in physical activities as ordered and tolerated to maintain or regain lost mobility from ICU admission.
- Perform intermittent suctioning ×10 to encourage airway secretion clearance.

VALVULAR HEART DISEASE

Overview

- Valvular disease is an umbrella term which describes mitral stenosis, mitral regurgitation, mitral prolapse, aortic stenosis, aortic regurgitation, and tricuspid or pulmonic valve stenosis. Stenosis describes a narrowing of the heart valve. Regurgitation describes the accumulation of leaflets on the valves which prevent complete closure and backward flow of blood. Prolapse describes a bulging of the valve which also prevents complete closure.
- Treatment of valvular heart disease ranges from medical management to open heart surgery.

Signs and Symptoms

- Dependent on the valve involved and type of impairment. Symptoms can include the following: Cardiogenic shock, dyspnea with or without exertion, fatigue, HF, heart sound changes, palpitations, peripheral edema, and pulmonary edema.

Labs
- Blood cultures
- CBC
- CMP

Diagnostic Testing
- 12-lead EKG
- Cardiac catheterization
- Continuous bedside monitoring
- Echocardiogram

NURSING PEARL

Sudden decrease or loss of pulse in extremities distal to arterial access sites can indicate serious complications and develop into a surgical emergency. If a decrease in perfusion is prolonged, loss of limb is possible. Therefore, it is essential that peripheral pulses and physical assessment be conducted at frequent and regular intervals.

POP QUIZ 2.11

If a patient transferred from the ICU becomes hemodynamically unstable, what should the nurse's next actions be?

COMPLICATIONS

Patients with valvular insufficiencies are at risk for developing HF. Timely identification, condition monitoring, and treatment are essential to improve patient outcomes. As conditions progress, patients may need surgery to replace or repair the valve to prevent further decompensation.

ALERT!

Acute mitral valve regurgitation can progress quickly to cardiogenic shock. Prompt identification and intervention are needed to prevent escalation of care.

Treatment

- Balloon valvuloplasty
- Fluid and sodium restriction
- Medications: Antibiotics are used if indicated in infective carditis or for rheumatic fever, antihypertensives such as beta blockers, anticoagulation, antidysrhythmic medications, diuretics, and vasodilators.
- Surgical valve replacement or repair

Nursing Interventions

- Administer medications as ordered.
- Assess surgical or insertion site for bleeding, hematoma, and signs of infection.
- Assess and treat pain with scheduled and as needed (PRN) medications.
- Improve activity tolerance.
- Maintain appropriate positioning to decrease cardiac workload: semi-Fowler's, HOB >30°.
- Monitor continuous telemetry and pulse oximetry.
- Monitor VS as ordered.
- Perform incentive spirometry.
- Perform detailed regular assessments, including auscultation of the heart and lungs, mental status, pain, and systemic perfusion and oxygenation.

NURSING PEARL

As valvular disease progresses, care may shift to managing HF, endocarditis, or dysrhythmia. These additional conditions may warrant additional interventions, including PICC line insertion for IV antibiotic administration, ICD, pacemaker, or ventricular assist device (VAD), depending on severity of condition.

Patient Education

- Adhere to heart healthy diet to limit sodium intake and decrease workload of the heart as recommended.
- Decrease alcohol intake to reduce cardiac strain.
- Monitor BP and HR daily.
- Monitor weight daily to assess for fluid retention.
- Pursue smoking cessation.
- Take coagulation and other medications as prescribed.
- Use prophylactic antibiotic treatment for dental or invasive procedures.

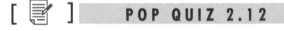

POP QUIZ 2.12

A patient with mitral valve stenosis has been newly diagnosed with atrial fibrillation. The nurse knows that atrial fibrillation can cause what complication if left untreated?

VASCULAR DISEASE

Overview

- Vascular disease includes coronary artery stenosis, arterial and venous occlusion, and peripheral vascular insufficiency.
- Symptom presentation and treatment differs for each condition; however, the overall goal is to improve circulation and perfusion.
- *Carotid artery stenosis* is an atherosclerotic disease that leads to partial blockage and causes ischemic stroke or transient ischemic attack (TIA)-like symptoms.
- *Arterial occlusion* is a medical emergency where arterial blood flow is stopped, resulting in ischemia of distal organs and tissues. ▶

COMPLICATIONS

Complications for vascular diseases include the development of nonhealing ulcers and wounds, tissue necrosis, pain, infection, embolism (deep vein thrombosis [DVT], PE, or stroke), and amputation. Appropriate medical management and lifestyle modifications must be implemented to prevent disease progression, which can result in vision changes, aphasia, and stroke.

Overview (*continued*)

- *Venous occlusion* occurs when a vein becomes narrowed, blocked, or pinched, resulting in tissue necrosis and death.
- *Peripheral vascular insufficiency* and disease is an atherosclerotic disease that leads to partial or total occlusion of the abdominal aorta, iliac arteries, lower limbs, and/or upper extremities.
- *Peripheral vascular insufficiency* can progress to both stenosis and/or occlusion of peripheral vessels. thereby resulting in renal vascular disease, ischemic bowel, and cerebral vascular disease, depending on the location of the occlusion.

Signs and Symptoms

- Carotid artery stenosis (stroke symptoms which resolve rapidly, within 48 hr of onset): cranial nerve deficits, limb weakness, slurred speech, and visual changes/disturbances
- Arterial occlusion: acute onset of skin color change consisting of white spots/nonblanchable areas, immediate or rapid onset, and severe and disproportionate pain
- Venous occlusion: blisters, pain (dull, delayed, or less severe as compared to arterial occlusions), pallor (red/bluish or purple skin coloration), pustules, and tissue necrosis
- Peripheral vascular insufficiency: bruits, coolness of extremity, intermittent claudication (cramping pain with exertion), nonhealing ulcers, organ ischemia depending on location of occlusion, pain in the calf and/or foot, renal or gastrointestinal (GI) dysfunction, and skin changes including hair loss to extremity

Diagnosis

Labs

- CBC (will usually show a decreased hematocrit)
- Coagulation studies may be elevated or decreased
  - Activated clotting time (ACT)
  - D-dimer
  - PT/INR
  - PTT
- BMP with magnesium
- Urinalysis, for proteinuria and hematuria

Diagnostic Testing

- Ankle-brachial index (ABI)
  - Normal 0.9 to 1.3
  - ABI <0.9 indicates peripheral artery disease
  - ABI <0.4 indicates severe ischemia
- CT angiography
- Doppler duplex ultrasonography
- MRA
- Peripheral angiography

 ALERT!

Risk factors for developing peripheral vascular insufficiency include age >50, BMI >30, type 1 and 2 diabetes, family history of cardiovascular disease, HIV, hypertension, hyperlipidemia, and tobacco use. The nurse should take note of risk factors upon obtaining patient history or examination and prepare for appropriate treatment.

[🌐] **NURSING PEARL**

The six Ps of peripheral arterial disease are pain, pallor, pulses that are absent or diminished, paresthesia, paralysis, and poikilothermia. If these signs and symptoms are identified during assessment, notify the provider immediately.

 ALERT!

Medication noncompliance, especially with anticoagulants, can place the patient at risk for thrombus and clot formation. Taking an accurate and thorough history and physical is essential to understanding the full clinical presentation and appropriate treatment plan.

Treatment

- Endovascular interventions:
  - Catheter-directed thrombectomy
  - Balloon angioplasty
  - Peripheral artery stenting
- Surgical interventions:
  - Carotid endarterectomy
  - Performed to decrease the risk of stroke
  - Femoral-popliteal bypass
- Medications:
  - Anticoagulation agents (Table 3.1)
  - Thrombolytics (Table 5.1)
  - Analgesics (Table A.2)
  - Vasodilators (Table 2.3)
  - Reversal agents (Vitamin K, Table 5.4)

Nursing Interventions

- Administer medications as ordered.
- Assess affected extremities for adequate circulation and perfusion.
- Assess and treat pain.
- Draw and monitor serial labs as ordered.
- If the patient undergoes a surgical or endovascular procedure to treat their peripheral vascular insufficiency, see the Cardiac Catheterization section for assessment and care of surgical sites. Hemodynamic changes include assessing EKG monitoring system for development of dysrhythmias and/or rate changes, monitoring BP, and monitoring for both hypotension and hypertension. Neurologic assessments should be performed frequently—especially for patients with carotid artery disease—to identify any serious changes. Oxygenation and positioning must also be monitored.

Patient Education

- Follow the DASH diet.
- Follow up as appropriate with outpatient appointments.
- Follow exercise and weight management recommendations.
- Follow diabetes management and treatment recommendations closely.
- Increase physical activity as recommended.
- If referred by provider, participate in cardiac rehab program.
- Pursue smoking cessation as advised.
- Take medications as prescribed.

[ ]   **NURSING PEARL**

Sudden decrease or loss of pulse in the extremities undetected by palpation and/or Doppler ultrasound is a serious complication and surgical emergency. If a decrease in perfusion is prolonged, tissue necrosis and loss of limb is possible. Therefore, it is essential that neurovascular and neuromotor checks be conducted at frequent and regular intervals in patients with vascular disease.

[ ]   **POP QUIZ 2.13**

A 60-year-old female patient is admitted to the PCU. Past medical history includes chronic A-fib, peripheral arterial disease (PAD), CAD, anxiety, and depression. She presents with an uncontrolled nosebleed. Laboratory studies are notable for an INR of 14. When interviewing the patient, she admits it is possible that she mixed her medication together and accidentally doubled her dose of Coumadin. The patient has nasal packing in place, and head CT results are pending. Vital signs are as follows: BP 113/75, HR 84, RR 16, T 98.4°F (36.9°C), and SpO$_2$ 94% on room air. What should the nurse's next action be?

RESOURCES

American Association of Critical Care Nurses. (2018). The cardiovascular system. In T. Hartjes (Ed.), *Core curriculum for high acuity, progressive care, and critical-care nursing* (7th ed., pp. 144–300). Elsevier.

American Heart Association. (2020). *Advanced cardiovascular life support provider manual* (pp. 123–142). Author.

American Heart Association. (n.d.). *Understanding blood pressure readings*. https://www.heart.org/en/health-topics/high-blood-pressure/understanding-blood-pressure-readings

Aronow, W. S. (2017, May 5). Treatment of hypertensive emergencies. *Annals of Translational Medicine, 5*, S5. https://www.ncbi.nlm.nih.gov/pmc/articles/PMC5440310

Fabre, V. (2019). *Endocarditis – Injection drug users*. Johns Hopkins ABX Guide. https://www.hopkinsguides.com/hopkins/view/Johns_Hopkins_ABX_Guide/540192/all/Endocarditis___injection_drug_users

Gopal, M., Bhaskaran, A., Khalife, W. I., & Barbagelata, A. (2009). Heart disease in patients with HIV/AIDS—An emerging clinical problem. *Current Cardiology Reviews, 5*(2), 149–154. https://www.ncbi.nlm.nih.gov/pmc/articles/PMC2805817

Hartung, H. P. (2008). Advances in the understanding of the mechanism of action of IVIG. *Journal of Neurology, 255*(S3), 3–6. https://doi.org/10.1007/s00415-008-3002-0

Medscape. (n.d.). Lanoxin [Drug information]. *Medscape*. https://reference.medscape.com/drug/lanoxin-digoxin-342432.

Moskowitz, A., Chen, K. P., Cooper, A. Z., Chahin, A., Ghassemi, M. M., & Celi, L. A. (2017). Management of atrial fibrillation with rapid ventricular response in the intensive care unit: A secondary analysis of electronic health record data. *Shock, 48*(4), 436–440. https://www.ncbi.nlm.nih.gov/pmc/articles/PMC5603354

National Heart, Lung, and Blood Institute. (n.d.-a). *Arrhythmia*. U.S. Department of Health and Human Services. https://www.nhlbi.nih.gov/health-topics/arrhythmia

National Heart, Lung, and Blood Institute. (n.d.-b). *Cardiogenic shock*. U.S. Department of Health and Human Services. https://www.nhlbi.nih.gov/health-topics/cardiogenic-shock

National Heart, Lung, and Blood Institute. (n.d.-c). *Heart inflammation*. U.S. Department of Health and Human Services. https://www.nhlbi.nih.gov/health-topics/heart-inflammation

Prescribers' Digital Reference. (n.d.-a). *Adenosine* [Drug information]. PDR Search. https://www.pdr.net/drug-summary/Adenosine-adenosine-24200

Prescribers' Digital Reference. (n.d.-b). *Aldactone* [Drug information]. PDR Search. https://www.pdr.net/drug-summary/Aldactone-spironolactone-978.2934

Prescribers' Digital Reference. (n.d.-c). *Atropine sulfate* [Drug information]. PDR Search. https://www.pdr.net/drug-summary/Atropine-Sulfate-Injection-atropine-sulfate-684

Prescribers' Digital Reference. (n.d.-d). *Bivigam (immune globulin intravenous (human)* [Drug information]. PDR Search. https://www.pdr.net/drug-summary/Bivigam-immune-globulin-intravenous--human--3477

Prescribers' Digital Reference. (n.d.-e). *Captopril* [Drug information]. PDR Search. https://www.pdr.net/drug-summary/Captopril-captopril-2348.4130

Prescribers' Digital Reference. (n.d.-f). *Cardene I.V. Premixed injection 20 mg* [Drug information]. PDR Search. https://www.pdr.net/drug-summary/Cardene-I-V--Premixed-Injection-20-mg-nicardipine-hydrochloride-2169.8386

Prescribers' Digital Reference. (n.d.-g). *Cardura (doxazosin mesylate)* [Drug information]. PDR Search. https://www.pdr.net/drug-summary/Cardura-doxazosin-mesylate-1849.6175

Prescribers' Digital Reference. (n.d.-h). *Coumadin (warfarin sodium)* [Drug information]. PDR Search. https://www.pdr.net/drug-summary/Coumadin-warfarin-sodium-106

Prescribers' Digital Reference. (n.d.-i). *Cozaar (losartan potassium)* [Drug information]. PDR Search. https://www.pdr.net/drug-summary/Cozaar-losartan-potassium-339.4526

Prescribers' Digital Reference. (n.d.-j). *Digoxin (digoxin)* [Drug information]. PDR Search. https://www.pdr.net/drug-summary/Digoxin-digoxin-724.8383

Prescribers' Digital Reference. (n.d.-k). *Diltiazem* [Drug information]. PDR Search. https://www.pdr.net/drug-summary/Diltiazem-Hydrochloride-Injection-diltiazem-hydrochloride-725

Prescribers' Digital Reference. (n.d.-l). *Diltiazem hydrochloride injection* [Drug information]. PDR Search. https://www.pdr.net/drug-summary/Diltiazem-Hydrochloride-Injection-diltiazem-hydrochloride-725

Prescribers' Digital Reference. (n.d.-m). *Dobutamine (dobutamine hydrochloride)* [Drug information]. PDR Search. https://www.pdr.net/drug-summary/Dobutamine-dobutamine-hydrochloride-3534.3469

Prescribers' Digital Reference. (n.d.-n). *Dopamine hydrochloride* [Drug information]. PDR Search. https://www.pdr.net/drug-summary/Dopamine-Hydrochloride-dopamine-hydrochloride-3710.3586

Prescribers' Digital Reference. (n.d.-o). *Effient (prasugrel)* [Drug information]. PDR Search. https://www.pdr.net/drug-summary/Effient-prasugrel-289.6190

Prescribers' Digital Reference. (n.d.-p). *Hydrochlorothiazide tablets* [Drug information]. PDR Search. https://www.pdr.net/drug-summary/Hydrochlorothiazide-Tablets-hydrochlorothiazide-1973.1942

Prescribers' Digital Reference. (n.d.-q). *Imuran (azathioprine)* [Drug information]. PDR Search. https://www.pdr.net/drug-summary/Imuran-azathioprine-745

Prescribers' Digital Reference. (n.d.-r). *Lasix (furosemide)* [Drug information]. PDR Search. https://www.pdr.net/drug-summary/Lasix-furosemide-2594.8405

Prescribers' Digital Reference. (n.d.-s). *Levophed (norepinephrine bitartrate)* [Drug information]. PDR Search. https://www.pdr.net/drug-summary/Levophed-norepinephrine-bitartrate-868

Prescribers' Digital Reference. (n.d.-t). *Lisinopril* [Drug information]. PDR Search. https://www.pdr.net/drug-summary/Prinivil-lisinopril-376.4115

Prescribers' Digital Reference. (n.d.-u). *Lovenox (enoxaparin sodium)* [Drug information]. PDR Search. https://www.pdr.net/drug-summary/Lovenox-enoxaparin-sodium-521.2354

Prescribers' Digital Reference. (n.d.-v). *Metoprolol tartrate (metoprolol tartrate)* [Drug information]. PDR Search. https://www.pdr.net/drug-summary/Metoprolol-Tartrate-metoprolol-tartrate-3114.5976

Prescribers' Digital Reference. (n.d.-w). *Micro-K 10 (potassium chloride)* [Drug information]. PDR Search. https://www.pdr.net/drug-summary/Micro-K-10-potassium-chloride-770

Prescribers' Digital Reference. (n.d.-x). *Minipress (prazosin hydrochloride)* [Drug information]. PDR Search. https://www.pdr.net/drug-summary/Minipress-prazosin-hydrochloride-999

Prescribers' Digital Reference. (n.d.-y). *Multaq (dronedarone)* [Drug information]. PDR Search. https://www.pdr.net/drug-summary/Multaq-dronedarone-522.1412

Prescribers' Digital Reference. (n.d.-z). *Nitroglycerin* [Drug information]. PDR Search. https://www.pdr.net/drug-summary/Nitroglycerin-in-5--Dextrose-nitroglycerin-1148

Prescribers' Digital Reference. (n.d.-aa). *Norpace/norpace CR (disopyramide phosphate)* [Drug information]. PDR Search. https://www.pdr.net/drug-summary/Norpace-Norpace-CR-disopyramide-phosphate-1182

Prescribers' Digital Reference. (n.d.-bb). *Norvasc (amlodipine besylate)* [Drug information]. PDR Search. https://www.pdr.net/drug-summary/Norvasc-amlodipine-besylate-1853.3578

Prescribers' Digital Reference. (n.d.-cc). *Plavix (clopidogrel bisulfate)* [Drug information]. PDR Search. https://www.pdr.net/drug-summary/Plavix-clopidogrel-bisulfate-525.3952

Prescribers' Digital Reference. (n.d.-dd). *Propranolol hydrochloride tablets (propranolol hydrochloride)* [Drug information]. PDR Search. https://www.pdr.net/drug-summary/Propranolol-Hydrochloride-Tablets-propranolol-hydrochloride-1400.8469

Prescribers' Digital Reference. (n.d.-ee). *Sodium nitroprusside* [Drug information]. PDR Search. https://www.pdr.net/drug-summary/Nitropress-sodium-nitroprusside-3404#12

Prescribers' Digital Reference. (n.d.-ff). *Valsartan (valsartan)* [Drug information]. PDR Search. https://www.pdr.net/drug-summary/Valsartan-valsartan-24321

Prescribers' Digital Reference. (n.d.-gg). *Vasotec (enalapril maleate)* [Drug information]. PDR Search. https://www.pdr.net/drug-summary/Vasotec-enalapril-maleate-2344.4124

Prescribers' Digital Reference. (n.d.-hh). *Verapamil hydrochloride injection (verapamil hydrochloride)* [Drug information]. PDR Search. https://www.pdr.net/drug-summary/Verapamil-Hydrochloride-Injection-verapamil-hydrochloride-2813.1935

ACUTE RESPIRATORY DISTRESS SYNDROME

Overview

- Acute respiratory distress syndrome (ARDS) is a form of acute respiratory failure that develops when there is damage to the alveolar–capillary membrane causing fluid buildup, hypoxemia, reduced lung compliance, and pulmonary infiltrates.
- ARDS is defined as a PaO_2/FiO_2 ratio of <300.
- It comprises three phases. *Exudative phase*: 7 to 10 days after exposure to lung injury, causing an inflammatory cascade. This cascade causes fluid and hemorrhage in the lung. *Proliferative phase*: Restoration of the epithelial and endothelial barriers is reestablished. *Fibrotic phase*: May not always occur but is associated with fibrous tissue formation, which can lead to prolonged mechanical ventilation and mortality.
- The most common cause of ARDS is systemic inflammatory response syndrome and/or sepsis.
- ARDS can lead to atelectasis, pulmonary edema, decreased pulmonary compliance, and difficulty breathing.
- Patients who develop ARDS cannot be effectively treated without intubation, and mechanical ventilation may need transfer to a higher level of care.

Signs and Symptoms

- Accessory muscle use
- Altered mental status (AMS)
- Chest pain
- Crackles
- Cyanosis
- Diaphoresis
- Dyspnea
- Fatigue
- Fever
- Hypotension
- Hypoxia
- Increasing oxygen demand
- Respiratory alkalosis
- Retractions
- Tachycardia
- Tachypnea
- Wheezes

COMPLICATIONS

Complications of ARDS include ventilator-associated pneumonia, barotrauma, atelectasis, pulmonary hypertension (HTN), lung scarring, multi-organ failure, and death. ARDS often presents with multiple other comorbidities and diagnoses (e.g., sepsis, multisystem trauma, acute pancreatitis, etc.), so collaborative care and management are essential to prevent permanent lung damage and death.

ALERT!

In patients transferred from the ICU who were mechanically ventilated with high positive end-expiratory pressure (PEEP) or increased tidal volumes, ARDS causes overdistention of the alveoli and increases the risk of developing barotrauma. In these transferred patients, watch for symptoms of pneumothorax, tension pneumothorax, and subcutaneous emphysema.

Diagnosis

Labs

- Arterial blood gas (ABG): Expected hypoxemia initially accompanied with acute respiratory alkalosis; severe ARDS is indicated through ABG progressing to hypercapnic respiratory acidosis.
- Complete metabolic panel (CMP): May reflect evidence of end-organ injury resulting from severe hypoxia, shock, or systemic inflammation.
- Complete blood count (CBC): May show elevated white blood cell (WBC) count if infection is present.

Diagnostic Testing

- Bronchoscopy
- Chest CT
- Chest x-ray
- Echocardiogram

Treatment

- Blood transfusion
- Medications (Table 3.1): antibiotics (Table A.1), anticoagulants, corticosteroids, and diuretics (Table 2.3)
- Nutrition and fluid support (Table A.3)
- Oxygen and ventilatory support: continuous positive airway pressure (CPPAP), bilevel positive airway pressure (BiPAP), and intubation and mechanical ventilation requiring transfer to higher level of care
- Physical therapy
- Positioning: head of bed (HOB) >30° to improve oxygenation and prevent risk of aspiration; patient is likely prone when transferred to the ICU

[⚡]   **ALERT!**

ARDS can be a complication of COVID-19, which is caused by the SARS-CoV-2 virus. Care parameters are continually evolving. For current information on caring for patients with COVID-19, consult the National Institute of Health (www.covid19treatmentguidelines.nih.gov) and the Centers for Disease Control and Prevention (CDC) (www.cdc.gov/coronavirus/2019-ncov/hcp/).

TABLE 3.1 Pulmonary Medications

INDICATIONS	MECHANISM OF ACTION	CONTRAINDICATIONS, PRECAUTIONS, AND ADVERSE EFFECTS
Anticholinergics (e.g., ipratropium)		
• Asthma, COPD, acute respiratory failure • Bronchospasm • Bronchoconstriction	• Block the effects of acetylcholine to help relax the muscles causing bronchoconstriction • Reduce the production of mucus • Inhibit cholinergic receptors in bronchial smooth muscle	• Medication is contraindicated in cross sensitivity to atropine or bromide. • Inhaled anticholinergics can produce a paradoxical bronchospasm, which can be life-threatening in some patients; however, it is rare and usually occurs with the first use of a new cannister. • Use caution in soy or peanut allergy, in patients with known dysrhythmia, or in BPH or urinary obstructions. • Adverse effects include hypotension, GI irritation, allergic reaction, headache, nervousness, dysrhythmia, and urinary retention.

(continued)

TABLE 3.1 Pulmonary Medications (*continued*)

INDICATIONS	MECHANISM OF ACTION	CONTRAINDICATIONS, PRECAUTIONS, AND ADVERSE EFFECTS
Anticoagulants (e.g., warfarin)		
• Blood clots such as DVTs and PEs	• Inhibit vitamin K availability to reduce the effects of clotting factors	• Patients taking warfarin are at increased risk of bleeding; ensure bleeding and fall precautions are maintained. • Clotting factors must be checked regularly.
Anticoagulants: Heparin, fractionated (enoxaparin)		
• Treatment and prophylaxis of thromboembolic disorders	• Prevent growth of existing thrombus • Prevent formation of new thrombus	• Medication is contraindicated in uncontrolled bleeding and severe thrombocytopenia. • Use caution in renal or hepatic disease, GI bleed/ulcerative disease, head injury, or bleeding disorders. • Adverse effects include bleeding.
Anticoagulants: Heparin, unfractionated (heparin)		
• PE, DVT • Postoperative antithrombotic prophylaxis	• Are used to treat and prevent the formation of blood clots by accelerating the activity of antithrombin III to inactivate thrombin	• Use cautiously in patients who have an increased risk for bleeding. • Medication is contraindicated for patients with severe thrombocytopenia. • Monitor CBC and clotting factors with special attention to PTT when administering as a continuous infusion. • Use cautiously in patients with hepatic disease, as they are often at higher risk of bleeding.
Beta-2 agonists/bronchodilators (albuterol)		
• Reverse and prevent airway obstruction related to COPD and asthma	• Relax airway smooth muscle and decrease obstruction and inflammation, resulting in improved airway clearance	• Use caution in patients with cardiac disease, diabetes, glaucoma, hyperthyroidism, and HTN. • Adverse effects include paradoxical bronchospasm, anxiety, nervousness, chest pain, dysrhythmia, and palpitations.
Corticosteroids (e.g., prednisone, dexamethasone, methylprednisolone)		
• Asthma, COPD, anaphylaxis, inflammatory states: ARDS, pneumonia, respiratory failure	• Inhibit steps in the inflammatory pathway to prevent inflammation of the lungs and reduce mucus production	• Patients receiving corticosteroids for an extended time or in high doses are at increased risk of immunosuppression, making them more prone to infection. • Avoid using in patients with Cushing's syndrome. • Use caution in untreated infection, diabetes, glaucoma, immunodepression, and liver disease. • Adverse effects include headache, hoarseness, diaphoresis, and bronchospasm. • Medication may reduce glucose tolerance, causing hyperglycemia in diabetic patients.

(*continued*)

TABLE 3.1 Pulmonary Medications (*continued*)

INDICATIONS	MECHANISM OF ACTION	CONTRAINDICATIONS, PRECAUTIONS, AND ADVERSE EFFECTS
Expectorants (e.g., dextromethorphan, guaifenesin)		
• Pneumonia, respiratory failure, ARDS	• Help alleviate congestion, reduce viscosity, and clear mucus from airways	• Do not give for persistent or chronic cough due to smoking, asthma, or COPD. • Medication is contraindicated in alcohol intolerance. • Use caution in prolonged cough accompanied by fever, rash, or headache and in diabetic patients. • Adverse effects include dizziness, headache, nausea, vomiting, diarrhea, and rash.
Prostacyclin analogs (e.g., epoprostenol, treprostinil, and iloprost)		
• Treatment of pulmonary atrial HTN	• Promote vasodilation and reduce pulmonary vascular resistance	• Medication is contraindicated in pulmonary edema. • Use caution in hypotension or patients at risk for bleeding. • Adverse effects include headache, flushing, tachycardia, nausea, vomiting, dizziness, and myalgia.

ARDS, acute respiratory distress syndrome; BPH, benign prostatic hyperplasia; CBC, complete blood count; COPD, chronic obstructive pulmonary disease; DVT, deep vein thrombosis; GI, gastrointestinal; HTN, hypertension; PE, pulmonary embolism; PTT, partial thromboplastin time.

Nursing Interventions

- Administer medication to achieve blood pressure (BP) goals.
- Assess and pad bony prominences and areas of skin.
- Consider the use of a diuretic to optimize fluid status.
- Consult physical and occupational therapy to assist the patient with ambulation.
- Consult with respiratory therapy to maintain adequate respiratory status.
- Draw labs as ordered.
- Encourage the patient to cough and deep breathe.
- Increase supplemental oxygen as needed to maintain O_2 SAT >90%.
- Maintain patient comfort.
- Monitor vital signs (VS).
- Obtain accurate intake and output (I/O).
- Obtain an ABG with any pulmonary changes.
- Perform daily oral care with chlorhexidine.
- Perform pulmonary hygiene and encourage the use of the incentive spirometer hourly.
- Position the patient appropriately for maximum ventilation and pressure ulcer prevention.

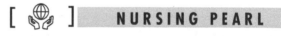 **NURSING PEARL**

Monitor laboratory values carefully and notify providers of any worsening trends. ARDS patients can decompensate quickly and require diligent monitoring and intervention if status worsens.

Patient Education

- Follow up with outpatient follow-up appointments, diagnostic tests, and laboratory draws.
- Participate in pulmonary rehab.
- Continue using incentive spirometry. ▶

Patient Education (*continued*)

- To use an incentive spirometer, place the mouthpiece facing the mouth. Exhale deeply, make a tight seal around the mouthpiece with the mouth and lips, and inhale as deeply as possible. Repeat 10 times every 1 to 2 hr.
- Engage in physical activity. Start small and work up to regain baseline functioning.
- Supplemental home oxygen may be required at time of discharge. Engage in safe oxygen therapy practices by avoiding smoking and avoiding open flames, flammable products, and heat sources. Avoid products with oil or petroleum, and keep a fire extinguisher close by.

POP QUIZ 3.1

Patients with ARDS who require mechanical ventilation in the ICU are at risk for developing barotrauma. How does barotrauma occur, and what are the clinical manifestations?

ASTHMA (SEVERE)

Overview

- Asthma is a chronic inflammatory disorder of the airway that affects both children and adults.
- Allergens, pollutants, food additives, occupational exposures, stress, exercise, cold air, viral upper respiratory infections (URIs), sinusitis, and menses can trigger severe asthma attacks.
- Airway inflammation in severe asthma attacks results in bronchoconstriction, hyperreactivity, and edema.
- Patients presenting with severe asthma attack usually present in the tripod position with accessory muscle use, anxiety or agitation, and/or wheezing with a respiration rate >30 and heart rate (HR) >120.

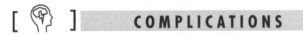

COMPLICATIONS

Patients who present with a severe asthma attack are at an increased risk of developing status asthmaticus. These patients should be urgently assessed and prepared for intubation. Without prompt identification and intervention, patients may experience respiratory failure or death.

Signs and Symptoms

- Anxiety
- Accessory muscle use
- Chest tightness
- Cough
- Cyanosis
- Diminished breath sounds
- Dyspnea
- Hypoxemia
- Tachycardia
- Tachypnea
- Wheezing

Diagnosis

Labs

- ABG: in asthma, reflect hypoxemia or hypercarbia
- CBC: in asthma, eosinophils elevated
- IgE levels (antibody that protects from bacteria, viruses, and allergens): in asthma attack, IgE elevated

ALERT!

ABG values should be used in conjunction with physical assessment and vital sign trends to determine whether transfer to a higher level of care for mechanical ventilation is indicated.

Diagnostic Testing
- Chest x-ray
- SpO$_2$ monitoring
- Peak expiratory flow rate

Treatment

- Medications (Table 3.1): inhaled anticholinergic agents, inhaled beta-2 adrenergic agonists, and corticosteroids
- Maintain patent airway.
- Oxygen and ventilatory support: intubation and mechanical ventilation, nasal cannula, nonrebreather, and simple mask
- Trigger removal (if allergic cause)
- Monoclonal antibody therapy in patients with positive skin tests

Nursing Interventions

- Administer medication as ordered.
- Administer supplemental oxygen; titrate up as appropriate on L/min and device.
- Prepare to call for a rapid response if the patient's condition rapidly deteriorates or a higher level of care is indicated.
- Closely trend ABG results.
- Closely monitor vital signs.
- Closely monitor for worsening signs of respiratory distress, including the following: increasing oxygen requirement with minimal response to medication or supplemental oxygen, hypoxemia, new inability to complete sentences or communicate verbally due to reduced oxygenation, retractions, and seated in the tripod position.
- Draw labs as ordered.
- Maintain patient comfort.
- Provide pain medication as needed.
- Perform daily oral care.
- Position patient appropriately for maximum ventilation and pressure ulcer prevention.
- Remove anxiety triggers if possible.

[🌐] NURSING PEARL

Patients experiencing severe asthma attack may experience anxiety. Provide therapeutic communication and support to acknowledge any feelings of anxiety. Worsening anxiety may worsen the severity of the asthma attack.

Patient Education

- After an acute asthma exacerbation, review the medication regimen with the provider.
- Review the asthma control plan: Keep rescue inhalers on hand in case of acute attack. Change one's occupation if allergen or trigger exposure is work related. Control asthma triggers by self-monitoring symptoms and removing from the source of allergen if possible. This may include avoiding tobacco, dust mites, animals, specific foods, or pollen. Ensure proper inhaler use. To use most inhalers, use thumb and fingers to hold the inhaler upright with the mouthpiece down, pointing toward the mouth. Remove the mouthpiece cover and gently shake. Hold the mouthpiece away from the mouth and exhale deeply. Use the inhalation method recommended by the provider (open mouth vs. closed mouth) and breathe in slowly (3 to 5 seconds) while pressing down at the top of the cannister to dispense medication. Hold breath for 10 seconds before removing the mouthpiece and exhaling slowly. Repeat this process for the recommended number of puffs. Once finished, wipe the mouthpiece and reapply the cap. ►

Patient Education (*continued*)

- Identify and control asthma triggers: Avoid allergen (e.g., tobacco, dust mites, animals, pollen) if possible. Get allergy testing if etiology is unknown. Self-monitor symptoms.
- Continuously review/educate on current situation and plan of care.
- Take medications as prescribed.
- Engage in weight reduction practices.
- Engage in smoking cessation protocols.

POP QUIZ 3.2

A patient experiencing a severe asthma exacerbation saw minimal improvement after Atrovent (ipratropium) administration. Throughout the shift, the patient's respiratory status progressively declined. What is the next intervention in severe asthma exacerbation?

CHRONIC OBSTRUCTIVE PULMONARY DISEASE EXACERBATION

Overview

- *Chronic obstructive pulmonary disease (COPD)* is a chronic restrictive airway disease classified by airflow limitation.
- COPD consists of both bronchitis (inflammation of the bronchioles) and emphysema (destruction of the alveoli secondary to irritant exposure such as smoke or particulates).
- COPD exacerbation can rapidly progress to acute respiratory failure requiring mechanical ventilation.
- Patients intubated due to a severe COPD exacerbation are likely to fail extubation.

Signs and Symptoms

- Accessory muscle use
- Chest tightness
- Chronic productive cough
- Central cyanosis
- Clubbing of the nails
- Dyspnea and tachypnea
- Hypercapnia
- Hypoxia
- Increased anteroposterior diameter
- Peripheral edema
- Low SpO_2
- Muscle atrophy
- Weight loss
- Wheezing

COMPLICATIONS

Complications of COPD include acute exacerbations, acute and/or chronic respiratory failure, pulmonary HTN, right-sided heart failure (HF), weight loss, and bacterial infections. Close monitoring and management of symptoms can help decrease the risk of developing these complications and improve quality of life.

ALERT!

Patients with no history of smoking or secondhand smoke inhalation who are diagnosed with COPD should be worked up for alpha-1 antitrypsin deficiency. This is a genetic disorder that can cause COPD and is the most common cause of COPD in nonsmokers.

NURSING PEARL

Typically, there are two findings seen in COPD:
- *Blue bloaters:* A patient whose skin appears ashen/blue and has a $PaCO_2$ >45 mmHg with PaO_2 <60 mmHg
- *Pink puffers:* A patient whose skin remains pink but seems to gasp (or puff) for air and whose $PaCO_2$ is normal and PaO_2 >60 mmHg

Diagnosis

Labs
- ABGs: May show hypercarbia or hypoxia.
- Blood and sputum cultures: May show organism growth.
- CBC: Elevated WBC possible if infection present.

Diagnostic Testing
- Chest CT
- Chest x-ray
- Pulmonary function tests

Treatment

- Airway suctioning as needed for secretions
- Chest physiotherapy
- Lung transplantation (end-stage treatment)
- Medications (Table 3.1): antibiotics, if indicated (Table A.1), anticholinergics, bronchodilators, corticosteroids
- Nutritional supplementation
- Pulmonary rehab
- Self-care: physical exercise, diaphragmatic breathing, and smoking cessation
- Supplemental oxygen and ventilatory support: nasal cannula, simple mask, nonrebreather, and intubation and mechanical ventilation

Nursing Interventions

- Administer medication as ordered.
- Administer noninvasive ventilation and mechanical ventilation, if necessary.
- Closely monitor ABGs and serial laboratory studies.
- Closely monitor vital signs.
- Maintain patient comfort by achieving patient pain goals.
- Perform chest physiotherapy.
- Prepare patient for intubation, if indicated.
- Position patient appropriately for maximum ventilation and pressure ulcer prevention.
- Remove anxiety triggers if necessary to improve ventilation.

Patient Education

- Attend pulmonary rehabilitation as ordered by provider.
- Avoid exposure to airway irritants.
- Use home oxygen therapy as indicated.
- Follow up with all scheduled appointments.
- Start smoking cessation program and avoid secondhand smoke.
- Take medications as ordered.
- Use supplemental oxygen as needed.
- Get vaccinated for seasonal flu and pneumonia.

[⚡]   **ALERT!**

Patients with COPD may have a baseline SpO_2 value <90%. This makes SpO_2 an unreliable diagnostic tool for assessing respiratory status. ABGs are a much more accurate indicator of respiratory status in this population; they accurately provide values for PaO_2, CO_2, and HCO_3, indicating acid–base imbalances and hypercapnia.

    NURSING PEARL

Chest physiotherapy can be delivered manually, with a vest, or with a programmable bed. Chest physiotherapy can help loosen airway secretions, which can be suctioned to maintain a patent airway.

    POP QUIZ 3.3

What is the most common cause of COPD in patients with no past history of smoking or history of exposure to secondhand smoke?

OBSTRUCTIVE SLEEP APNEA

Overview

- Obstructive sleep apnea (OSA) occurs when the airway becomes fully or partially occluded while the patient is sleeping, resulting in an obstruction of airflow.
- This occurs when there is not sufficient space to accommodate airflow in a portion of the upper airway.
- Complications of sleep apnea can range from poor, nonrestorative sleep to significant long-term effects on cardiovascular (CV) health, mental illness, and quality of life.
- Risk factors for sleep apnea include obesity, alcohol use, smoking, anatomic structure, male gender, use of sedatives, habitual snoring, use of sedatives, and family history.
- There are many treatment options for OSA, ranging from lifestyle modifications to surgical procedures.

Signs and Symptoms

- Apnea during sleep
- Daytime fatigue
- Decreased attention and concentration
- Dry mouth and headache
- Frequent loud snoring
- Gasping for air while sleeping
- Nocturia
- Sexual dysfunction

Diagnosis

Diagnostic Testing

- Sleep studies

Treatment

- Lifestyle modifications: diet modification to achieve healthy body mass index (BMI); healthy sleeping habits; physical activity; smoking cessation program, if indicated
- Airway devices: CPAP; mouth pieces
- Surgical procedures: nerve stimulator implant, orofacial therapy, tonsillectomy, and tracheostomy

Nursing Interventions

- Apply supplemental oxygen for an SpO_2 goal >90%.
- Consult with respiratory therapist.
- Develop sleep plan and schedule with patient.
- Encourage consistent use of oral or nasal airway device.
- Encourage lifestyle modifications to improve OSA.
- Perform sleep hygiene.
- Monitor and treat complications.
- Monitor continuous SpO_2 values while patient is sleeping.

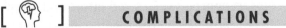

COMPLICATIONS

Complications of untreated OSA include atrial fibrillation (A-fib), cancer, cardiac and vascular disease (myocardial infarction [MI], HF, stroke), metabolic disorders (type 2 diabetes and glucose intolerance), and glaucoma. OSA has a high mortality rate and should be treated seriously when diagnosed to prevent further complications and systemic damage.

ALERT!

Sleep studies are the gold standard to diagnose OSA. Additionally, lab values can be helpful to rule out other contributing medical or metabolic conditions.

NURSING PEARL

CPAP compliance is low; over 50% of patients do not continue usage after the first month. However, patients who are compliant with CPAP have better outcomes compared to those who do not use CPAP.

Patient Education

- Encourage compliance with airway devices. Follow the user instructions to assemble a CPAP home device. Insert appropriately sized filters and attach the CPAP hose to the mask. Program CPAP pressure settings as determined by the results of a sleep study test and provider. Set up the humidifier and be sure to use distilled water. Fit the CPAP to face and secure snuggly with the straps. Turn on the device and enjoy a restful sleep. Be sure to clean CPAP regularly.
- Modify diet as ordered by provider.
- Maintain healthy sleep patterns.
- Maintain physical activity as ordered by provider.
- Begin smoking cessation plan if needed.

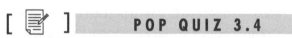

POP QUIZ 3.4

What medications should be avoided overnight in patients with OSA?

PLEURAL SPACE COMPLICATIONS

Overview

- Pleural space complications include chylothorax, empyema, hemothorax, pneumothorax, and pleural effusion.
- *Chylothorax* is an accumulation of chyle in the pleural area of the lung. Chyle is a milky white substance that is produced in the small intestine. This can be absorbed by the lymphatic system and deposited in the lung. Often, this is the result of thoracic trauma, neoplasm, or infection.
- *Empyema* is the collection of pus in the pleural area of the lung.
- *Hemothorax* is the presence of blood in the pleural space, usually caused by trauma.
- *Pneumothorax* is the presence of air in the pleural space. Pneumothorax can be further classified as spontaneous or traumatic/tension.
- *Pleural effusion* is defined as the excessive buildup of fluid in the pleural area. Often, this can result from pneumonia, HF, malignancy, cirrhosis, and/or ascites.

Signs and Symptoms

- Small or large chylothorax: Small chylothorax is asymptomatic and detected through nonrelated imaging. Large chylothorax is usually unilateral and most common in the right lung. Possible symptoms include chest pressure, decreased breath sounds, dullness to percussion, decreased exercise capacity, and progressive dyspnea.
- Empyema symptoms are consistent with pneumonia but linger for an extended period of time: cough; crackles; dullness to percussion; egophony; increased palpable fremitus; fever; pleuritic, sharp chest pain on inspiration and sputum production.
- Hemothorax: absent or decreased breath sounds, chest wall asymmetry, cardiac arrest, hypoxia, hypotension, respiratory distress and arrest, tachypnea, and tracheal deviation. ▶

COMPLICATIONS

If significant, hemothorax can result in hemodynamic instability, shock, hypoxia, and death. Complications of pneumothorax include pneumoperitoneum, pneumopericardium, pulmonary edema, empyema, respiratory failure or arrest, cardiac arrest, and pleural effusion complications include empyema, sepsis, and pneumothorax.

ALERT!

Any accumulation of fluid or air in the pleural space can compromise lung function, placing the patient at risk for adverse events. Treatment requires early identification and evacuation of invading fluid or air from the pleural space.

ALERT!

Alert the provider if absence of breath sounds is noted on assessment, especially in the context of vital sign changes or increasing oxygen demand. These findings require immediate intervention.

Signs and Symptoms (*continued*)

- Pleural effusion can be asymptomatic or present with the following: cough, decreased tactile fremitus, dullness noted on percussion, dyspnea on exertion, egophony, fever, pleural rub, and sharp pain with breathing or cough.
- With spontaneous pneumothorax, symptoms may include the following: absent chest wall movement, asymmetric lung expansion, acute dyspnea with increased work of breathing, cyanosis, decreased tactile fremitus or breath sounds, hyperresonance on percussion, jugular vein distention (JVD), pulsus paradoxus, sharp pleuritic ipsilateral chest pain, respiratory failure, tachycardia, tachypnea, and acute respiratory failure and hemodynamic instability (tension/traumatic pneumothorax).

Diagnosis

Labs

- ABG to show respiratory compromise, acidosis, or hypercarbia
- CBC to show elevated WBC

Diagnostic Testing

- Chest CT
- Chest x-ray
- Ultrasound

Treatment

- Supplemental oxygen with titration as needed to maintain oxygen saturation >90%
- Medications as ordered: analgesics (Table A.2); antibiotics, if indicated (Table A.1); and diuretics, if indicated (Table 2.3)
- Chest tube inserted into chest wall to drain air or fluid
- Thoracentesis: procedure in which large-bore needle is inserted into the pleural wall space and drains accumulating fluid
- Needle decompression: emergency procedure used to stabilize patients with tension pneumothorax
- Thoracotomy: open surgical procedure to gain access to the pleural space so surgeons can remove fluid from around the lungs and insert drains as needed to stabilize the patient

Nursing Interventions

- Assess and maintain chest tube integrity. Assess for air leak. Attach to low wall suction or water seal as ordered. Maintain clean, dry, and occlusive chest tube dressings. Change chest tube dressing per facility protocol (usually every 72 hr or when soiled). Monitor chest tube output volume, color, and consistency. Notify the provider for any rapid increase in drainage amount.
- Promote pulmonary hygiene. Titrate oxygen and delivery device as needed. Turn, cough, and take a deep breath. Use incentive spirometer. Move patient out of bed to chair.
- Promote hemodynamic stability: Administer blood transfusion. Administer medications (Table 3.1). Administer IV fluids. ▶

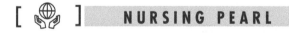
NURSING PEARL

Indications for an urgent thoracotomy for a hemothorax include 300 to 500 mL/hr of output for 2 to 4 consecutive hr after chest tube insertion, or >1,500 mL over 24 hr. This is a complication of hemothorax and may indicate active bleeding of a great vessel injury, chest wall injury, or cardiac tamponade. These conditions indicate active bleeding. Notify the provider immediately and prepare for transfer to higher level of care.

Nursing Interventions (*continued*)

- Notify the provider if the patient's oxygen saturation does not improve, despite increasing supplemental oxygen. Prepare for transfer to a higher level of care.
- Update the patient and/or family on current clinical status, plan of care, and upcoming procedures.

Patient Education

- Ask questions about the purpose of external medical devices including bedside telemetry, chest tube systems, and incentive spirometer. Ask questions about medication for hemothorax, chylothorax, pleural effusion, or empyema.
- Notify the nurse immediately if any of the following occurs: bleeding, drainage, or pain around the chest tube insertion sites; chest pain; dyspnea; or feelings of anxiety or impending doom.

POP QUIZ 3.5

When discussing treatment options for a hemothorax, the nursing student states a needle decompression can be used to treat a hemothorax. How should the nurse respond?

PNEUMONIA

Overview

- Pneumonia is defined as an acute inflammation of the lungs caused by a variety of agents that may lead to alveolar consolidation.
- Pneumonia may be categorized by the following: aspiration of foreign substance, food, or liquid into lung causing injury; bacterial infection; viral infection; or fungal infection.

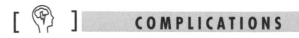

COMPLICATIONS

Untreated pneumonia can progress to sepsis, empyema, lung abscess, multiple organ dysfunction syndrome, and respiratory failure. Timely diagnosis and treatment can prevent progression to any of these complications.

Signs and Symptoms

- Accessory muscle use
- Bronchial or diminished breath sounds
- Chest pain
- Fever and chills
- Productive cough
- Tachycardia
- Weakness, malaise

Diagnosis

Labs

- ABG to indicate hypoxia or acidosis.
- Blood and sputum cultures to identify organism present and guide treatment through antibiotic susceptibility.
- CBC: Elevated WBC counts indicate infectious process presence.

Diagnostic Testing

- Bronchoscopy with bronchoalveolar lavage
- Chest x-ray
- Chest CT scan
- Thoracentesis

Treatment

- IV fluids as needed (Table A.3)
- Supplemental oxygen and ventilatory support
- Identify/treat cause: If aspiration, use antibiotics (Table A.1); if bacterial, use antibiotics; if fungal, use antifungals; and if viral, use antivirals and lung support.
- Adjunct medications as indicated (Table 3.1): anticholinergics, bronchodilators, corticosteroids, expectorants, and antipyretics (Table A.2)
- Adequate nutrition through oral by mouth (PO) intake or tube feeding alternatives as necessary

Nursing Interventions

- Administer antibiotics as ordered.
- Apply supplemental oxygenation if needed. Titrate oxygen and delivery device as needed.
- Collect blood, sputum, and urine cultures.
- Encourage activity, mobility, and incentive spirometer use to help improve recovery.
- Frequently monitor airway patency.
- Monitor and follow up on labs as ordered.
- Monitor fever curve and provide cooling interventions as needed.
- Perform chest physiotherapy.
- Position patient in an upright position to promote adequate ventilation.
- Promote hemodynamic stability. Administer intravenous (IV) fluids, if indicated. Support BP as needed.
- Promote pulmonary hygiene. Encourage cough and deep breathing. Encourage incentive spirometer.
- Pulmonary toileting, secretion mobilization, and clearance are essential to help improve oxygenation and perfusion.

Patient Education

- Vaccinate against flu and pneumonia at discharge if available or in outpatient setting before the start of flu season.
- Work with primary care provider to identify resources or medications to support smoking cessation.
- In cases of aspiration pneumonia, restrict diet as ordered. This may include preparing thicker consistency meals.
- If diagnosed with aspiration pneumonia, follow up with a swallow study, speech therapy consults, and swallowing rehab.

PULMONARY EMBOLISM

Overview

- A *pulmonary embolism (PE)* is a partial or complete blockage of the pulmonary arteries due to a blood clot, fat, air, or foreign material.
- If the PE is caused by a blood clot, the origin of the clot most often comes from a deep vein thrombosis (DVT) in the leg or a venous clot.
- Fat emboli are usually a complication secondary to a long bone or pelvic fracture. ▶

POP QUIZ 3.6

What is one essential daily intervention that should be performed to prevent the development of ventilatory-associated pneumonia?

COMPLICATIONS

Complications of a PE are severe and include the following:
- Cardiac arrest
- Dysrhythmia
- Pulmonary infarction
- Pulmonary HTN
- Respiratory arrest
- Death

Overview (*continued*)

- Air emboli may occur after surgery or through an IV or central line.
- Septic emboli may occur if the patient experiences a bacterial or viral infection.

Signs and Symptoms

- Chest pain
- Cough
- Crackles
- Dyspnea
- Feelings of impending doom
- Fever
- Hemoptysis
- Hypoxemia
- Mental status changes
- Petechiae on truck and head of body (fat emboli)
- Pleural friction rub
- Pulmonary HTN
- Right ventricular hypertrophy
- Syncope
- Tachycardia

Diagnosis

Labs

- ABG: Expect hypoxemia or hypercarbia.
- CBC: May show elevated platelet counts.
- Coagulation studies: D-dimer, international normalized ratio (INR), prothrombin time (PT), and partial thromboplastin time (PTT)
- Troponins

Diagnostic Testing

- Chest x-ray
- Chest CT scan with and without contrast
- Pulmonary angiography
- Venous ultrasound
- Ventilation and perfusion lung scan
- CT angiography
- Echocardiogram

Treatment

- Medication (Table 3.1): fibrinolytic agents (Table 5.1), heparin (Table 3.1), low-molecular-weight heparin, warfarin (Table 3.1), opioids (Table A.2), and oxygen and ventilatory support
- Surgery: inferior vena cava filter, pulmonary embolectomy

[⚡]   **ALERT!**

Risks for PE include DVT/venous thromboembolism (VTE), A-fib, MI, cerebrovascular accident (CVA), surgery, trauma, prolonged immobilization, pregnancy, hormonal birth control, smoking, and obesity.

[🌐]   **NURSING PEARL**

First-choice anticoagulants include unfractionated or low-molecular-weight heparin for inpatient treatment. Patients are usually bridged to warfarin when ready for discharge.

Nursing Interventions

- Administer medications as ordered.
- Discuss potential procedures, such as chest tube insertion and surgery.
- Educate on follow-up care after discharge.
- Monitor and follow up on labs as ordered.
- Patients on a heparin drip will have serial PTTs drawn until a therapeutic level is obtained.
- Monitor for dysrhythmia on continuous cardiac monitoring.
- Monitor for hematoma or signs of bleeding due to anticoagulation therapy.
- Notify healthcare team of worsening status or condition: anxiety, chest pain, dyspnea, and position patient in semi-Fowler's position.
- Promote adequate oxygenation. Titrate supplemental oxygen as needed. Continuous SpO_2 monitoring.
- Promote hemodynamic stability. Administer blood transfusion, if indicated. Support BP as needed.
- Support patient's emotional well-being.

Patient Education

- Ambulate and exercise as tolerated and ordered.
- Anticoagulation medication increases risk for bleeding. Take precautions to fall-proof the home environment by wearing appropriate footwear or nonskid socks, removing rugs and other tripping hazards, installing handrails, and using nonslip mats in bathrooms or other areas of concern.
- Continue outpatient lab draws to monitor long-term anticoagulation therapy as needed.
- Take precautions to prevent DVT, specifically postsurgery: Ambulation as allowed; elevate lower extremities when not ambulatory; and wear graduated compression stockings or sequential compression devices (SCDs).

PULMONARY HYPERTENSION

Overview

- *Pulmonary HTN* occurs when the pressure in the blood vessels that carry blood from the heart to the lungs is higher than normal.
- Pulmonary HTN often presents with right-sided HF.
- Though drug therapy has advanced to improve quality of life, there is no cure.

Signs and Symptoms

- Ascites
- Cardiac murmurs and gallops
- Chest pain and dyspnea on exertion
- Fatigue and lethargy
- Ortner's syndrome: hoarseness, cough, and hemoptysis
- Peripheral edema
- JVD
- Pleural effusion
- Right ventricular dysfunction
- Syncopal episodes

ALERT!

Monitor patients with long bone fractures closely. Severe long bone fractures can leak fat emboli into the vascular space, which can travel to the lungs and result in a PE and respiratory compromise in an otherwise stable patient.

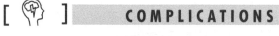

COMPLICATIONS

Complications of pulmonary HTN include PE, HF, pericardial effusion, hepatic damage, dysrhythmia, bleeding, and anemia. With no curative treatment, careful medical management is required to keep the patient's condition from progressing.

Diagnosis

Labs

- ABG to show hypoxemia
- B-type natriuretic peptide (BNP) to show elevation, indicating right ventricular overload (end-organ damage)
- CMP to show elevated liver and kidney function tests (end-organ damage)
- CBC to show low hemoglobin (Hgb) or hematocrit (Hct) due to medication therapy

Diagnostic Testing

- Chest x-ray
- Chest CT scan
- Cardiac catheterization: pulmonary artery pressure >25 mmHg, cardiac output, and left ventricular filling pressure
- Echocardiogram
- Pulmonary function tests
- Pulmonary angiography
- Ventilation and perfusion lung scan

Treatment

- Oxygen and ventilatory support
- Medications: diuretics (Table 2.3), anticoagulation (Table 2.3), calcium channel blockers (Table 2.3), and prostacyclin analogs (Table 3.1)
- Surgery: atrial septostomy, pulmonary thromboendarterectomy, and lung transplant

Nursing Interventions

- Administer medications as ordered.
- Maintain patient comfort.
- Monitor and follow up on labs as ordered.
- Monitor for dysrhythmia on continuous monitoring.
- Position patient in semi-Fowler's position.
- Promote hemodynamic stability and oxygenation via medication management.
- Titrate oxygen and delivery device as needed to maintain oxygen saturation >90% or to ordered goal.

Patient Education

- Adhere to medication schedule and watch for signs and symptoms of complications.
- Attend all follow-up care after discharge.
- Be able to identify signs and symptoms of complications and know when to seek medical expertise.
- Maintain care of peripherally inserted central catheter (PICC) or port if discharged with an invasive line.
- Notify healthcare team of worsening condition: chest pain, dyspnea ►

[⚡]   ALERT!

Pulmonary HTN has either an unknown etiology or a genetic component. Currently, other causes of pulmonary HTN are unknown. This, in combination with vague nonspecific symptoms, makes diagnosis difficult.

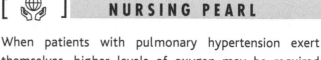

[🌐]   NURSING PEARL

When patients with pulmonary hypertension exert themselves, higher levels of oxygen may be required for support. Consider preemptively increasing oxygen supplementation before physical exertion such as ambulating to the bedside commode or working with PT.

[📝]   POP QUIZ 3.7

What treatment options exist for patients whose pulmonary HTN is unresponsive to conventional medical management?

Patient Education (*continued*)

- Supplemental home oxygen may be required at time of discharge. Engage in safe oxygen therapy practices by avoiding smoking, open flames, flammable products, and heat sources. Avoid products with oil or petroleum and keep a fire extinguisher close by.
- Take medications as prescribed and do not discontinue without speaking with provider.

RESPIRATORY DEPRESSION

Overview

- Respiratory depression can result from certain medical conditions (chronic lung disease or OSA), trauma to the head or chest, medications, severe obesity, alcohol abuse, or drug abuse.
- Reversal of respiratory depression depends on the cause of the respiratory depression.

Signs and Symptoms

- AMS
- Cyanosis
- Dyspnea
- Fatigue
- Headache
- Slow, shallow breathing

Diagnosis

Labs

- ABG to indicate hypoxia or hypercarbia

Diagnostic Testing

- Chest x-ray
- Pulse oximetry
- Sleep study
- Pulmonary function tests (PFTs)

Treatment

- Oxygen and ventilatory support
- Medication: flumazenil, naloxone

Nursing Interventions

- Administer reversal medications as ordered.
- Continuously monitor pulse oximetry.
- Frequently assess the rate and rhythm of the patient's respirations.
- Frequently monitor airway patency.
- Insert an oral airway if needed to maintain an open, patent airway. ▶

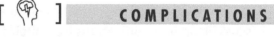

COMPLICATIONS

Respiratory depression can lead to respiratory failure and death. Early identification and treatment of causative factors is essential to prevent complications and death.

ALERT!

Medication-induced respiratory depression can rapidly progress to respiratory failure and arrest. Naloxone and flumazenil are common reversal agents for narcotics and benzodiazepines, which can cause respiratory depression.

NURSING PEARL

Naloxone has a short half-life. Patients experiencing medication-induced respiratory depression may need multiple doses to overcome the sedating effect.

Nursing Interventions (*continued*)

- Monitor and follow up on labs as ordered.
- Monitor VS, especially respiratory rate (RR) and BP.
- Position patient in an upright position to promote adequate ventilation.
- Promote hemodynamic stability and support BP as needed.
- Promote oxygenation.
- Titrate oxygen and delivery device as needed.

Patient Education

- Avoid drinking and taking narcotics or other respiratory depressants together.
- Discuss lifestyle modifications if alcohol/drug induced.
- Engage in diet modification and physical activity if overweight.
- If diagnosed with OSA, wear CPAP device nightly.

RESPIRATORY FAILURE

Overview

- *Acute respiratory failure* occurs when the lungs are unable to exchange oxygen and CO_2 to oxygenate the body, resulting in hypoxia and/or hypercapnia.
- This usually occurs rapidly due to the buildup of fluid in the lung.
- Respiratory failure can be broken down into two categories. *Hypoxic respiratory failure* occurs when there is not enough oxygen circulating in the blood. Hypoxic respiratory failure can be caused by pneumonia, ARDS, asthma, PE, or edema. *Hypercapnic respiratory failure* occurs when too much CO_2 builds up in the blood. This can be caused by central nervous system (CNS) depression due to drug or alcohol use, COPD, Guillain-Barre syndrome, multiple sclerosis (MS), myasthenia gravis, or an increase in intracranial pressure (ICP).

Signs and Symptoms

- Accessory muscle use
- AMS
- Anxiety/agitation
- Cyanosis
- Diaphoresis
- Dyspnea
- Retractions
- Slow, shallow breathing

Diagnosis

Labs

- ABG: typically reveal hypoxia and/or hypercapnia
- Blood and sputum cultures
- Basic metabolic panel (BMP)
- CBC

[📝] **POP QUIZ 3.8**

A patient presents to the progressive care unit (PCU) from the post-anesthesia care unit (PACU). The patient is complaining of 10/10 pain at the incision site and requests additional pain medication, but quickly falls asleep and frequently needs sternal rubs to provide responses to the nurse's questions. The patient's vital signs are as follows: HR 92, BP 115/82 mmHg, RR: 8, SpO_2 92% on 4LNC, and T 96.8°F (36.0°C). What should the nurse's next action be?

[🧠] **COMPLICATIONS**

Respiratory failure causes impaired gas exchange and systemic oxygen deprivation. Complications include cerebral ischemia, renal failure, MI, cardiac arrest, and death. Recognizing respiratory decompensation and initiating emergency therapy is essential to improving patient outcome.

Diagnostic Testing
- Bronchoscopy
- Chest CT
- Chest x-ray
- Echocardiogram
- PFTs
- Possible other tests to determine underlying conditions that may have caused the acute respiratory failure

Treatment

- Correct hypoxemia, respiratory acidosis, and hypercapnia using supplemental oxygen and ventilation therapy: noninvasive positive pressure ventilation, mechanical ventilation and extracorporeal membrane oxygenation (ECMO), and immediate transfer to higher level of care
- Medications (Table 3.1): antibiotics (Table A.1), anticholinergics, bronchodilators, and corticosteroids

Nursing Interventions

- Administer medications as ordered.
- Assess vital signs frequently, specifically the patient's respiration rate and SpO_2.
- Consult with respiratory therapist to provide adequate ventilation.
- Frequently monitor airway patency.
- Maintain continuous pulse oximetry.
- Monitor and follow up on labs as ordered.
- Pad bony prominences on the patient's face prior to placing a CPAP or BiPAP mask to prevent pressure ulcers.
- Perform chest physiotherapy to loosen and remove secretions.
- Perform frequent pulmonary assessments.
- Position patient in an upright position to promote adequate ventilation.
- Promote oxygenation. Titrate oxygen and delivery device as needed.
- Position patient appropriately to maximize ventilation with HOB >30° or prone, depending on clinical condition.
- Turn every 2 hr.

Patient Education

- Acute respiratory failure can occur quickly, often due to other comorbid conditions. Do not delay contacting a medical professional if concerns regarding care or status arise.
- Discuss pulmonary rehabilitation.
- Maintain pulmonary toileting and airway secretion clearance during recovery.
- Seek emergency medical care if experiencing worsening or difficult breathing that is unrelieved by any intervention. Educate on follow-up care with primary care or pulmonology.
- Take medications as prescribed.

[⚡]   ALERT!

Be alert to changes in the patient's work of breathing such as tachypnea, tripod positioning, worsening dyspnea, difficulty responding to questions in full sentences, retractions, accessory muscle use, and/or anxiety. Be proactive and initiate appropriate noninvasive positive pressure ventilation before complete decompensation and respiratory failure.

[⚡]   ALERT!

BiPAP is contraindicated in patients who are unable to maintain their airway or remain conscious. If BiPAP is initiated, careful assessment and monitoring of the patient's mental status and alertness is necessary to ensure ventilation is effective.

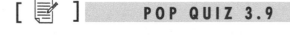

[📝]   POP QUIZ 3.9

How can patients in severe respiratory failure benefit from being positioned?

THORACIC SURGERY

Overview

- Thoracic surgery includes any surgical procedure that occurs on the organs of the chest, including the lungs, heart, esophagus, and trachea.
- Any thoracic surgery has the potential to require intensive monitoring due to the nature of the surgery or complications that occur during the surgery.
- Patients who have had thoracic surgeries such as video-assisted thoracoscopic surgery (VATS), lobectomy, and pneumonectomy are commonly admitted into the PCU. VATS procedures can be used for diagnostic and therapeutic purposes, including biopsy collection, cancer staging, fluid drainage, and tissue resection. Lobectomy is the removal of a lobe of the lung. Pneumonectomy is the removal of the entire lung.
- Other thoracic surgery patients transferred to PCUs include those who have had esophagectomy, pneumonectomy, decortication, pleurectomy, and lung transplants.

Diagnosis

Labs

- Labs to identify the patient's status prior to the procedure and postoperatively include ABG; CBC; clotting factors such as PT, PTT, and INR; CMP; and type and screen.

Diagnostic Testing

- Bronchoscopy with lavage
- Chest x-ray
- Chest CT scan
- Ultrasound

Treatment

- Postoperative analgesia (Table A.2)
- Postoperative supplemental oxygen as needed

Nursing Interventions

- Ambulate once cleared from bedrest.
- Assess and manage postoperative pain with medication and nonpharmacologic interventions. Medication intervention may include continuous IV infusion of fentanyl, hydromorphone, or morphine. Patients may also receive epidurals or thoracic blocks with combinations of bupivacaine/hydromorphone or bupivacaine/fentanyl. Ketorolac or acetaminophen may be adjunctive medications to assist with pain management. Incisional pain may be managed with ice packs or lidocaine patches. Nonpharmacologic interventions for pain management include massage, acupressure, music therapy, pet therapy (if allowed by institution and patient condition), or methods of distraction using conversation, relaxation techniques, meditation, television, or any other calming activity. ▶

COMPLICATIONS

Thoracic surgery has many complications, including agitation after anesthesia, anxiety, cyanosis, decreased ventilation, diaphoresis, dyspnea, increased oxygen requirements or work of breathing, tachycardia, tachypnea, cardiac dysrhythmias, atelectasis, pneumonia, respiratory failure, and death. Close monitoring of ventilatory and hemodynamic status postprocedure can help identify complications and initiate treatment.

[⚡]   ALERT!

Atelectasis following thoracic surgery can be an emergency requiring intubation or emergent chest tube placement.

NURSING PEARL

Always assess chest tubes from the insertion site at the patient to the atrium to ensure there are no kinks in the line. Also check that suction is on (if ordered). Note and report any air leaks to the provider.

Nursing Interventions (*continued*)

- Assess, clean, and maintain chest tubes and drains.
- Assess drain output for increasing and/or change in output (e.g., increasing volumes, drainage that changes from dark to bright/frank blood).
- Assess surgical site for symptoms of infection including redness, swelling, purulent and/or foul-smelling drainage, and systemic changes (hypotension, tachycardia, and fever).
- Assist patient with cough and deep breathing exercises. Splint and support surgical sites as needed.
- Collect blood and sputum cultures when an infection is suspected.
- Encourage the use of incentive spirometry, if possible, postoperatively.
- Engage in DVT/VTE prophylaxis per institutional protocol. This usually includes anticoagulation, SCDs, ambulation, and bed mobility (q2h turns, calf pumps, leg lifts, etc.).
- Maintain oral hygiene care per institutional protocol.
- Maintain pulmonary hygiene with oral suctioning.
- Trend lactate, ABG, CBC, and BMP.

Patient Education

- Ambulate and engage in physical activity as early as possible.
- Discuss need for follow-up care after discharge. Keep scheduled appointments and lab draws to monitor health status.
- Maintain care of surgical incision. Monitor for new pain, redness, swelling, or warmth to touch around surgical site. Also monitor for new or purulent drainage.
- Maintain proper pulmonary toileting and airway clearance.

POP QUIZ 3.10

When discussing care of a patient following thoracic surgery with a nursing student, the student describes atelectasis as an emergency, requiring chest tube placement and possible intubation and transfer. How should the nurse respond?

RESOURCES

Centers for Disease Control and Prevention. (n.d.). *Healthcare workers: Information on COVID-19*. https://www .cdc.gov/coronavirus/2019-ncov/hcp

Lewis, S. M. (2011). *Medical-surgical nursing: Assessment and management of clinical problems*. Mosby.

National Heart, Lung, and Blood Institute. (2019). *Acute respiratory distress syndrome*. U.S. Department of Health and Human Services. https://www.nhlbi.nih.gov/health-topics/acute-respiratory-distress-syndrome

National Heart, Lung, and Blood Institute. (2020). *Asthma*. U.S. Department of Health and Human Services. https:// www.nhlbi.nih.gov/health-topics/asthma

National Heart, Lung, and Blood Institute. (n.d.-a). *Pleural disorders*. U.S. Department of Health and Human Services. https://www.nhlbi.nih.gov/health-topics/pleural-disorders

National Heart, Lung, and Blood Institute. (n.d.-b). *Pulmonary hypertension*. U.S. Department of Health and Human Services. https://www.nhlbi.nih.gov/health-topics/pulmonary-hypertension

National Heart, Lung, and Blood Institute. (n.d.-c). *Sleep apnea*. U.S. Department of Health and Human Services. https://www.nhlbi.nih.gov/health-topics/sleep-apnea

National Institutes of Health. (n.d.). *COVID-19 treatment guidelines*. https://www.covid19treatmentguidelines .nih.gov

OpenAnesthesia. (n.d). *ABG: COPD*. https://www.openanesthesia.org/abg_copd

Prescribers' Digital Reference. (n.d.-a). *Albuterol sulfate* [Drug information]. PDR Search. https://www.pdr.net/ drug-summary/Albuterol-Sulfate-Inhalation-Solution-0-5--albuterol-sulfate-1426.4211

Prescribers' Digital Reference. (n.d.-b). *Alteplase* [Drug information]. PDR Search. https://www.pdr.net/drug-summary/Activase-alteplase-1332.3358

Prescribers' Digital Reference. (n.d.-c). *Amphotericin B* [Drug information]. PDR Search. https://www.pdr.net/drug-summary/Amphotericin-B-amphotericin-B-3117.3010

Prescribers' Digital Reference. (n.d.-d). *Clopidogrel bisulfate* [Drug information]. PDR Search. https://www.pdr.net/drug-summary/Plavix-clopidogrel-bisulfate-525.3952

Prescribers' Digital Reference. (n.d.-e). *Dextromethorphan hydrobromide/guaifenesin* [Drug Information]. PDR Search. https://www.pdr.net/drug-summary/Robitussin-Maximum-Strength-Cough-Chest-Congestion-DM-dextromethorphan-hydrobromide-guaifenesin-3199.2055

Prescribers' Digital Reference. (n.d.-f). *Enoxaparin sodium* [Drug information]. PDR Search. https://www.pdr.net/drug-summary/Lovenox-enoxaparin-sodium-521.2354

Prescribers' Digital Reference. (n.d.-g). *Epoprostenol sodium* [Drug information]. PDR Search. https://www.pdr.net/drug-summary/Flolan-epoprostenol-sodium-188.3624

Prescribers' Digital Reference. (n.d.-h). *Fluconazole* [Drug information]. PDR Search. https://www.pdr.net/drug-summary/Diflucan-fluconazole-1847.3044

Prescribers' Digital Reference. (n.d.-i). *Flumazenil* [Drug information]. PDR Search. https://www.pdr.net/drug-summary/Flumazenil-flumazenil-1729

Prescribers' Digital Reference. (n.d.-j). *Guaifenesin* [Drug information]. PDR Search. https://www.pdr.net/drug-summary/Maximum-Strength-Mucinex-guaifenesin-1642.1918

Prescribers' Digital Reference. (n.d.-k). *Heparin sodium* [Drug information]. PDR Search. https://www.pdr.net/drug-summary/Heparin-Sodium-Injection-heparin-sodium-1263.107

Prescribers' Digital Reference. (n.d.-l). *Iloprost* [Drug information]. PDR Search. https://www.pdr.net/drug-summary/Ventavis-iloprost-1709

Prescribers' Digital Reference. (n.d.-m). *Ipratropium bromide* [Drug Information]. PDR Search . https://www.pdr.net/drug-summary/Atrovent-HFA-ipratropium-bromide-1743

Prescribers' Digital Reference. (n.d.-n). *Methylprednisolone sodium succinate* [Drug information]. PDR Search. https://www.pdr.net/drug-summary/Methylprednisolone-Sodium-Succinate-methylprednisolone-sodium-succinate-24315

Prescribers' Digital Reference. (n.d.-o). *Morphine sulfate* [Drug information]. PDR Search. https://www.pdr.net/drug-summary/Morphine-Sulfate-Oral-Solution-morphine-sulfate-1228

Prescribers' Digital Reference. (n.d.-p). *Naloxone hydrochloride* [Drug information]. PDR Search. https://www.pdr.net/drug-summary/Narcan-naloxone-hydrochloride-3837

Prescribers' Digital Reference. (n.d.-q). *Prednisone* [Drug information]. PDR Search. https://www.pdr.net/drug-summary/Prednisone-Tablets-prednisone-3516.6194

Prescribers' Digital Reference. (n.d.-r). *Treprostinil* [Drug information]. PDR Search. https://www.pdr.net/drug-summary/Remodulin-treprostinil-1004.3120

Prescribers' Digital Reference. (n.d.-s). *Warfarin sodium* [Drug information]. PDR Search. https://www.pdr.net/drug-summary/Coumadin-warfarin-sodium-106

Robriquet, L., Georges, H., Leroy, O., Devos, P., D'escrivan, T., & Guery, B. (2006). Predictors of extubation failure in patients with chronic obstructive pulmonary disease. *Journal of Critical Care, 21*(2), 185–190. https://doi.org/10.1016/j.jcrc.2005.08.007

Siegel, M. D. (2020). Acute respiratory distress syndrome: Clinical features, diagnosis, and complications in adults. *UpToDate*. https://www.uptodate.com/contents/acute-respiratory-distress-syndrome-clinical-features-diagnosis-and-complications-in-adults

Tarbox, A. K., & Swaroop, M. (2013). Pulmonary embolism. *International Journal of Critical Illness and Injury Science, 3*(1), 69–72. https://doi.org/10.4103%2F2229-5151.109427

Yale School of Medicine. (n.d.). *Common tests for patients with pulmonary hypertension*. https://medicine.yale.edu/intmed/pulmonary/clinical/pvdp/tests

DIABETES MELLITUS TYPE 1

Overview

- Diabetes mellitus (DM) type 1 is caused by an autoimmune response in which the body attacks and destroys pancreatic cells that produce insulin.
- This results in a failure to produce insulin, which leads to uncontrolled hyperglycemia.
- Typically, DM type 1 develops in childhood or adolescence.
- Risk factors for developing DM type 1 are not well understood, but are thought to have a genetic component.

Signs and Symptoms

- Symptoms of patients with DM type 1 may include blurred vision; fatigue; impaired wound healing; mood changes (more common with uncontrolled, undiagnosed, or fluctuating blood glucoses); polydipsia; polyuria; polyphagia; recurrent infections; unexplained weight loss prior to diagnosis; and weakness.
- Refer to the sections on hypo- and hyperglycemia for signs and symptoms of those specific disorders.

Diagnosis

Labs

- Fasting blood glucose—nothing by mouth (NPO) for at least 8 hr before the test. Normal: <100 mg/dL. Prediabetes: 100 to 125 mg/dL. Diabetes: 126 mg/dL or higher.
- HbA1c indicates the average bloodsugar for the past 2 to 3 months. Normal: <5.7%. Prediabetes: 5.7% to 6.5%. Diabetes: 6.5% or higher.
- Two-hr oral glucose tolerance test—checks blood sugar levels before and 2 hr after a sweet drink. Normal: <140 mg/dL. Prediabetes: 140 mg/dL to 199 mg/dL. Diabetes: 200 mg/dL or higher.
- Random plasma glucose in a patient with classic symptoms of hyperglycemia or hyperglycemic crisis: ≥200 mg/dL
- Urinalysis: positive glucose, positive ketones.
- Basic metabolic panel (BMP) to assess electrolyte abnormalities and kidney function.

[ ] **COMPLICATIONS**

Complications of type 1 DM include:

- Hypoglycemic episodes, which can lead to loss of consciousness and/or seizures
- Ketoacidosis
- Nephropathy
- Neuropathy
- Retinopathy
- Systemic vascular damage, which causes decreased blood circulation due to narrowed blood vessels. This can lead to impaired wound healing

[ ] **ALERT!**

HbA1c provides evidence about a patient's average blood glucose levels during the previous 2 to 3 months, which is the predicted half-life of red blood cells. This value is checked in both type 1 and type 2 diabetes and should be <6.5%. Follow-up with regularly scheduled appointments and lab draws to appropriately monitor this value.

Treatment

■ Lifestyle modifications: 30 minutes or more of daily physical activity, frequent daily blood glucose monitoring, follow low-carbohydrate diet, and long-term plans to achieve and maintain a healthy weight and body mass index (BMI)
■ Medications: insulin replacement (Table 4.1 and Figure 4.1)

TABLE 4.1 Endocrine Medications

INDICATIONS	MECHANISM OF ACTION	CONTRAINDICATIONS, PRECAUTIONS, AND ADVERSE EFFECTS
Alpha-glucosidase inhibitors (acarbose and miglitol)		
• Hyperglycemia • Type 2 diabetes	• Taken with meals to prevent hyperglycemia by slowing down carbohydrate digestion and absorption	• Medication is contraindicated in hypoglycemia, type 1 diabetes, and dual therapy with other oral antidiabetic medications and in patients with chronic intestinal disease or creatinine >2 mg/dL. • Adverse effects include GI disturbances.
Biguanides (e.g., metformin)		
• Hyperglycemia • First-line treatment for type 2 diabetes	• Decrease hepatic gluconeogenesis production • Decrease intestinal absorption of glucose • Increase peripheral uptake and utilization	• Medication is contraindicated in patients with renal or liver failure, unstable heart failure, acidosis, severe alcohol abuse, and DKA. • Adverse effects include decreased B_{12} levels, GI disturbances, metallic taste, and weight loss. • Use caution in concurrent use with IV contrast, as medication has a nephrotoxic effect; hold metformin 48 hr prior to and after any procedure using IV contrast.
Dextrose injection, 50% (D50) (also available as 5% dextrose in water, 240 mL [D5W])		
• Parenteral (IV) treatment of hypoglycemia	• Glucose replacement and supplementation	• Medication is contraindicated in hyperglycemia. • Adverse effects include hyperglycemia.
DPP-4 inhibitors (e.g., alogliptin and sitagliptin)		
• Taken daily to prevent hyperglycemia by increasing insulin production • Type 2 diabetes	• Stimulate insulin secretion and suppress glucagon secretion • Inhibit gastric emptying	• Medication is contraindicated in type 1 diabetes, DKA, and patients with pancreatitis. • Use caution in older adult patients and those with renal impairment. • Adverse effects include hypoglycemia.
Glycogenolytic agents (glucagon)		
• Parenteral (IM) treatment of hypoglycemia	• Stimulate hepatic production of glucose from glycogen stores	• Medication is contraindicated in hypersensitivity and pheochromocytoma. • Use caution in insulinoma or pheochromocytoma history, starvation, and adrenal insufficiency. • Adverse effects include anaphylaxis, hypotension, nausea, and vomiting.

(continued)

TABLE 4.1 Endocrine Medications (*continued*)

INDICATIONS	MECHANISM OF ACTION	CONTRAINDICATIONS, PRECAUTIONS, AND ADVERSE EFFECTS
Incretin mimetics (exenatide)		
• Blood glucose control in type 2 diabetes	• Mimic the action of incretin and promote endogenous insulin secretion	• Medication is contraindicated in hypersensitivity, type 1 diabetes, DKA, ESRD, and severe GI disease. • Use caution in pediatric populations. • Adverse effects include pancreatitis, nausea, vomiting, and diarrhea.
Insulin: Intermediate-acting (NPH)		
• Hyperglycemia control • Can be used in both type 1 and type 2 diabetes	• Bind to a glycoprotein receptor specific to insulin on surface of target cells • Onset 1–2 hr • Duration 12 hr	• Adverse effects include hypoglycemia and lipohypertrophy (with long-term use).
Insulin: Long-acting (e.g., glargine)		
• Hyperglycemia control • Once-daily dosing • Can be used in both type 1 and type 2 diabetes	• Bind to a glycoprotein receptor specific to insulin on the surface of a target cell • Onset 1.5–2 hr • Duration 12–24 hr	• Use caution in infection, stress, and changes in diet. • The most common adverse effect is hypoglycemia. • Long-term use may cause lipohypertrophy.
Insulin: Rapid-acting (e.g., lispro and aspart)		
• Treatment of hyperglycemia • Given to correct elevated blood glucose prior to meals or preemptively before carbohydrate intake • Can be used in both type 1 and type 2 diabetes	• Bind to a glycoprotein receptor specific to insulin on the surface of a target cell • Onset 5–15 min • Duration 4–6 hr	• Contraindications include hypoglycemia. • Use caution in infection, stress, and changes in diet. • The most common adverse effect is hypoglycemia. • Medication is given subcutaneously. • Long-term use may cause lipohypertrophy.
Insulin: Short-acting (e.g., regular insulin)		
• Treatment of hyperglycemia • Can be used in both type 1 and type 2 diabetes • Can be used as an IV infusion to treat DKA and HHS	• Bind to a glycoprotein receptor specific to insulin on the surface of the target cell • Onset 30–60 min • Duration 6–8 hr	• Contraindications include hypoglycemia. • Use caution in infection, stress, and changes in diet. • The most common adverse effect is hypoglycemia.
Meglitinides (e.g., repaglinide and nateglinide)		
• Taken with meals to prevent hyperglycemia by stimulating the body to produce more insulin • Type 2 diabetes	• Stimulate insulin secretion by the pancreatic beta cells	• Contraindications include hypoglycemia, type 1 diabetes, and dual therapy with other oral antidiabetics. • Use caution in patients with infections, liver and cardiovascular disease, lactic acidosis, and in the geriatric population. • Adverse effects include hypoglycemia.

(continued)

TABLE 4.1 Endocrine Medications (*continued*)

INDICATIONS	MECHANISM OF ACTION	CONTRAINDICATIONS, PRECAUTIONS, AND ADVERSE EFFECTS
Sodium-glucose cotransporter-2 inhibitors (SGLT2) (e.g., canagliflozin, dapagliflozin, and empagliflozin)		
• Blood glucose control in type 2 diabetes	• Prevent reabsorption of glucose filtered in the tubular lumen of the kidney through inhibiting SGLT2	• Medication is contraindicated in patients with severe rental impairments or who are on dialysis. • Use caution in DKA, type 1 DM, dehydration, hypotension, infection, or in geriatric populations. • Adverse effects include hypoglycemia, yeast infection, frequent urination, electrolyte imbalances, dehydration, nausea, and weakness.
Sulfonylureas (e.g., glyburide and glipizide)		
• Hyperglycemia • Second-line treatment for type 2 diabetes	• Stimulate endogenous insulin secretion by native pancreatic cells, increasing the body's sensitivity to its own insulin	• Medication can be used in combination with other oral hypoglycemic agents in patients who fail initial therapy with lifestyle interventions and metformin. • There is risk for potential allergic reactions in patients with a history of sulfa allergies. • Use caution in patients with chronic kidney disease as it is renally excreted. • Adverse effects include hypoglycemia.
Thiazolidinediones (e.g., rosiglitazone and pioglitazone)		
• Hyperglycemia • Third-line treatment for type 2 diabetes	• Improve sensitivity to insulin and decrease insulin resistance	• Medication is contraindicated in patients with heart failure or any evidence of fluid overload, history of fracture, or at high risk for fracture, acute liver disease, type 1 diabetes, and pregnancy. • Adverse effects include heart failure, elevated liver enzymes, anemia, and fractures. • Pioglitazone is contraindicated in patients with a history of or active bladder cancer.

DKA, diabetic ketoacidosis; DM, diabetes mellitus; ESRD, end-stage renal disease; GI, gastrointestinal; HHS, hyperosmolar hyperglycemic syndrome; IV, intravenous; NPH, neutral protamine Hagedorn.

Nursing Interventions

- Administer appropriate insulin or oral medication dosages as directed by the provider based on the patient's blood glucose.
- Assess the skin for nonhealing or open wounds, especially on the patient's feet.
- Check the patient's blood glucose before meals and at bedtime (ACHS). ▶

[ ]   **NURSING PEARL**

Diabetes can cause problems during pregnancy for women and their developing babies. Women who want to become pregnant should consult a diabetes nurse educator and/or endocrinologist to formulate a care plan that promotes a healthy pregnancy and newborn.

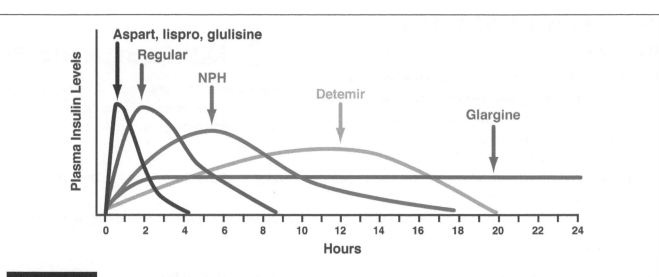

FIGURE 4.1 Insulin onset, peak, and duration.

NPH, neutral protamine Hagedorn.

Source: Reproduced with permission of Leslie DeGroot, MD, Editor-in-chief, Endotext.org from Hirsch, IB, Skyler, JS. The management of type 1 diabetes. www.endotext.org. Version of December 18, 2015, published by MDTEXT.COM INC. South Dartmouth, MA 02748.

Nursing Interventions (*continued*)

- Monitor and follow-up on labs as ordered.
- Monitor daily carbohydrate intake.
- Monitor vital signs (VS).
- Refer to social worker to ensure patient has accessibility to medications and blood glucose monitoring supplies.

Patient Education

- After discharge, monitor blood glucose before meals, at bedtime, and when feeling symptomatic.
- Conduct daily skin assessments at home. If unable to visualize areas of skin, use mirrors or seek assistance from another person in the house.
- Eat a low-carbohydrate diet and keep track of daily carbohydrate intake.
- Engage in exercise or physical activity for at least 30 minutes a day.
- Rotate insulin injection site, which may include the abdomen, upper arm, thigh, lower back, hips, or buttocks.
- Understand the signs of hyper- and hypoglycemic episodes and how to care for each. Early hypoglycemic symptoms include behavioral changes (anxiety and irritability), diaphoresis, fatigue, hunger, palpitations, and tachycardia. Late hypoglycemic symptoms include confusion, lethargy, slurred speech, seizures, and coma. Hyperglycemic symptoms may manifest as altered mental status (AMS), abdominal pain, fatigue and lethargy, frequent urination and thirst, and vomiting. Monitor blood glucose daily before meals, at bedtime, and when feeling symptomatic using a home blood glucose monitoring device. Treat elevated blood glucose values with a prescribed diabetes management plan. This may include increasing short-acting insulin dose or diet to manage hyperglycemia.

[📝] **POP QUIZ 4.1**

What should family be instructed to do if they find their diabetic family member symptomatic for hypoglycemia or in an altered or unresponsive state, unable to take anything by mouth?

DIABETES MELLITUS TYPE 2

Overview

- DM type 2 occurs when the cells in the body become resistant to insulin and the pancreas cannot make enough insulin to meet the body's demands, leading to an accumulation of glucose.
- It was once thought that DM type 2 was a disorder that affected adults only. However, with an increasing prevalence of childhood obesity, DM type 2 is now seen in pediatric populations as well.
- DM type 2 is the most prevalent form of diabetes and can be directly related to BMI, diet, and exercise.

Signs and Symptoms

Refer to the Diabetes Mellitus Type 1, Hyperglycemia, and Hypoglycemia sections.

Diagnosis

Labs

- Fasting blood glucose—NPO for at least 8 hr before the test. Normal: <100 mg/dL. Prediabetes: 100 to 125 mg/dL. Diabetes: 126 mg/dL or higher.
- HbA1c—measures average blood sugar for the past 2 to 3 months. Normal: <5.7%. Prediabetes: 5.7% to 6.5%. Diabetes: 6.5% or higher.
- Two-hr oral glucose tolerance test—checks blood sugar levels before and 2 hr after a sweet drink. Normal: <140 mg/dL. Prediabetes: 140 mg/dL to 199 mg/dL. Diabetes: 200 mg/dL or higher.
- Random plasma glucose test in a patient with classic symptoms of hyperglycemia or hyperglycemic crisis: ≥200 mg/dL
- Urinalysis: positive glucose, positive ketones
- BMP to assess electrolyte abnormalities and kidney function

Treatment

- Lifestyle modifications: 30 minutes or more of daily physical activity, blood glucose monitoring with meals and at bedtime, long-term plans to achieve and maintain a healthy weight and BMI, and low-carbohydrate dietary choices
- Medications (see Table 4.1): alpha-glucosidase inhibitors, biguanides, DPP-4 inhibitors, incretin mimetics, insulin replacement, sulfonylureas, meglitinides, and thiazolidinediones

Nursing Interventions

- Administer appropriate insulin or oral medication dosages as directed by the provider based on the patient's blood glucose.
- Assess the skin for nonhealing or open wounds, especially on the patient's feet.
- Conduct frequent blood glucose checks and monitor for both hypoglycemia and hyperglycemia. ▶

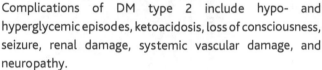

COMPLICATIONS

Complications of DM type 2 include hypo- and hyperglycemic episodes, ketoacidosis, loss of consciousness, seizure, renal damage, systemic vascular damage, and neuropathy.

ALERT!

Patients diagnosed with prediabetes may be able to reverse blood glucose to normal ranges with lifestyle modifications. The American Diabetes Association (ADA) recommends weight loss and 30 minutes of moderate exercise 5 days a week as methods to reduce the risk of type 2 diabetes in patients diagnosed with prediabetes. Prior to discharge, refer patients to a diabetes educator or other appropriate resources for assistance in making these lifestyle modifications.

NURSING PEARL

When patients order their first meal following a type 2 diabetes diagnosis, they may need assistance in interpreting what they can and cannot eat. Be prepared to offer guidance and consult a diabetes nurse educator to assist with education.

Nursing Interventions (*continued*)

- Monitor and follow-up on labs as ordered.
- Monitor daily carbohydrate intake.
- Monitor VS.

Patient Education

- Conduct daily skin assessments at home. If unable to visualize areas of skin, use mirrors or seek assistance from another person.
- Count grams of carbohydrate intake and follow the recommended low-carbohydrate diet.
- Engage in daily physical activity of at least 30 minutes.
- Monitor blood glucose before meals, at bedtime, and when feeling symptomatic.
- Rotate site of insulin injections as applicable. Various injection sites may include the abdomen, upper arm, thigh, lower back, hips, or buttocks.
- Understand the signs of hyper- and hypoglycemic episodes and how to care for each.

[📝] **POP QUIZ 4.2**

A patient admitted to the progressive care unit (PCU) has a fasting glucose of 157. What should be considered with this finding?

DIABETIC KETOACIDOSIS

Overview

- Diabetic ketoacidosis (DKA) is a life-threatening condition characterized by extreme hyperglycemia, ketosis, and acidosis.
- DKA develops when insulin levels are low, causing the body to respond by converting stores of fat and protein into glucose. This releases ketones into the bloodstream, resulting in severely elevated blood glucose levels.
- DKA is most common in patients with type 1 diabetes, but it has the potential to develop in any poorly controlled diabetic patient.

[🧠] **COMPLICATIONS**

DKA is a life-threatening condition. Complications of DKA include diabetic coma, dysrhythmia development, and cardiac arrest. Careful management and replacement of volume and insulin are needed to reverse DKA progression.

Signs and Symptoms

- Abdominal pain
- Anorexia
- Confusion
- Dehydration
- Dry mucous membranes
- Fruity breath
- Hypotension
- Increased thirst
- Kussmaul respirations
- Lethargy
- Normal or elevated serum osmolality
- Polyuria and nocturia
- Poor skin turgor ▶

Signs and Symptoms (*continued*)

- Severe hyperglycemia
- Tachycardia
- Weakness
- Vomiting

Diagnosis

Labs

- ABG: acidosis with pH <7.3
- Blood glucose: profound hyperglycemia with blood glucose >250
- Complete metabolic panel (CMP): anion gap >10, bicarbonate >18 mEq, hypernatremia, hyperkalemia, hypermagnesemia, hyperphosphatemia
- Urinalysis: positive for glucose and ketones

[⚙] **ALERT!**

Frequent monitoring of laboratory values is essential to appropriately manage and reverse metabolic imbalances. Consider drawing from central or arterial line to decrease the number of peripheral sticks the patient will receive.

Treatment

- Continuous insulin infusion is titrated based on blood glucose levels and facility protocol.
- DKA patients are profoundly dehydrated and require careful fluid resuscitation.
- Electrolyte replacement: potassium, magnesium, bicarbonate, and phosphate lab values are drawn frequently and treated per provider order.
- Intravenous (IV) fluids: First hr: 0.9% NaCl at 15 to 20 mL/kg as ordered by provider. Fluid replacement after first hr depends on hemodynamic and hydration status and electrolyte values: Patients with hypernatremia receive 0.45% NaCl at 4 to 14 mL/kg/hr (250 to 500 mL/hr), whereas patients with hyponatremia continue receiving 0.9% NaCl at 4 to 14 mL/kg/hr (250 to 500 mL/hr) per physician order.
- Possible transfer to ICU is needed for close monitoring (depends on facility).
- Switch to subcutaneous insulin injection when blood glucose level is <200 and two of the following laboratory values are met: Serum bicarbonate ≥15 mEq/L, venous pH >7.3, and/or calculated anion gap ≤12 mEq/L.

Nursing Interventions

- Administer medications, IV insulin, IV fluid, and electrolyte replacement as ordered based on laboratory values.
- Monitor blood glucose hourly (or per institution policy).
- Monitor VS.
- Monitor and follow-up on labs as ordered.
- Monitor intake and output (I/O).
- Promote adequate nutrition. If patients are receiving IV insulin, keep NPO for glucose control. If insulin drip is discontinued and the patient is transitioning to oral by mouth (PO) intake, monitor carbohydrate counts for all orally ingested foods.

[🌐] **NURSING PEARL**

Blood glucose should be monitored hourly while a patient is on an insulin drip. However, blood glucose checks can be extended to q2h per facility protocol if the patient's blood glucoses are stable and the drip has consistently remained at the same rate. Hypoglycemia can occur rapidly if not closely monitored.

Patient Education

- Assess blood glucose before meals and at bedtime (or more frequently as needed).
- If administering subcutaneous insulin, rotate injection site.
- If DKA is suspected at home, consider using a urine dipstick to detect ketones and check blood glucose; seek care as appropriate.
- Monitor for warning signs and symptoms of possible DKA, including signs of hyperglycemia accompanied by fruity breath, deep respirations, and confusion.
- Postdischarge care: Anticipate fluctuations in blood glucose if sick or undergoing stress. Be sure to monitor for symptoms of hypoglycemia, which include confusion, diaphoresis, hunger, irritability, tachycardia, and lightheadedness. Monitor for symptoms of hyperglycemia, which include dyspnea, headache, dehydration, excessive thirst, frequent urination, weakness, and nausea.

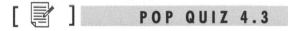

POP QUIZ 4.3

A patient was admitted for DKA last night. This morning, they are found to have a Na+ value of 152. They are receiving a continuous insulin infusion at 7 units/hr and 0.9% normal saline (NS) at 125 mL/hr. What should the nurse's next action be?

HYPERGLYCEMIA

Overview

- Hyperglycemia can be a manifestation of insulin resistance or pancreatic insufficiency to produce insulin as seen in both type 1 and type 2 diabetes. Medications are often necessary to lower blood glucose.
- A high blood glucose may also be seen in critically ill patients, even in the absence of preexisting diabetes, due to infection, certain medications (steroids), chronic disease, or nutrition given through an IV or feeding tube.

COMPLICATIONS

Prolonged hyperglycemia can be a symptom of uncontrolled diabetes. Prolonged uncontrolled blood glucose values can result in both microvascular and systemic damage including neuropathy, ophthalmic damage (retinopathy), renal damage (nephropathy), coronary artery disease (CAD), peripheral vascular disease (PVD), and cerebrovascular disease. This systemic damage can ultimately result in renal failure, cardiac dysfunction, blindness, limb ischemia, and death.

Signs and Symptoms

- AMS
- Abdominal pain
- Fatigue
- Lethargy
- Polydipsia
- Polyuria
- Vomiting
- Weight loss

Labs

- BMP
- Fasting blood glucose: >126 mg/dL
- Point of care blood glucose check: >140 mg/dL
- Random plasma glucose: >200 mg/dL
- Urinalysis: positive glucose

Treatment

- Medications (Table 4.1): If hyperglycemia is due to critical illness, infections, or glucose-increasing medications (steroids): Chronic disease or tube feeding/total parenteral nutrition (TPN) treat with insulin. If hyperglycemia is due to type 1 diabetes: Insulin replacement. If hyperglycemia is due to type 2 diabetes: Alpha-glucosidase inhibitors, biguanides, DPP-4 inhibitors, incretin mimetics, insulin replacement, meglitinides, sulfonylureas, and thiazolidinediones.
- Lifestyle modifications: 30 minutes or more of daily physical activity, achieve and maintain healthy weight and BMI, daily blood glucose monitoring (or more frequently, as needed), and low-carbohydrate diet with supportive services as needed.

Nursing Interventions

- Administer medications as ordered based on etiology and laboratory values.
- Assess skin for open or nonhealing wounds, paying special attention to the patient's feet.
- Check the patient's blood glucose after administration of insulin or another antihyperglycemic agent. Monitor for symptoms of both hypoglycemia and hyperglycemia.
- Monitor and follow-up on labs as ordered.
- Monitor VS.
- Notify the provider if the patient's blood glucose remains elevated despite intervention.
- Perform an ophthalmic examination if the patient complains of vision changes.
- Promote adequate nutrition by monitoring carbohydrate intake.

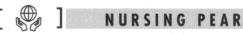 **NURSING PEARL**

Consultation with a diabetes nurse educator and dietician may be helpful for newly diagnosed patients with diabetes. This can also be helpful for the family who will support their care.

Patient Education

- Conduct daily skin assessments at home. If unable to visualize areas of skin, use mirrors or seek assistance from another person.
- Count grams of carbohydrate intake and follow the recommended low-carbohydrate diet.
- Engage in daily physical activity of at least 30 minutes.
- Follow-up with appropriate providers, which may include a primary care doctor, endocrinologist, eye doctor, and podiatrist.
- Monitor blood glucose before meals, at bedtime, and when feeling symptomatic.
- Recognize the symptoms of hyperglycemic episodes.
- Rotate site of insulin injections as applicable.

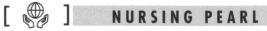 **POP QUIZ 4.4**

Describe the vascular complications associated with prolonged, untreated, or uncontrolled hyperglycemia.

HYPOGLYCEMIA

Overview

- Hypoglycemia is defined as a blood glucose lower than 70 mg/dL; however, symptoms may not manifest until blood glucose drops below 55 mg/dL.
- While uncommon in patients who do not have diabetes, hypoglycemia can occur transiently after long periods without eating, during severe illness, or following insulin overcorrection or overdose.

COMPLICATIONS

Untreated hypoglycemia can result in seizure, coma, or death. It is essential to identify and treat hypoglycemia before patients progress to these severe complications.

Signs and Symptoms

- Early: behavioral changes such as anxiety and irritability, diaphoresis, fatigue, hunger, palpitations, and tachycardia
- Late: coma, confusion, lethargy, seizure, and slurred speech

Labs

- Blood glucose check: <70 mg/dL
- BMP
- HbA1C
- Liver function test

Treatment

- Medications (Table 4.1): D50 or D5W IV if patient is NPO or unable to tolerate oral intake; glucagon intramuscularly (IM)
- PO intake of a readily absorbable carbohydrate if the patient is able to tolerate oral intake

Nursing Interventions

- Administer a dextrose medication or a 15-g carbohydrate snack.
- If the patient is NPO, consider adding maintenance IV fluids with dextrose until the patient is able to tolerate PO intake.
- Monitor and follow-up on labs as ordered.
- Monitor VS.
- Promote adequate nutrition. Check to make sure the patient is adequately eating meals.
- Perform frequent blood glucose checks 15 minutes after an intervention. If blood glucose remains below 70 mg/dL, repeat with another intervention.
- Be sure to follow institutional protocol, as hypoglycemia treatments may vary.
- Continue to check blood glucose hourly thereafter until the blood glucose has stabilized.
- Notify the provider, who may alter the patient's treatment plan.

Patient Education

- Always carry a carbohydrate snack or glucose tablet.
- Be sure to monitor blood glucose levels closely at home.
- Consider wearing a diabetic alert bracelet.
- Discuss frequent follow-up care with endocrinology postdischarge.
- Monitor disease progress through regularly scheduled checkups and careful glucose monitoring.
- Understand the signs and symptoms of hypoglycemic episodes and how to intervene.

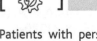

[ ]   **ALERT!**

Patients with persistent hypoglycemia may learn to live and function with a lower blood glucose. This means that a patient may be asymptomatic with a blood glucose <70 mg/dL. This can be very dangerous and can cause a delay in recognition of the condition until late signs/symptoms develop. Notify the provider of any low glucose level even if the patient is asymptomatic.

[ ]   **NURSING PEARL**

Patients with hypoglycemia may need a consult with a dietician to evaluate diet choices or eating patterns. If a new diagnosis of type 1 or type 2 diabetes is made, a consult to a diabetes nurse educator should be made.

[ ]   **POP QUIZ 4.5**

A patient is admitted with a blood glucose of 58 mg/dL. After being treated with 4 oz of orange juice, the patient's repeat blood glucose is 65. What should the nurse's next action be?

RESOURCES

American Diabetes Association. (n.d.-a). *Diagnosis*. https://www.diabetes.org/a1c/diagnosis

American Diabetes Association. (n.d.-b). *Hypoglycemia (low blood glucose)*. https://www.diabetes.org/healthy-living/medication-treatments/blood-glucose-testing-and-control/hypoglycemia

Deglin, J. H., Vallerand, A. H., & Sanoski, C. A. (2011). *Davis's drug guide for nurses*. F.A. Davis.

DiMeglio, L. A., Evans-Molina, C., & Oram, R. A. (2018). Type 1 diabetes. *Lancet, 391*(10138), 2449–2462. https://doi.org/10.1016/S0140-6736(18)31320-5

Gosmanov, A. R., Gosmanova, E. O., & Dillard-Cannon, E. (2014). Management of adult diabetic ketoacidosis. *Diabetes, Metabolic Syndrome and Obesity: Targets and Therapy, 7*, 255–264. https://doi.org/10.2147/DMSO.S50516

Huether, S. E., & McCance, K. L. (2012). *Understanding pathophysiology*. Elsevier/Mosby.

Lewis, S. M. (2011). *Medical-surgical nursing: Assessment and management of clinical problems*. Mosby.

Prescribers' Digital Reference. (n.d.-a). *Acarbose* [Drug Information]. PDR Search. https://www.pdr.net/drug-summary/Precose-acarbose-1315

Prescribers' Digital Reference. (n.d.-b). *Canagliflozin* [Drug Information]. PDR Search. https://www.pdr.net/drug-summary/Invokana-canagliflozin-3094

Prescribers' Digital Reference. (n.d.-c). *Exenatide* [Drug Information]. PDR Search. https://www.pdr.net/drug-summary/Byetta-exenatide-61

Prescribers' Digital Reference. (n.d.-d). *Glucagon rDNA origin* [Drug Information]. PDR Search. https://www.pdr.net/drug-summary/Glucagon-glucagon--rDNA-origin--290.2553

Prescribers' Digital Reference. (n.d.-e). *Insulin aspart rDNA origin* [Drug Information]. PDR Search. https://www.pdr.net/drug-summary/NovoLog-insulin-aspart--rDNA-origin--456.3612

Prescribers' Digital Reference. (n.d.-f). *Insulin glargine* [Drug Information]. PDR Search. https://www.pdr.net/drug-summary/Basaglar-insulin-glargine-3870.8201

Prescribers' Digital Reference. (n.d.-g). *Insulin lispro* [Drug Information]. PDR Search. https://www.pdr.net/drug-summary/Humalog-insulin-lispro-291.3757

Prescribers' Digital Reference. (n.d.-h). *Miglitol* [Drug Information]. PDR Search. https://www.pdr.net/drug-summary/Glyset-miglitol-1872

Prescribers' Digital Reference. (n.d.-i). *NPH, human insulin isophane rDNA origin* [Drug Information]. PDR Search. https://www.pdr.net/drug-summary/Humulin-N-NPH--human-insulin-isophane--rDNA-origin--2911.4411

Prescribers' Digital Reference. (n.d.-j). *Pioglitazone* [Drug Information]. PDR Search. https://www.pdr.net/drug-summary/Actos-pioglitazone-556.397

Prescribers' Digital Reference. (n.d.-k). *Regular, human insulin rDNA origin* [Drug Information]. PDR Search. https://www.pdr.net/drug-summary/Humulin-R-regular--human-insulin--rDNA-origin--2912.3423

Prescribers' Digital Reference. (n.d.-l). *Rosiglitazone maleate* [Drug Information]. PDR Search. https://www.pdr.net/drug-summary/Avandia-rosiglitazone-maleate-175.404

Prescribers' Digital Reference. (n.d.-m). *Saxagliptin* [Drug Information]. PDR Search. https://www.pdr.net/drug-summary/Onglyza-saxagliptin-111.5959

Sommerfield, A. J., Deary, I. J., & Frier, B. M. (2004). Acute hyperglycemia alters mood state and impairs cognitive performance in people with type 2 diabetes. *Diabetes Care, 27*(10), 2335–2340. https://doi.org/10.2337/diacare.27.10.2335

5 HEMATOLOGY

ANEMIA

Overview

- Anemia indicates a reduction in the number or volume of red blood cells (RBCs), or a reduction in hemoglobin (Hgb) and hematocrit (Hct) circulating throughout the body.
- Anemia primarily causes a reduction in blood oxygen-carrying capacity, resulting in hypoxia.
- Sickle cell anemia is a common inherited form of anemia. Hallmark findings include a crescent or "sickle" shaped RBC which has decreased oxygen-carrying capacity and can obstruct blood flow to other areas of the body.
- Timely recognition and intervention are key to prevent severe complications.
- Three etiologies of anemia are (Table 5.1) blood loss, reduced RBC production, and increased RBC destruction.

COMPLICATIONS

Severe untreated anemia can affect age groups differently. In younger populations, impaired neurologic development may occur. In pregnancy, severe anemia can lead to early labor and premature birth. Complications for severe anemia, such as multiorgan failure or death, are more common in the geriatric population due to preexisting comorbidities in this population.

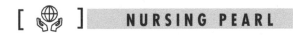

NURSING PEARL

Preparation for a stem cell transplant causes anemia, but low RBCs persist following the transplant until the new bone marrow is able to produce the appropriate number of RBCs.

TABLE 5.1 Conditions That Cause Anemia

BLOOD LOSS	INCREASED RBC DESTRUCTION	REDUCED RBC PRODUCTION
• Acute • Chronic • May be related to: ◦ Coagulopathies ◦ Frequent phlebotomy ◦ Surgery ◦ Trauma	• Damage by artificial valves • Immune destruction (e.g., hemolytic transfusion reaction) • Inherited disorders (e.g., sickle cell) • RBC membrane defects • Splenic destruction	• Aplastic anemia • Bone marrow malignancies • Chemotherapy or radiation • Chronic inflammatory conditions • Chronic kidney disease • Nutritional deficiencies: ◦ B_{12} ◦ Folate ◦ Iron • Stem cell transplant

RBC, red blood cell.

Signs and Symptoms

- Mild anemia may be asymptomatic.
- Severe anemia symptoms may include any of the following: altered mental status (AMS); brittle nails; chest pain; decreased exertional tolerance; delayed growth; dizziness; dyspnea, especially on exertion; fatigue, weakness, and lethargy; hair loss; headache; hypotension; jaundice; koilonychia (spooning nails); pallor; petechiae; pica; splenomegaly or hepatomegaly; and tachycardia.
- Symptoms specific to sickle cell may include any of the following: acute and/or chronic pain, dactylitis (swelling of hands and feet), infections and fevers, priapism, and vision problems.

Diagnosis

Labs

- Vitamin B$_{12}$: <180 ng/L
- Blood films/smears: May show abnormally sized RBCs.
- Bilirubin: May be >1.2 mg/dL in hemolytic anemia.
- Complete blood count (CBC): Hemoglobin may be <13 g/dL in men and <12 g/dL in women, whereas hematocrit may be <38% in men and <35% in women.
- Coombs' test: May be positive.
- Iron/ferritin: <30 ng/mL
- Folate: <2.7 ng/mL
- High-performance liquid chromatography (sickle cell)
- Reticulocyte count: <0.5%
- Serum iron: May be <60 mcg/dL
- Stool, guaiac test: May be positive.
- Total iron-binding capacity

[⚙] **ALERT!**

Sickle cell anemia may present in the inpatient setting as a sickle cell crisis, which may be triggered by infection, hypoxia, acidosis, dehydration, and other stressors. Sickle cell crises may present in a combination of three categories (Table 5.2). Identification of appropriate phase of crisis can help guide treatment.

[⚙] **ALERT!**

If severe anemia results in angina, myocardial infarction (MI), heart failure (HF), or dysrhythmias, cardiology should be consulted immediately for evaluation.

TABLE 5.2 Manifestations of Sickle Cell Crisis

Hematologic aplastic crisis	• Exacerbation of anemia with significant drop in hemoglobin • Sickle cells have a 10- to 20-day half-life • Sickle cells frequently sequestered by spleen • Symptomatic anemia
Infectious crisis	• Elevated risk of secondary infections (e.g., pneumonia, bloodstream infections, meningitis, and osteomyelitis) • Sickle cell occlusions in the spleen reduce immunologic function
Vaso-occlusive crisis	• Microvascular occlusions caused by sickled RBCs • Severe pain possible in abdomen, chest, bones, and joints • Tissue and organ ischemia

RBCs, red blood cells.

TABLE 5.3 Vitamin and Mineral Related Anemias

ANEMIA	VITAMIN/MINERAL DEFICIENCY
Iron deficient anemia	Iron deficiency
Megaloblastic anemia	Folate deficiency
Pernicious anemia	B_{12} deficiency

Diagnostic Testing
- Chest x-ray
- CT
- Upper endoscopy (if suspected gastrointestinal [GI] hemorrhage)
- Pelvic ultrasound

Treatment

- Treatment is dependent on etiology (Table 5.3).
- Deficiency: vitamin B_{12}, iron, or folate—oral by mouth (PO) or intravenous (IV) replacement of B_{12}, folate, or iron (Table 5.4) and blood transfusion (Table 5.3)
- Aplastic anemia: bone marrow transplant
- Chronic disease: If renal failure, use erythropoietin (Table 5.4); if autoimmune or rheumatologic conditions, manage the causative disease.
- Red blood destruction (hemolytic anemia): sickle cell—blood transfusions, exchange transfusions, antibiotics, opioids, hydroxyurea, IV hydration, oxygen therapy, and stem cell/bone marrow transplant; medication mediated—discontinue medication immediately (if possible); disseminated intravascular coagulation (DIC)—antifibrinolytic agents (Table 5.4); faulty mechanical valves—valve replacement surgery; persistent despite treatment—splenectomy may be indicated.

TABLE 5.4 Hematology, Immunology, and Oncology Medications

INDICATIONS	MECHANISM OF ACTION	CONTRAINDICATIONS, PRECAUTIONS, AND ADVERSE EFFECTS
Antifibrinolytic therapy (tranexamic acid)		
• DIC, bleeding after trauma, hemorrhage	• Hemostatic agent to bind to the lysine binding site for fibrin on the plasmin molecule	• Antifibrinolytic therapy is contraindicated in intracranial bleed and thrombolytic disease. • Use caution in renal impairment, seizure disorders, and surgery. • Adverse effects include thrombosis, thromboembolism, pulmonary embolism, renal thrombosis, visual impairments, and seizures.

(continued)

TABLE 5.4 Hematology, Immunology, and Oncology Medications (*continued*)

INDICATIONS	MECHANISM OF ACTION	CONTRAINDICATIONS, PRECAUTIONS, AND ADVERSE EFFECTS
Antihistamine (diphenhydramine hydrochloride)		
• Treatment of allergic reactions, including transfusion reactions • Anaphylaxis	• Competitively inhibit the effects of histamine on H1-receptor sites in the GI tract, large blood vessels, and bronchial muscle suppressing the formation of edema and itching resulting from histaminic activity	• Antihistamine is contraindicated in asthma and COPD. • Use caution in closed angle glaucoma, increased intraocular pressure, bladder obstruction, GI obstruction, ileus, urinary retention, and hepatic or cardiac disease. • Adverse effects include oversedation, seizure, hemolytic anemia, agranulocytosis, dermatitis, confusion, dysarthria, euphoria, neuritis, constipation, blurred vision, urinary retention, and wheezing.
Antimetabolites/antineoplastic agents (hydroxyurea)		
• Treatment of abnormally shaped hemoglobin	• Increase hemoglobin F or fetal hemoglobin, which is larger and more flexible than other forms of hemoglobin • Decrease propensity of sickle cells to form clots	• Women who are pregnant or might become pregnant should not handle the medication. • Individuals touching the medication should wear disposable gloves. • It is recommended to use effective contraception while taking hydroxyurea and for females to discontinue if planning to become pregnant in the next 3 months. • Live vaccines should not be administered while taking hydroxyurea, as they can cause life-threatening infection.
Corticosteroids (e.g., hydrocortisone)		
• Allergic reactions including anaphylaxis • Drug hypersensitivities	• Decrease formation and release of endogenous inflammatory mediators including prostaglandins, kinins, and histamine	• Avoid abrupt discontinuation, which may result in Cushing's syndrome. • Monitor for secondary fungal infections. • Monitor for secondary infections related to immunosuppression.
Direct thrombin inhibitor (argatroban, bivalirudin)		
• Anticoagulant option for HIT and DIC	• Inhibit and neutralize the actions of thrombin, including thrombin trapped within established clots	• Direct thrombin inhibitors are contraindicated in active bleeding, spinal anesthesia, diverticulitis, endocarditis, aneurysm, hypertension, inflammatory bowel disease, lumbar puncture, and hepatic disease. • Do not abruptly discontinue. • Use caution in patients with angina and/or prolonged PTT. • Adverse effects include bleeding, dysrhythmias including A-fib, bradycardia, V-tach and cardiac arrest, pulmonary edema, chest pain, MI, and thrombosis.

(continued)

TABLE 5.4 Hematology, Immunology, and Oncology Medications (*continued*)

INDICATIONS	MECHANISM OF ACTION	CONTRAINDICATIONS, PRECAUTIONS, AND ADVERSE EFFECTS
Erythropoietin agents (epoetin alfa)		
• Anemia associated with CKD, malignancy, renal failure, or medication therapy in HIV-infected patients	• Stimulate bone marrow to make more RBCs	• Erythropoietin agents are contraindicated in albumin or mammalian cell-derived product hypersensitivity and uncontrolled hypertension. • Use caution in history of seizures. • Adverse effects include seizures, CHF, MI, stroke, and hypertension.
Folic acid supplements		
• Prevention and treatment of megaloblastic and macrocytic anemia	• Supplementation to assist with protein synthesis and RBC function • Stimulate production of RBCs, WBCs, and platelets to restore normal hematopoiesis	• Antianemics are contraindicated in pernicious, aplastic, or normocytic anemias. • Use caution in undiagnosed anemias. • Adverse effects include rash, irritability, difficulty sleeping, malaise, confusion, and fever.
Iron supplements (e.g., ferrous sulfate, ferumoxytol, iron sucrose injection, etc.)		
• Low hemoglobin • Inadequate iron reserves	• Increase hemoglobin production • Allow for transportation of oxygen via hemoglobin	• Administer on empty stomach with orange juice to increase absorption. • Iron supplements are contraindicated in dialysis, hypotension, anaphylaxis, hemochromatosis, hemoglobinopathy, hemosiderosis, 24 hr prior to an MRI, hepatic or gastric disease, and during pregnancy/lactation. • Adverse effects include angioedema, cyanosis, wheezing, hypotension, constipation, black tarry stools, peripheral edema, chest pain, dyspnea, tachycardia, and hypertension. • To prevent teeth color staining, rinse mouth with water or brush teeth after taking liquid form. • Administer iron 2 hr prior or 4 hr after calcium or antacids for optimal iron absorption. • Iron may decrease concentration of levothyroxine. Administer iron 4 hr after levothyroxine.
Vitamin B$_{12}$ supplements (cyanocobalamin)		
• Vitamin B$_{12}$ deficiency, pernicious anemia	• Vitamin supplementation to assist in metabolic processes including fat and carbohydrate metabolism and protein synthesis, cell production, and hematopoiesis	• Medication is contraindicated in cobalt hypersensitivity. • Use caution in renal dysfunction, folic or iron deficiency, polycythemia vera, hypokalemia, bone marrow suppression, and uremia. • Adverse effects include pulmonary edema, HF, aluminum toxicity, thrombosis, thrombocytosis, hypokalemia, and polycythemia.

(*continued*)

TABLE 5.4	Hematology, Immunology, and Oncology Medications (*continued*)	
INDICATIONS	**MECHANISM OF ACTION**	**CONTRAINDICATIONS, PRECAUTIONS, AND ADVERSE EFFECTS**
Vitamin K (phytonadione)		
• Hyperprothrombinemia	• Has identical action to vitamin K: Facilitates binding of proteins to help blood coagulate	• Medication is less effective in patients with hepatic disease. • Frequently monitor coagulation lab values to prevent overcorrection.

A-fib, atrial fibrillation; CHF, congestive heart failure; CKD, chronic kidney disease; COPD, chronic obstructive pulmonary disease; DIC, disseminated intravascular coagulation; GI, gastrointestinal; HF, heart failure; HIT, heparin-induced thrombocytopenia; MI, myocardial infarction; PTT, partial thromboplastin time; RBCs, red blood cells; V-tach, ventricular tachycardia; WBCs, white blood cells.

Nursing Interventions

- Administer oxygen, medications (Table 5.4), IV hydration (Table A.3), and blood products as ordered.
- Assess airway, breathing, and circulation.
- Assess for signs of hemorrhage or occult bleeding.
- Assess for signs of infection.
- Assess for signs of respiratory distress or hypoperfusion.
- Assess for worsening signs of fatigue, weakness, and lethargy.
- Draw and monitor serial CBCs to assess RBC, Hgb, and Hct.
- Elevate extremities to prevent swelling.
- Monitor electrolyte and blood levels following transfusion of blood products.
- Monitor perfusion and oxygenation.
- Monitor vital signs (VS) for signs of worsening condition.
- Position patient with head of bed (HOB) at 30° or higher to improve oxygenation and perfusion.
- Prepare patient for administration of blood transfusion for severe anemia
- Promote appropriate diet choices for deficiency anemias.
- Provide therapeutic communication and support; discuss condition specific to anemia diagnosis and assess for willingness to accept blood transfusions.

Patient Education

- After discharge, avoid extreme temperatures and changes in altitudes that could cause a vaso-occlusive crisis.
- Avoid smoking due to nicotine's ability to attach to hemoglobin and cause decreased oxygen delivery.
- Avoid offending drug or drug class if hemolytic anemia is a result of medication therapy.
- Follow up regularly with hematologist for routine monitoring.
- Identify iron-rich foods: dark green leafy vegetables; dried fruit; iron-fortified cereals, breads, and pastas; legumes; red meat, pork, or poultry; and seafood. ▶

NURSING PEARL

If patient is experiencing iron deficiency anemia, there is an increased risk of constipation and black tarry stools with iron replacement therapy.

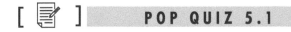

POP QUIZ 5.1

A patient with iron deficiency anemia receiving IV iron infusions is admitted to the progressive care unit (PCU) from the emergency department (ED) with abdominal pain, fatigue, and weakness. The patient's baseline VS included heart rate (HR) 80 and blood pressure (BP) 120/70 mmHg; however, the BP is now 90/62 mmHg and HR is 130. The patient urgently requests a bedpan and has a bowel movement: 300 mL of black tarry loose watery stool that has a strong odor. Patient states this is not consistent with usual bowel movements. What could be the cause of this large volume black tarry stool?

Patient Education (*continued*)

- Incorporate vitamin C-containing foods to enhance iron absorption (iron deficiency anemia): broccoli, grapefruit, kiwi, leafy green vegetables, melons, and oranges.
- If compromised spleen, follow infection prevention techniques: handwashing, staying up to date on vaccinations, and taking prophylactic antibiotics as prescribed.
- Recognize an increased risk of black tarry stools and constipation with iron replacement therapy.
- Recognize fortified foods are necessary to treat vitamin B_{12} deficiency.
- Self-monitor for symptoms of worsening anemia.
- Take medications and iron or vitamin supplements as indicated by provider.

BLOOD PRODUCT ADMINISTRATION

Overview

- Transfusion of blood products includes whole blood, RBCs, platelets, and plasma.
- Any consenting adult over the age of 18 is able to refuse blood transfusions.
- In nonemergent situations, patients should have an active type and screen prior to receiving blood.
- Once administered, monitor VS frequently to assess for a possible blood transfusion reaction.

 COMPLICATIONS

Complications of blood product transfusion include allergic reaction, circulatory overload, transfusion-related lung injury, infections (HIV, hepatitis B, and hepatitis C), electrolyte abnormalities, DIC, renal failure, hemolysis, and death. Frequent monitoring and assessment are needed to identify and treat any transfusion reaction.

Signs and Symptoms

Signs and symptoms of a blood product transfusion reaction include:

- Chills
- Dyspnea
- Fever
- Hypotension
- Hypothermia
- Itching
- Respiratory distress
- Urticaria

Diagnosis

Labs

- Labs diagnostic for transfusion reaction or need for transfusion (Table 5.5) include bilirubin, basic metabolic panel (BMP), CBC, haptoglobin, negative ABO: Test for other antibodies, type and screen, lactate dehydrogenase (LDH), and urinalysis.

 ALERT!

If a transfusion reaction is suspected, stop the transfusion, notify the provider, administer IV fluids, obtain patient labs, and send the blood product back to the blood bank for additional testing.

Treatment

- Blood product administration for any disease process or condition resulting in blood volume loss or depletion, such as anemia, cancer, surgery, or trauma.
- Administration of blood products requires large bore IV (20 gauge or larger), active type and screen, and consent.

TABLE 5.5 General Indications for Blood Product Transfusion	
CONDITION	**TREATMENT**
• Patients with Hgb <7 g/dL	• Packed RBCs
• Patients with platelets <20,000/μL • Platelets <50,000/μL and actively bleeding	• Platelets
• Plasma coagulation factors deficient • Reversal of anticoagulation	• Fresh frozen plasma
• Diagnosis of DIC • Factor VIII replacement • Fibrinogen levels <100 mg/dL	• Cryoprecipitate

Note: Transfusion criteria and target lab levels may vary in different types of patient populations.

DIC, disseminated intravascular coagulation; Hgb, hemoglobin; RBCs, red blood cells.

Treatment (*continued*)

■ If a transfusion reaction is suspected, immediately stop the blood transfusion. Disconnect the blood tubing from the patient's IV. Draw back to remove blood from the IV or central line tubing. Flush the IV line with 0.9% saline flush. Administer maintenance fluid (usually 0.9% normal saline [NS]) at ordered rate (Table A.3). Support ventilation with oxygen supplementation as needed. Notify the provider. Obtain VS and labs. Send the blood product back to the blood bank for additional testing. If itching/urticaria, administer antihistamine as ordered.

Nursing Interventions

■ Apply supplemental oxygen as needed.
■ Assess for worsening signs of transfusion reaction.
■ Monitor vitals for signs of worsening condition related to transfusion reaction.
■ Monitor perfusion and oxygenation.
■ Position patient with HOB at 30° or higher to improve oxygenation.
■ Provide therapeutic communication and support by addressing and managing anxiety experienced by patients after experiencing a reaction.

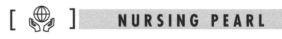

NURSING PEARL

If a patient experiences a blood transfusion reaction, notify the patient and/or family members and advise them to notify any medical providers in the future that they have experienced a transfusion reaction.

Patient Education

■ Self-monitor for symptoms of worsening or delayed transfusion reaction.
■ Follow diet and lifestyle recommendations under the Anemia: Patient Education section to prevent worsening anemia.
■ Follow up with all outpatient lab draws and appointments as scheduled.
■ Take prescribed medications after discharge to help restore and maintain RBCs or deficient vitamins/minerals to baseline values.

POP QUIZ 5.2

A 45-year-old patient with a history of end-stage renal disease (ESRD) is admitted to the PCU with worsening abdominal pain, nausea, and vomiting. He has a left arm fistula and a 22 gauge IV in the right hand. On admission, the patient started vomiting black coffee ground emesis. The patient was later found to have a GI bleed. The provider orders two units of packed RBCs. What is the first action to administer these blood products?

MEDICATION-INDUCED COAGULOPATHIES

Overview

- A coagulopathy is any alteration in baseline hematologic function that results in impaired clot formation.
- Anticoagulation medications including warfarin, platelet inhibitors, and heparin can result in coagulopathies, which can range from abnormal lab results to a medical emergency.
- Close monitoring of coagulation lab results is necessary to effectively titrate continuous anticoagulation medication infusions to prevent over-anticoagulation.
- Heparin coagulopathy can progress to a state known as heparin-induced thrombocytopenia (HIT). Patients with HIT are in an extremely hypercoagulable state and have a 30% mortality rate.

Signs and Symptoms

- Shared symptoms of coagulopathies induced by warfarin, platelet inhibitors, and heparin include bleeding, exfoliative dermatitis, or skin necrosis.
- Symptoms are specific to platelet inhibitors and HIT (Table 5.6).

Diagnosis

Labs

- BMP
- CBC: platelets <150,000/mcL ▶

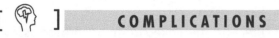

COMPLICATIONS

Complications of medication-induced coagulopathies include hemorrhage and bleeding anywhere in the body. Symptoms range from mild (petechiae and ecchymosis) to severe and life-threatening (intracranial hemorrhage, GI bleed, retroperitoneal bleed, etc.). Appropriate diagnosis and treatment are necessary to prevent further deterioration of condition.

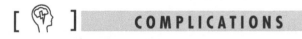

COMPLICATIONS

Onset of thrombocytopenia HIT is typically 5 to 10 days following initiation of therapy; however, symptoms can begin in <24 hr if the patient has antibodies due to prior heparin exposure.

TABLE 5.6 Platelet Inhibitors and HIT Symptoms

PLATELET INHIBITORS	HIT
• Agranulocytosis	• Chest pain
• Angioedema	• Chills
• Aplastic anemia	• Development of new blood clot
• Bronchospasm	• Dyspnea
• Erythema multiforme	• Ecchymosis
• Hepatic failure	• Enlargement or extension of blood clot
• Pancreatitis	• Fever
• Pancytopenia	• Hypertension
• Peptic ulcer	• Sudden onset of pain, redness, and swelling of an arm or leg
• Thrombotic thrombocytopenic purpura	• Rash or sore around injection site
• Stevens–Johnson syndrome	• Tachycardia
	• Weakness, numbness, painful extremity movement

HIT, heparin-induced thrombocytopenia.

Labs (continued)

■ Coagulation: May be elevated due to decreased platelet counts, prothrombin time/international normalized ratio (PT/INR), partial thromboplastin time (PTT), or D-dimer.
■ Fibrinogen
■ PF4 enzyme-linked immunosorbent assay (ELISA) (HIT)
■ Serotonin release assay (HIT)
■ Thromboelastography (TEG)

Diagnostic Testing

■ 4Ts score for HIT: 4Ts scoring system includes screening for the four hallmark signs of HIT: magnitude of thrombocytopenia, timing of thrombocytopenia with respect to heparin exposure, thrombosis or other sequelae of HIT, and likelihood of other causes of thrombocytopenia. The patient will receive a score between 0 and 2 for each category. A score of 0 to 3 indicates low probability, 4 to 5 indicates intermediate probability, and 6 to 8 indicates a high probability of HIT.
■ Spleen ultrasound can be used.
■ Other imaging helpful to identify potential hemorrhage, bleeding, or thrombosis includes a CT scan, MRI, and ultrasound.

Treatment

■ Warfarin-induced coagulopathy: vitamin K administration
■ Platelet inhibitor-induced coagulopathy: No specific antidote, time for drug to wear off, and symptom treatment as needed
■ HIT: discontinuation/removal of heparin administration and heparin-dosed agents from patient (heparin-flushed lines, etc.); alternate anticoagulation medications: enoxaparin, argatroban, and bivalirudin

Nursing Interventions

■ Apply supplemental oxygen if indicated.
■ Assess abdomen for potential signs of retroperitoneal bleeding, such as abdominal or back pain or bruising on flanks.
■ Assess airway, breathing, and circulation.
■ Assess for coffee ground emesis or black stool.
■ Assess neurologic status for potential change, possibly indicative of intracranial bleed.
■ Draw and monitor CBC and clotting factor laboratory trends.
■ Maintain activity precautions until coagulopathy is reversed.
■ Monitor perfusion and oxygenation.
■ Monitor VS for changes related to hypovolemia or excessive bleeding, such as tachycardia and hypotension.
■ Position patient with HOB at 30° or higher to assist with improved oxygenation and perfusion.
■ Provide therapeutic communication and support to allow the patient to express possible feelings of anger, fear, or anxiety from medication-induced coagulopathy.

Patient Education

■ Follow activity orders based on coagulopathy levels.
■ If due to an accidental medication overdose at home, use an organizational system to prevent medication errors in the future. ▶

POP QUIZ 5.3

A patient diagnosed with a pulmonary embolism (PE) is receiving a continuous heparin infusion and develops HIT. What would the nurse anticipate would be the next order from the provider?

Patient Education (*continued*)

- If HIT develops, notify all future providers of a previous history of a reaction to heparin.
- Self-monitor for symptoms of bleeding; notify provider immediately for any new signs of bleeding.

RESOURCES

Harewood, J. (2021, July 18). Hemolytic transfusion reaction. *StatPearls*. StatPearls Publishing. https://www.ncbi
.nlm.nih.gov/books/NBK448158

Laposata, M. (2019, January 17). Coagulopathies and bleeding disorders; hemorrhage, clotting abnormalities,
microvascular bleeding. *Cancer Therapy Advisor*. https://www.cancertherapyadvisor.com/home/decision
-support-in-medicine/critical-care-medicine/coagulopathies-and-bleeding-disorders-hemorrhage-clotting
-abnormalities-microvascular-bleeding

National Heart, Lung, and Blood Institute. (n.d.). *Blood transfusion*. U.S. Department of Health and Human Services.
https://www.nhlbi.nih.gov/health-topics/blood-transfusion#:~:text=Four%20types%20of%20blood%20
products,given%20by%20volunteer%20blood%20donors

Prescribers' Digital Reference. (n.d.-a). *Argatroban* [Drug information]. PDR Search. https://www.pdr.net/drug
-summary/Argatroban-Injection-in-0-9--Sodium-Chloride-argatroban-1458

Prescribers' Digital Reference. (n.d.-b). *Coumadin* [Drug information]. PDR Search. https://www.pdr.net/drug
-summary/Coumadin-warfarin-sodium-106#11

Prescribers' Digital Reference. (n.d.-c). *Droxia (hydroxyurea)* [Drug information]. PDR Search. https://www.pdr
.net/drug-summary/Droxia-hydroxyurea-898

Prescribers' Digital Reference. (n.d.-d). *Epogen (epoetin alfa)* [Drug information]. PDR Search. https://www.pdr.net/
drug-summary/Epogen-epoetin-alfa-2887

Prescribers' Digital Reference. (n.d.-e). *Feraheme* [Drug information]. PDR Search. https://www.pdr.net/drug
-summary/Feraheme-ferumoxytol-1201.3477#14

Prescribers' Digital Reference. (n.d.-f). *Folic acid tablets (folic acid)* [Drug information]. PDR Search. https://www
.pdr.net/drug-summary/Folic-Acid-Tablets-folic-acid-1634

Prescribers' Digital Reference. (n.d.-g). *Heparin sodium injection* [Drug information]. PDR Search. https://www.pdr
.net/drug-summary/Heparin-Sodium-Injection-heparin-sodium-1263.107

Prescribers' Digital Reference. (n.d.-h). *Lysteda* [Drug information]. PDR Search. https://www.pdr.net/drug-summary/
Lysteda-tranexamic-acid-1247.8307

Prescribers' Digital Reference. (n.d.-i). *Nascobal* [Drug information]. PDR Search. https://www.pdr.net/drug
-summary/Nascobal-cyanocobalamin-2286

Prescribers' Digital Reference. (n.d.-j). *Plavix* [Drug information]. PDR Search. https://www.pdr.net/drug-summary/
Plavix-clopidogrel-bisulfate-525.3952

Prescribers' Digital Reference. (n.d.-k). *Venofer* [Drug information]. PDR Search. https://www.pdr.net/drug
-summary/Venofer-iron-sucrose-805#14

Suddock, J. T. (2021, August 11). Transfusion reactions. *StatPearls*. StatPearls Publishing. https://www.ncbi.nlm.nih
.gov/books/NBK482202

UW Medicine Pharmacy Services. (n.d.). *Pre-test probability scoring for HIT*. https://depts.washington.edu/anticoag/
home/content/pre-test-probability-scoring-hit-0

ENCEPHALOPATHY

Overview

- *Encephalopathy* is an umbrella term that describes any diffuse disease that alters brain function or structure.
- There are many underlying causes of encephalopathy. *Hypoxic-ischemic brain injury* most often results from injuries such as cardiac arrest, stroke, or head trauma. *Toxic-metabolic brain injury* most often results from poisoning, illicit drug use, excessive alcohol intake, exposure to heavy metals or solvents, or severe metabolic abnormalities caused by organ failure. *Infectious brain injury* can occur from bacteria, viruses, or fungi, which may cause meningitis or encephalitis. *Hepatic brain injury* most often results from elevated ammonia levels seen in severe liver failure.
- While some causes of encephalopathy can be treated, others are progressive and can result in severe complications.

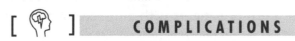 **COMPLICATIONS**

Encephalopathy can result in permanent brain damage, coma, seizures, altered mental status (AMS), dementia, or death. Early intervention and treatment are essential.

Signs and Symptoms

- Hypoxic/ischemic encephalopathy: myoclonic activity or status epilepticus; poor neurologic examination (patient typically unresponsive or brain-dead)
- Toxic-metabolic encephalopathy (hypoglycemic, hypercapnic, uremic, vitamin deficiency, and dialysis related): asterixis, Cheyne–Stokes respiration, generalized central nervous system (CNS) depression, muscle tone loss, pupillary changes (constricted but reactive), and seizures
- Infectious encephalopathy: behavioral changes, cognitive decline, hallucinations, lymphadenopathy (Epstein–Barr virus [EBV] encephalitis), microcephaly (prenatal exposure to the Zika virus), rash (herpes simplex virus [HSV] encephalitis), and splenomegaly (EBV encephalitis)
- Hepatic encephalopathy: behavioral changes, decreased awareness or level of consciousness or coma, difficulty concentrating, and mental status changes

Diagnosis

Labs

- Arterial blood gas (ABG): May indicate acidosis, hypercarbia, or hypoxia.
- Ammonia: May be typically elevated >45 units/dL.
- Blood cultures: May be positive with infection.
- Complete blood count (CBC): May be elevated white blood cell (WBC) count if an infection is present.
- Comprehensive metabolic panel (CMP): May show electrolyte abnormalities or decreased renal or liver function.

Diagnostic Testing
- EEG
- Brain MRI
- Head CT scan
- Spinal fluid culture

[⚙] **ALERT!**

Cerebrospinal fluid (CSF) findings indicative of viral encephalopathy include normal glucose levels, moderately elevated proteins, and lymphocytosis.

Treatment

- All encephalopathy forms primary therapy. General supportive and preventative care includes antipsychotics, such as haloperidol, for agitation or severe behavior changes (Table 11.1); medications to prevent progression depending on etiology (specific treatments in the following section for each etiology); physical, occupational, and speech therapy in addition to cognitive retraining to assist the patient in regaining baseline functioning, and seizure management medications.
- Specific treatment is dependent on etiology.
- For hypoxic/ischemic encephalopathy, correct the cause if possible: Correct metabolic abnormalities; if septic, administer antibiotics; if toxic ingestion or overdose, deliver antidote if available; and stabilize hemodynamics. For therapeutic-induced hypothermia, set a target temperature 89.6°F to 93.2°F (32°C–34°C) in the initial hr after cardiac arrest to improve neurologic outcome of resuscitated patients.
- For toxic-metabolic encephalopathy, treatment varies due to the underlying etiology: Review/discontinue medications with potential toxicity to the central nervous system (CNS), and administer thiamine (Table 11.1) for patients with a history of alcoholism, malnutrition, cancer, hyperemesis gravidarum, or renal failure on hemodialysis.
- For infectious encephalopathy, predisposing condition correction is needed. Use appropriate medication regimen for etiology of infectious encephalopathy. Antimicrobial or antifungal therapy is used with no delay, if possible. For amoebic encephalitis, there is no definitive treatment; however, over 90% of cases can be treated with miltefosine, azole antifungals, and pentamidine. For bacterial encephalitis or meningitis, use ampicillin, cephalosporins (cefotaxime, ceftriaxone, cefepime), vancomycin, meropenem, or dexamethasone, if applicable or fungal encephalitis or meningitis, use high dose, intravenous antifungal medications; the duration of treatment is dependent on the patient's immune system and type of fungus causing the infection. Viral encephalitis can be treated with acyclovir for HSV encephalopathy, ganciclovir for CMV encephalopathy, or foscarnet for CMV ganciclovir-resistant encephalopathy. (Table 6.1)
- For hepatic encephalopathy, predisposing condition correction involves medications such as lactulose or rifaximin (Table 7.1) to lower blood ammonia levels.

Nursing Interventions

- Administer medications as prescribed.
- Assess for changes in behavior or mood.
- Assess for worsening signs of CNS depression.
- Assess vital signs for signs of worsening condition or respiratory compromise.
- Maintain sleep hygiene.
- Monitor for changes in perfusion and oxygenation.
- Monitor for changes in neurologic status. Frequently reorient to environment, time, date, and situation as needed.
- Monitor for diarrhea (expected side effect from lactulose) and resultant electrolyte imbalances and dehydration.
- Position patient with head of bed (HOB) at 30° or higher. ▶

TABLE 6.1 Neurologic Medications

INDICATIONS	MECHANISM OF ACTION	CONTRAINDICATIONS, PRECAUTIONS, AND ADVERSE EFFECTS
Alkylphosphocholines (miltefosine)		
• Amoebic encephalitis	• Interact with membrane lipids at the site of the organism, inhibiting mitochondrial process to result in cell death	• Medication is contraindicated in pregnancy and Sjogren-Larsson syndrome. • Medication may impact male fertility. • Use caution in renal or hepatic disorders. • Contraception is required during treatment and for 5 months following the last dose to protect from possible risk to fetal development. • Adverse effects include nausea, vomiting, dizziness, headache, testicular pain, abdominal pain, and itching.
Anticonvulsants: Benzodiazepines (e.g., alprazolam, clonazepam, diazepam, lorazepam, midazolam)		
• Seizure treatment and management	• Potentiate the effect of GABA to increase inhibition of the reticular activating system	• Do not abruptly discontinue. • Adverse effects include fatigue, nausea, vomiting, weight changes (loss or gain), sexual dysfunction, agitation, unsteady gait, slurred speech, or sedation. • Use caution in use with active suicidal ideation, psychosis or bipolar disorder, CNS depression, pulmonary disease, alcoholism or substance abuse, liver or renal disease, and geriatric populations.
Anticonvulsants (e.g., valproate, levetiracetam, phenytoin)		
• Seizure management	• Decrease excitation • Enhance inhibition of neurons and/or alter electrical activity by affecting ion channels in the cell membrane	• Adverse effects include CNS depression, drowsiness, diplopia, ataxia, nystagmus, cognitive function changes, and rash.
Antivirals (acyclovir)		
• HSV encephalitis	• Prevent replication of HSV DNA through competitive inhibition, inactivating viral DNA, and terminating growing HSV DNA	• Medication is contraindicated in milk protein hypersensitivity. • Use caution in dehydration, renal impairment, seizures, electrolyte imbalance, hepatic disease, hypoxemia, and neurologic diseases. • Adverse effects include seizures, renal failure, tissue necrosis, angioedema, visual impairment, DIC, vasculitis, psychosis, hepatitis, jaundice, hypotension, and coma.

(continued)

TABLE 6.1 Neurologic Medications (*continued*)

INDICATIONS	MECHANISM OF ACTION	CONTRAINDICATIONS, PRECAUTIONS, AND ADVERSE EFFECTS
Antivirals (foscarnet)		
• Ganciclovir-resistant CMV encephalitis infections in transplant recipients or patients with AIDS	• Prevent viral DNA replication at binding sites	• Use caution in anemia, neutropenia, cardiomyopathy, nephrotoxicity, renal failure, sodium restriction, dehydration, cardiac disease, electrolyte imbalance, and seizure.
Antivirals (ganciclovir)		
• CMV encephalitis	• Inhibit viral DNA synthesis by competitive inhibition	• Use caution in anemia, bone marrow suppression, chemotherapy, leukopenia, neutropenia, thrombocytopenia, dehydration, and renal failure/impairment.
Fibrinolytic therapy (e.g., alteplase, streptokinase, tenecteplase, reteplase)		
• Known clot in ischemic stroke • ACS	• Breaks up and dissolves clot	• Contraindications include active internal bleeding (hemorrhagic stroke), history of CVA, recent surgery, bleeding disorders, and uncontrolled hypertension. • Use caution in patients with recent surgery or trauma, severe hepatic or renal disease, and concurrent anticoagulation therapy. • Adverse effects include generalized risk for bleeding (most notably in intracranial hemorrhage), GI bleeding, and retroperitoneal bleeding.
HMG-CoA reductase inhibitors/statins (e.g., atorvastatin, simvastatin)		
• Treatment of hypercholesterolemia, including hyperlipidemia, hyperlipoproteinemia, or hypertriglyceridemia • Myocardial infarction prophylaxis • Stroke prophylaxis	• Inhibit HMG-CoA reductase to lower amount of mevalonate (precursor of sterols including cholesterol), which reduces cholesterol in hepatic cells, increases hepatic uptake of LDL cholesterol from circulation, and reduces total cholesterol, LDL cholesterol, and serum triglycerides	• Medication is contraindicated in active hepatic disease, including cholestasis, hepatic encephalopathy, hepatitis, jaundice, or unexplained persistent elevations in serum aminotransferase concentrations. • Myopathy is a potential serious side effect; discontinue if patient develops elevated CPK or rhabdomyolysis. • Adverse reactions include hepatic failure, myoglobinuria, myalgia, diarrhea, nausea, and dyspepsia.
Mineral and electrolyte replacement (zinc)		
• Supplementation in zinc deficiency related to hepatic encephalopathy	• Replace in deficient states • Assist with enzymatic reactions required for normal growth and tissue repair	• Use caution in renal failure. • Adverse effects include gastric irritation, nausea, and vomiting.

ACS, acute coronary syndrome; CMV, cytomegalovirus; CNS, central nervous system; CPK, creatine phosphokinase; CVA, cerebrovascular accident; DIC, disseminated intravascular coagulation; GABA, gamma-aminobutyric acid; GI, gastrointestinal; HSV, herpes simplex virus; LDL, low-density lipoprotein.

Nursing Interventions (*continued*)

- Provide a safe, calm environment. Consider using 1:1 sitter for patient safety. Observe patient frequently. Physically restrain patient as the last resort. Place patient in a low bed. Provide a fall mat. Use a bed/chair alarm.
- Provide family counseling.

Patient Education

- Follow up outpatient with neurology or primary team responsible for care during hospitalization.
- If applicable, pursue alcohol and drug cessation. Seek additional support through Alcoholics Anonymous (AA), therapist, or other supportive programs.
- Self-monitor for symptoms or worsening condition, if possible.

SEIZURES

Overview

- A *seizure* is a sudden change in behavior or awareness, and/or abnormal movements caused by the uncontrolled and excessive electrical discharge of neurons in the brain.
- Largely a clinical diagnosis, seizures can occur due to an underlying medical condition or independently. A thorough history, physical and neurologic examinations, and additional tests are needed to identity an underlying cause.

Signs and Symptoms

- Presentation dependent on the type of electrolyte disturbance
- Generalized seizures: absence seizure, atonic seizures, clonic seizures, myoclonic, tonic-clonic seizures, or tonic
- Partial seizures: complex partial seizures or simple partial seizures

Diagnosis

Labs

There are no labs specific to diagnose seizures; however, the following may be helpful to rule out metabolic or infectious causes:

- Basic metabolic panel (BMP)
- Calcium
- CBC
- Magnesium
- Liver function tests (LFTs)
- Rapid point-of-care glucose (checked at first seizure)
- Toxicology screens

POP QUIZ 6.1

A patient with hepatic encephalopathy is refusing lactulose this morning. Their ammonia level is 62 µ/dL. Their neurologic status has improved; however, they are still only oriented to person and place. What should the nurse's next step be?

COMPLICATIONS

Seizures can progress to status epilepticus, which is a constant state of seizure activity without return to consciousness. This may result in permanent brain damage and death.

Diagnostic Testing

- Brain MRI
- ECG
- EEG
- Head CT scan
- Lumbar puncture if suggestive of an acute infectious process

Treatment

- Consult to neurology.
- Medications (Table 6.1): Antiseizure medication therapy dependent on factors including probability that event represented seizure, suspected or confirmed cause of seizure based on initial evaluation, stability of patient, and estimated risk of recurrent seizure; most seizures remit spontaneously within 2 minutes. Rapid administration of a benzodiazepine or antiseizure medication is usually not required. In critically ill patients with an acute symptomatic seizure, administer antiseizure medications intravenously. Administer antiseizure medications prophylactically to high-risk patients.
- Surgery may be an option.
- Treat the underlying condition, if possible
- Stimulate the vagal nerve.

[⚡]   **ALERT!**

Vagal nerve stimulation is an alternative to medication therapy. Vagal nerve stimulation can prevent seizures by preventing excessive neuron discharge.

Nursing Interventions

- Administer medications as ordered.
- Assess airway, breathing, and circulation.
- Assess the need for noninvasive oxygen or intubation in severe situations.
- Continuously assess vital signs.
- During a witnessed seizure, do not insert anything in the mouth. Remove harmful objects near the patient. Turn the patient on their side if able. Protect the patient's head from injury.
- If the seizure was unwitnessed by the progressive care unit (PCU) staff, ask the patient or family member for a detailed description of the event, postictal period, any triggers, family history of seizures, and any prior seizures.
- Maintain patent intravenous (IV) access.
- Provide a safe environment and initiate seizure precautions: Place the bed in the lowest position with bed rail padding, floor mats, and suction and oxygen setup/available.

Patient Education

- Avoid swimming alone or working at high elevations.
- Avoid operating heavy machinery or automobiles until seizures are considered controlled as determined by a physician per state guidelines. This may result in feelings of loss of independence and decreased self-esteem. Seek support as needed.
- Decrease stressors if possible.
- Follow up with scheduled appointments and lab draws.
- Keep a seizure calendar to keep a record of seizure events. ▶

[📝]   **POP QUIZ 6.2**

The nurse is performing a morning assessment when the patient stops responding to questions and has a blank stare, then makes myoclonic jerking movements. The next step during a seizure is to do what?

Patient Education (*continued*)

- Educate friends, families, and/or coworkers on condition. If a seizure lasts longer than 5 minutes or consciousness is not regained, call 911.
- Modify lifestyle to ensure safety in the event of a seizure. Keep bathroom doors unlocked, take showers instead of baths, and consider replacing glass with safety glass.
- Take prescribed seizure medication as instructed. Do not skip a dose. Take a forgotten dose as soon as possible. If more than one dose is forgotten, follow up with provider for guidance.
- Understand the triggers for seizure including sleep deprivation, alcohol intake, medications, infections, or systemic illness.

STROKE

Overview

- A *stroke* occurs when there is a sudden loss or blockage of blood circulation to an area of the brain, causing neurologic dysfunction.
- Three classifications of stroke are ischemic, hemorrhagic, and a transient ischemic attack (TIA). An

[🧠] **COMPLICATIONS**

Severe ischemia or hemorrhage can cause diffuse and devastating irreversible brain damage and cell death. This can result in brain death, herniation, and death.

ischemic stroke is caused by an occlusion of a cerebral artery that interferes with the overall blood flow to the brain. This can result from myocardial infarction (MI), atrial fibrillation (A-fib), deep vein thrombosis (DVT), surgical procedures, and certain genetic blood clotting disorders (Factor V Leiden). A *hemorrhagic stroke* occurs when there is bleeding into the brain due to the rupture of a blood vessel. It can be classified as an intracerebral or subarachnoid hemorrhage. Hemorrhagic stroke is caused by an arteriovenous malformation, hypertension, trauma, anticoagulation, and illicit drug use. *Transient ischemic attack (TIA)* is defined as a brief disruption of blood flow to the brain and is not associated with permanent neurologic disability. TIAs are similar to ischemic strokes, but the symptoms of TIAs are temporary.

Signs and Symptoms

- Possible symptoms of acute ischemic or hemorrhagic stroke: aphagia; ataxia; dysarthria; facial droop; hypertension (HTN; systolic blood pressure >220 mmHg); ocular abnormalities; rapid change in level of consciousness; rapid neurologic decline; sudden, altered alertness or obtundation; weakness or paresis that may affect a single extremity, half of the body, or all four extremities; or unequal pupils.
- TIA is a temporary period of symptoms similar to those of an ischemic stroke.

Diagnosis

Labs

- ABG if hypoxia is suspected
- Blood glucose to rule out mental status changes related to hypoglycemia
- CMP to rule out mental status changes related to electrolyte, renal, or liver function abnormalities
- Cardiac biomarkers if a cardiac event is suspected
- CBC: WBC may be elevated if infection is present. Elevated platelet count may indicate high potential for clot formation and possible cause of ischemic stroke.
- Prothrombin time/international normalized ratio (PT/INR) and partial thromboplastin time (PTT): Likely elevated if taking anticoagulants
- Pregnancy test for women of childbearing age
- Toxicology screen

Diagnostic Testing
- Brain MRI
- Carotid duplex scanning
- EEG
- Non-contrast head CT scan
- Lumbar puncture

Treatment

- Ischemic stroke: Alteplase (Table 6.1) is first-line therapy if initiated within 4.5 hr of symptom onset or time of last known well; antithrombotic therapy with aspirin (Table 2.3) is initiated within 48 hr of stroke onset and continued at discharge; blood pressure reduction occurs after the acute phase of ischemic stroke has passed; mechanical thrombectomy, lipid-lowering therapy with high-intensity statin (Table 6.1), and prophylaxis for DVT and pulmonary embolism (PE) (Table 3.1) may also be used.

- Hemorrhagic stroke: For blood pressure management, discontinue all anticoagulant and antiplatelet drugs; attempt hemorrhage extension prevention with appropriate medications or reversal agents (such as vitamin K, fresh frozen plasma [FFP], prothrombin complex concentrate [PCC] for warfarin, and protamine sulfate for heparin); attempt management of elevated intracranial pressure (ICP), which will require higher level of care; follow seizure management/prophylaxis; and consider surgical intervention.

- General care: Continuous monitoring of blood coagulation studies (PT, PTT, INR); IV fluids are the agent of choice for intravascular fluid repletion and maintenance fluid therapy is isotonic saline without dextrose (Table A.3). Other general care includes speech, physical, and occupational therapy, and supplemental oxygen or rapid sequence intubation (RSI) and transfer to higher level of care if indicated (stroke or neuro ICU).

ALERT!

Contraindications for tissue plasminogen activator (TPA) administration include acute intracranial hemorrhage, history of intracranial hemorrhage, severe uncontrolled HTN (systolic >185 mmHg and diastolic >110 mmHg), severe head trauma within the last 3 months, thrombocytopenia (platelet count >100,000/mm3), hyper-coagulability (INR >1.7 or PT >15 seconds), heparin administration within the last 24 hr, severe hypo- or hyperglycemia, advanced age, recent major surgery to any area of the body, recent gastrointestinal (GI) hemorrhage, and seizures.

Nursing Interventions

- Assess airway, breathing, and circulation.
- Assess blood glucose levels and treat as ordered.
- Assess for elevated or low blood pressure (BP), fluid retention, and electrolyte imbalances.
- Assess for fever and manage as ordered.
- Assess the need for noninvasive oxygen.
- Aspiration precautions: Complete bedside swallow study if patient meets criteria to assess for safe swallowing, and consult speech language pathology if there is a concern for dysphagia.
- Discuss current status and plan of care.
- Draw serial labs as ordered (blood glucose, CBC, PT, PTT, and INR).
- Implement fall prevention interventions including nonslip socks, bed/chair alarms, call bell within reach, bed in the lowest position, frequent assistance with voiding/bowel movements (BM), and peri care.
- Perform serial neurologic examinations and Glasgow Coma Scale (GCS) as indicated per provider and unit guidelines.
- Perform National Institutes of Health Stroke Scale (NIHSS) upon admission, every 12 hr, if there are any neurologic changes, and/or per institutional guidelines.
- Prevent pressure injuries.

Patient Education

- Adhere to diet and food regimens as ordered by the provider (Mediterranean diet).
- Attend any follow-up tests or procedures.
- Engage in physical exercise and weight reduction to maintain a healthy lifestyle.
- Follow activity orders.
- Pursue smoking cessation if indicated.
- Take medications as prescribed.
- Work with physical and occupational therapy, especially if there is residual weakness or paralysis, to learn how to complete activities of daily living (ADLs) and work toward getting back to baseline.

[📝]   POP QUIZ 6.3

A 63-year-old male is transferred to the PCU following ICU admission for ischemic stroke. Residual symptoms have started to resolve; however, the patient still experiences left-sided weakness, left-sided facial droop, and ataxia. The patient's daughter has visited for the first time today, bringing the patient's favorite dessert, a chocolate milkshake. Before giving the patient the chocolate milkshake, what should the nurse confirm has taken place?

RESOURCES

Centers for Disease Control and Prevention. (n.d.-a). *Parasites*. U.S. Department of Health and Human Services. https://www.cdc.gov/parasites/naegleria/treatment.html

Centers for Disease Control and Prevention. (n.d.-b). *Stroke*. U.S. Department of Health and Human Services. https://www.cdc.gov/stroke/types_of_stroke.htm#hemorrhagic

Ferenci, P. (2017, April 18). Hepatic encephalopathy. *Gastroenterology Report*, 5(2), 138–147. https://doi.org/10.1093/gastro/gox013

Fugate, J. E., & Rabinstein, A. A. (2015, July). Absolute and relative contraindications to IV RT-PA for acute ischemic stroke. *The Neurohospitalist*, 5(3), 110-121. https://www.ncbi.nlm.nih.gov/pmc/articles/PMC4530420/

Hashburn, R., Tunkel, A., & Mitty, J. (n.d). Initial therapy and prognosis of bacterial meningitis in adults. *UptoDate*. https://www.uptodate.com/contents/initial-therapy-and-prognosis-of-bacterial-meningitis-in-adults#H13

National Institute of Neurological Disorders and Stroke. (n.d.). Encephalopathy information page. U.S. Department of Health and Human Services. https://www.ninds.nih.gov/Disorders/All-Disorders/Encephalopathy-Information-Page

Parija, S. C., Dinoop, K., & Venugopal, H. (2015). *Management of granulomatous amebic encephalitis: Laboratory diagnosis and treatment*. Tropical Parasitology, 5, 23–28. https://www.ncbi.nlm.nih.gov/pmc/articles/PMC4326989

Prescribers' Digital Reference. (n.d.-a). *Acyclovir* [Drug information]. PDR Search. https://www.pdr.net/drug-summary/Acyclovir-acyclovir-sodium-670#10

Prescribers' Digital Reference. (n.d.-b). *Alteplase* [Drug information]. PDR Search. https://www.pdr.net/drug-summary/Activase-alteplase-1332.3358

Prescribers' Digital Reference. (n.d.-c). *Cytovene* [Drug information]. PDR Search. https://www.pdr.net/drug-summary/Cytovene-ganciclovir-sodium-1025#11

Prescribers' Digital Reference. (n.d.-d). *Depakene* [Drug information]. PDR Search. https://www.pdr.net/drug-summary/Depakene-valproic-acid-979

Prescribers' Digital Reference. (n.d.-e). *Depakote tablets* [Drug information]. PDR Search. https://www.pdr.net/drug-summary/Depakote-Tablets-divalproex-sodium-1075.5693

Prescribers' Digital Reference. (n.d.-f). *Enulose* [Drug information]. PDR Search. https://www.pdr.net/drug-summary/Enulose-lactulose-635#14

Prescribers' Digital Reference. (n.d.-g). *Foscavir* [Drug information]. PDR Search. https://www.pdr.net/drug-summary/Foscavir-foscarnet-sodium-3639#11

Prescribers' Digital Reference. (n.d.-h). *Impavido (miltefosine)* [Drug information]. PDR Search. https://www.pdr.net/drug-summary/Impavido-miltefosine-3607

Prescribers' Digital Reference. (n.d.-i). *Keppra injection* [Drug information]. PDR Search. https://www.pdr.net/drug-summary/Keppra-Injection-levetiracetam-1055.6058

Prescribers' Digital Reference. (n.d.-j). *Klonopin* [Drug information]. PDR Search. https://www.pdr.net/drug-summary/Klonopin-clonazepam-3064.5869

Prescribers' Digital Reference. (n.d.-k). *Lyrica* [Drug information]. PDR Search. https://www.pdr.net/drug-summary/Lyrica-pregabalin-467.8329

Prescribers' Digital Reference. (n.d.-l). *Phenytoin sodium injection* [Drug information]. PDR Search. https://www.pdr.net/drug-summary/Phenytoin-Sodium-Injection-phenytoin-sodium-1151.8322

Prescribers' Digital Reference. (n.d.-m). *Plavix* [Drug information]. PDR Search. https://www.pdr.net/drug-summary/Plavix-clopidogrel-bisulfate-525.3952

Prescribers' Digital Reference. (n.d.-n). *Simvastatin* [Drug information]. PDR Search. https://www.pdr.net/drug-summary/Zocor-simvastatin-402.3285

7 GASTROINTESTINAL SYSTEM

BOWEL OBSTRUCTION

Overview

- A bowel obstruction involves a partial or complete blockage of forward motility of bowel contents in the small or large intestine. Mechanical causes include obstruction tumors, strictures, adhesions, volvulus, impaction, or intussusception. Functional causes include paralytic ileus, inflammatory disease, or prior intestinal surgeries that alter regular bowel function. Other risk factors for obstruction include hypokalemia, peritonitis, sepsis, opiate or barium intake, hernia, and diverticulitis.
- Obstruction prevents the absorption of water, vitamin synthesis, and breakdown of bilirubin, in the large bowel, which can lead to further complications.

Signs and Symptoms

- Small bowel obstruction: abdominal pain; bloating; bowel sounds from hyperactive to absent, depending on severity of obstruction; decreased appetite; distended abdomen; frequent bilious vomiting; focal abdominal tenderness; and severe constipation
- Large bowel obstruction: Bowel sounds from hyperactive to absent, depending on severity of obstruction; constant abdominal pain; constipation; diffuse abdominal tenderness; distended abdomen; decreased appetite; and intermittent feculent vomiting

Diagnosis

Labs

- Basic metabolic panel (BMP): May show hyperkalemia (K >5.0 mmol/L) in severe obstruction or bowel necrosis.
- Blood cultures (if concern for peritonitis/sepsis)
- Complete blood count (CBC): White blood cell (WBC) counts may be elevated in infection; hemoglobin and hematocrit (H/H) may be decreased with bleeding
- Lactate: >2 mmol/L.

Diagnostic Testing

- Abdominal ultrasound with Doppler
- Kidneys, ureter, bladder (KUB)
- Abdominal CT scan

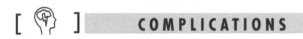

COMPLICATIONS

Strangulation leading to ischemic bowel is a major complication of bowel obstructions. Patients with ischemic bowel are at risk to develop tissue necrosis or bowel perforation, putting them at an increased risk for peritonitis and sepsis.

ALERT!

Patients with an ischemic or perforated bowel will have a markedly elevated lactate. This is due to decreased blood flow to the ischemic or perforated area resulting in anaerobic metabolism, thus elevating lactate.

Treatment

- Bowel rest
- Comorbid condition management
- Foley catheter for strict urinary output monitoring
- Intravenous (IV) fluids (Table A.3) and electrolyte replacement (Table 8.3), if indicated
- Nasogastric (NG) tube for bowel decompression and emesis control
- Nothing by mouth (NPO)
- Pain control (Table A.2)
- Surgery consultation if bowel obstruction caused by hernia (nonemergency surgery will reduce hernia) or bowel obstruction caused by strangulated or nonreducible hernia (immediate surgical consult and emergency surgery indicated)

Nursing Interventions

- Assess airway, breathing, and circulation.
- Assess for signs of hypoperfusion and sepsis.
- Draw and monitor serial labs as ordered.
- Monitor for the presence of flatus.
- Maintain NG tube to low-intermittent wall suction as ordered.
- Maintain strict intake and output (I/O).
- Monitor the volume of NG tube output.
- Note for any occurrence of bowel movements.
- Perform serial abdominal examinations. Note for any of the following: Firm or rigid abdomen, increased size/distention, or increased abdominal pain.
- Position patient with head of bed (HOB) at 30° or higher to prevent risk of aspiration.
- Provide therapeutic communication and support.

Patient Education

- Ambulate/change positions as ordered and tolerated to decrease risk of deep vein thrombosis (DVT) and increase gastrointestinal (GI) motility.
- Adhere to diet orders: NPO, clear liquids, and so on.
- Maintain DVT prevention/prophylaxis protocols, anticoagulation, and sequential compression devices (SCDs).
- Self-assess and identify potential lifestyle or dietary choices that may contribute to bowel obstruction. Diet or lifestyle modifications to prevent bowel obstructions include increasing daily fiber and water intake.
- Self-monitor for symptoms or worsening condition, if possible.
- Take laxatives as prescribed by provider to prevent recurrence of bowel obstruction and improve GI motility.

[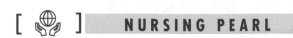]   **NURSING PEARL**

Strangulated or ischemic bowel that is unnoticed or untreated has nearly a 100% mortality rate. Detailed assessment and prompt communication of condition to the surgical team can decrease the mortality rate to <10% after timely intervention.

[ ]   **POP QUIZ 7.1**

A patient is admitted to the progressive care unit (PCU) for a bowel obstruction with complaints of abdominal pain, constipation, and intermittent vomiting of feculent nature. Based on the patient's presentation, which type of bowel obstruction is suspected?

DIABETIC GASTROPARESIS

Overview

- Gastroparesis is delayed gastric emptying without evidence of obstruction.
- Gastroparesis is a common finding in poorly controlled diabetic patients, which results in dysfunction of the autonomic nervous system, neurons, pacemaker cells of the stomach, intestines, and smooth muscle of the GI tract.

Signs and Symptoms

- Abdominal distention
- Bloating
- Early satiety
- Halitosis
- Neuropathy
- Postprandial fullness
- Poor glycemic control
- Vomiting: Often contains undigested, chewed food
- Weight changes

Diagnosis

Labs

- Labs are not diagnostic for diabetic gastroparesis; labs are to confirm poorly controlled diabetes through elevated point-of-care blood glucose values and HbA1c >7%.

Diagnostic Testing

- Abdominal CT scan
- Endoscopy
- Scintigraphy gastric emptying test

Treatment

- Lifestyle modifications: avoiding carbonated beverages; decreasing alcohol use; diet and exercise to achieve stricter glycemic control; small, frequent meals; smoking cessation
- Medications (Table 7.1; Table 4.1 [for diabetes medications])
- Tube placement: G-tube; G/J-tube; NG tube
- Surgery: partial gastrectomy with Roux-en-Y, gastrojejunostomy, and gastric resection

Nursing Interventions

- Administer medications as ordered.
- Assess airway, breathing, and circulation.
- Assess for signs of worsening symptoms. ▶

 COMPLICATIONS

Complications of diabetic gastroparesis include malnutrition, aspiration pneumonia, and worsening diabetes, which may progress to hypoglycemia, diabetic ketoacidosis (DKA), or a hyperosmolar hyperglycemic state. Prompt treatment is needed to prevent progression of the condition.

 ALERT!

Little data exist on surgical treatments for diabetic gastroparesis. Therefore, surgery to treat diabetic gastroparesis should be the last treatment option and should be recommended by a gastroenterologist.

TABLE 7.1 Gastrointestinal Medications

INDICATIONS	MECHANISM OF ACTION	CONTRAINDICATIONS, PRECAUTIONS, AND ADVERSE EFFECTS
Antibiotics: Rifamycins (rifaximin)		
• Hepatic encephalopathy	• Reduce ammonia-producing bacteria in the colon, thus reducing ammonia burden	• Monitor for signs of worsening hepatic disease. • Monitor for bleeding or worsening coagulation tests.
Anticonstipation: Contact/stimulant laxatives (sennosides)		
• Treatment of constipation	• Irritates the sensory nerve endings stimulating colonic motility • Reduces colonic water absorption to alleviate constipation	• Medication is contraindicated in patients with bowel or other GI obstruction. • Use caution in pregnancy. • Adverse effects include diarrhea, fecal urgency, abdominal pain, and flatulence.
Anticonstipation: Osmotic laxatives (lactulose)		
• Hepatic encephalopathy • Constipation	• Increases osmotic pressure to cause fluid accumulation that breaks down stool • Ionizes ammonia in the colon to the ammonium ion, preventing ammonia diffusion into the bloodstream, which can lower serum ammonia levels by 25% to 50%	• Monitor for hypernatremia, hypokalemia, and metabolic acidosis.
Anticonstipation: Softeners, emollients, enemas for constipation (docusate sodium)		
• For the prevention or treatment of constipation	• Decreases surface tension to allow water and lipids to penetrate the stool, hydrating it and allowing it to be passed	• Use caution in patients experiencing abdominal pain of unknown origin, GI bleeding, or vomiting. • Adverse reactions include diarrhea.
Antidiarrheal (loperamide)		
• Control diarrhea	• Interferes with peristalsis by direct action on the circular and longitudinal muscles of the intestinal wall to slow motility	• Contraindications include dysentery, fever, gastroenteritis, infection, pseudomembranous colitis, cardiac dysrhythmia, constipation, toxic megacolon, UC, and AIDS. • Use caution in hepatic disease. • Adverse effects include ileus, toxic megacolon, angioedema, lethal dysrhythmias and cardiac arrest, constipation, rash, respiratory depression, and QT prolongation.

(continued)

TABLE 7.1 Gastrointestinal Medications (*continued*)

INDICATIONS	MECHANISM OF ACTION	CONTRAINDICATIONS, PRECAUTIONS, AND ADVERSE EFFECTS
H2 receptor antagonists (famotidine)		
• GI disorders such as peptic ulcers and GERD	• Inhibit binding of histamine to H2 receptors on gastric cells decreasing gastric acid secretions	• Use caution in gastric cancer, GI bleed, infection, hepatic disease, QT prolongation, renal impairment, PKU, vitamin B_{12} deficiency, and smoking. • Adverse effects include seizures, angioedema, dysrhythmia, agranulocytosis, pancytopenia, rhabdomyolysis, constipation, liver impairment, renal impairment, delirium, confusion, and hallucinations.
Propulsive (metoclopramide)		
• Diabetic gastroparesis	• Inhibits dopamine receptors in the chemoreceptor trigger zone • Decreases sensitivity of the visceral afferent nerves that transmit from the GI system to the vomiting center in the chemoreceptor trigger zone	• Medication is contraindicated in paraben and procainamide hypersensitivity. • Use caution in GI bleed, obstruction or perforation, Parkinson's disease, seizures or tardive dyskinesia, cardiac disease, HF, HTN, hepatic disease, renal failure, breast cancer, and malignant hyperthermia. • Adverse effects include seizure, suicidal ideation, tardive dyskinesia, dysrhythmia, hepatotoxicity, angioedema, serotonin syndrome, depression, confusion, or hepatic and renal disease.
Pancreatic enzymes (pancrelipase)		
• Management of exocrine pancreatic insufficiency	• Release lipase, amylase, and protease at high levels, assisting with hydrolysis of fats, breakdown of starches into sugars, and breakdown of proteins into peptides	• Use caution in patients with porcine protein hypersensitivity, gout, renal impairment, and hyperuricemia. • Adverse effects include abdominal pain, elevated hepatic enzymes, hyperuricemia, nausea, and vomiting.
Phenothiazine antiemetics (e.g., promethazine, Compazine)		
• Nausea	• Block H1 receptors causing anticholinergic actions, resulting in reduced CNS stimulation of nausea and motion sickness	• Monitor for oversedation. • Monitor IV side for extravasation and tissue necrosis. • Use caution in patients with hepatic disease.

(*continued*)

TABLE 7.1 Gastrointestinal Medications (*continued*)

INDICATIONS	MECHANISM OF ACTION	CONTRAINDICATIONS, PRECAUTIONS, AND ADVERSE EFFECTS
Proton pump inhibitors (pantoprazole, omeprazole)		
• GERD; empirically used for upper GI bleeds	• Suppress gastric acid secretion by inhibiting gastric ATPase enzyme pump, decreasing acid	• Contraindications include interstitial nephritis. • Use caution in hepatic disease, gastric cancer, colitis, diarrhea, vitamin B_{12} and zinc deficiency, bone fractures, osteopenia/osteoporosis, hypomagnesemia, prolonged QT interval, and lupus. • Adverse reactions include GI bleeding, seizures, MI, dysrhythmias, elevated hepatic enzymes, interstitial nephritis, anemias, headache, nausea, and abdominal pain.
Serotonin receptor antagonists (ondansetron)		
• Diabetic gastroparesis • Nausea and vomiting	• Block the serotonin 5-HT3 receptors at the peripheral vagal nerve terminals in the intestines, blocking signal transmission to the CNS to antagonize the effect of serotonin and decrease the presence of nausea and vomiting	• Use caution with hepatic disease, PKU, GI obstruction or ileus, any cardiac dysrhythmia, electrolyte imbalance, malnutrition, MI, and thyroid disease. • Adverse effects include bradycardia, bronchospasm, hepatic failure, dysrhythmia, angioedema, laryngeal edema, laryngospasm, constipation, urinary retention, hypokalemia, and hypotension.
Vasoactive medications (somatostatin, octreotide)		
• Treating variceal bleeding by inhibiting vasodilatory hormone release	• Bind to somatostatin receptors • Lead to smooth muscle contraction in blood vessels	• Use caution in pancreatitis, hepatic or renal disease, DM, biliary obstruction, goiter, hypothyroidism, vitamin deficiency, alcoholism, and cardiac dysrhythmia and disease. • Adverse effects include bradycardia and dysrhythmia, GI bleeding or obstruction, hyperglycemia, constipation, goiter, edema, jaundice, ascites, nausea, abdominal pain, and rash.

CNS, central nervous system; DM, diabetes mellitus, HF, heart failure; HTN, hypertension; GERD, gastroesophageal reflux disease; GI, gastrointestinal; MI, myocardial infarction; PKU, phenylketonuria; UC, ulcerative colitis.

Nursing Interventions (*continued*)

- Assess the skin, securement, and placement of tube site if present.
- Draw and monitor serial labs as ordered.
- If performing gastric decompression with an NG tube, assess color, quantity, and consistency of gastric contents.
- Measure gastric residuals prior to medication or tube feed administration. Re-instill gastric contents back to patient to not cause electrolyte imbalances.
- Check the patient's blood glucose before meals and at bedtime.
- Administer appropriate insulin dosages as directed by the provider based on the patient's blood glucose.
- Provide therapeutic communication and support.

Patient Education

- Achieve glycemic control as evidenced by HbA1c <6%.
- Adhere to a low-carbohydrate diet and keep track of daily carbohydrate intake.
- Eat small, frequent meals. Do not rush while eating, and avoid large quantities of fluid at one time to decrease likelihood of developing nausea.
- Limit alcohol intake.
- Maintain daily physical activity of at least 30 minutes.
- Monitor blood glucose before meals, at bedtime, and when feeling symptomatic.
- Monitor for daily bowel movements.
- Pursue smoking cessation.
- Refer to social worker to ensure accessibility to medications and blood glucose monitoring supplies.
- Rotate insulin injection site, which may include the abdomen, upper arm, thigh, lower back, hips, or buttocks.
- Take medications as prescribed.
- Understand the signs of hyper- and hypoglycemic episodes and how to care for each.

[📝] **POP QUIZ 7.2**

A patient in the PCU has been admitted for diabetic gastroparesis. He has an NG tube and is receiving intermittent tube feedings, 200 mL every 3 hr as tolerated. What should the first step be prior to administering his tube feeding?

GASTROESOPHAGEAL REFLUX DISEASE

Overview

- Gastroesophageal reflux disease (GERD) is the backwards flow of stomach contents into the esophagus.
- Although there is no clear cause for GERD, possible causes include hiatal hernia, impaired esophageal mucosal defense against gastric reflux, impaired lower esophageal sphincter, and poor esophageal peristalsis.

Signs and Symptoms

- Belching
- Dysphagia
- Epigastric pain
- Heartburn
- Nausea
- Regurgitation

[🧠] 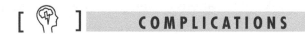 **COMPLICATIONS**

Complications of GERD include Barrett's esophagus (an erosive esophagitis), esophageal strictures, and esophageal adenocarcinoma. Early identification, treatment, and appropriate management can prevent these complications.

Diagnosis

Diagnostic Testing

There are no diagnostic tests specific to diagnose GERD. However, the following may be helpful to rule out complications:

- Esophagogastroduodenoscopy (EGD)
- Barium swallow study

Treatment

- Weight loss and diet modification: Eliminate acidic foods and improve dietary choices to enable weight loss.
- Exercise
- Eating pattern and frequency: Avoid large meals; avoid spicy or fried foods, onions, garlic, caffeine, and carbonated beverages; eat small, frequent meals; eat at least 3 hr before bedtime; and take medication as instructed (Table 7.1).
- Surgery: bariatric surgery, laparoscopic Nissen fundoplication

Nursing Interventions

- Assess airway, breathing, and circulation.
- Assess for worsening symptoms.
- Avoid foods that are high in fat, salts, or spices including fatty meats, processed snacks, cheese, greasy or fried foods, or spicy foods.
- Avoid acidic foods like tomato sauces, citrus, chocolate, peppermints, or carbonated beverages.
- Encourage ambulation and/or movement as tolerated.
- Encourage foods that are high in fiber (whole grains, root vegetables, or green vegetables), are alkaline (melons, cauliflowers, nuts, bananas, etc.), or have high water content (tea, celery, lettuce, broth-based soups, etc.).
- Maintain HOB 30° or greater at mealtimes and while sleeping.
- Promote exercise with physical therapy (PT).

Patient Education

- Engage in appropriate dietary modifications.
- Engage in physical activity.
- Keep up to date on current status and plan of care.
- Pursue a smoking and/or alcohol cessation program.
- Sleep with extra pillows or a wedge pillow under head or shoulders for elevation to decrease the risk of reflux.
- Take medications as prescribed (omeprazole, pantoprazole, or famotidine).

GASTROINTESTINAL BLEED

Overview

- GI bleed can be categorized as upper or lower, each with different symptoms and presentation.
- Causes for an upper GI bleed include peptic ulcer disease, varices, postsurgical bleeds, GI tumors, gastritis, duodenitis, and esophagitis. ▶

COMPLICATIONS

GI bleed, regardless of upper or lower, can result in respiratory distress, myocardial infarction (MI), infection, hypovolemic shock, and death. Early identification and treatment are needed to prevent deterioration of condition.

Overview (*continued*)

■ Causes for a lower GI bleed include diverticulosis, infectious or ischemic colitis, inflammatory bowel disease, hemorrhoids, colon cancer, anal fissures, and postsurgical bleeds.

Signs and Symptoms

■ Upper GI bleed: abdominal tenderness; decreased pulse pressure; epigastric pain; hematemesis, bright red or coffee ground; hyperactive bowel sounds; hypotension; melena; nausea and vomiting; orthostatic hypotension; pale skin or mucous membranes; and/or presyncope/syncope

■ Lower GI bleed: abdominal cramping or discomfort; diarrhea; hematochezia, often bright or dark red, that may pass clots with stool; hypotension; orthostatic hypotension; pale skin or mucous membranes; and/or presyncope/syncope

ALERT!

Risk factors for GI bleeding include varices, portal hypertension, alcohol or tobacco use, ulcers, Helicobacter pylori, diverticulitis, hemorrhoids, inflammatory bowel disease, nonsteroidal anti-inflammatory drugs (NSAIDs), and anticoagulation and antiplatelet agents. Complete a thorough physical and health history to identify potential risk factors.

Diagnosis

Labs

■ Active type and screen
■ CBC: decreased hemoglobin (<13.5 g/dL in men and 12.0 g/dL in women) and hematocrit (<41% in men and 36% in women)
■ Coagulation may be increased: prothrombin time (PT) >13.5 seconds/international normalized ratio (INR) >1.1, partial thromboplastin time (PTT) >35 seconds.
■ Guaiac test: GI contents and stool
■ *H. pylori* test: May be positive.
■ Lactate (>2.2 mmol/L)
■ Liver function tests (LFTs): Elevated LFTs (aspartate aminotransferase [AST] >40 u/L and alanine transaminase [ALT] >56 u/L) may cause increased clotting times contributing to increased blood loss.
■ Stool culture: *Clostridium difficile* and *Escherichia coli* may be detected.

Diagnostic Testing

■ CT angiography
■ Colonoscopy
■ Endoscopy

Treatment

■ Blood products as needed/ordered (Table 5.5)
■ Balloon tamponade (requires transfer to higher level of care)
■ *IV fluid resuscitation*: lactated Ringer's (LR) or normal saline (NS; Table A.3)
■ Medications as needed (Table 7.1)
■ NPO
■ Oxygen support: Avoid noninvasive positive pressure ventilation (NIPPV) with ongoing vomiting. Prepare for intubation if patient's mental status becomes altered or they are unable to protect the airway.
■ Placement of at least two large-bore peripheral IVs or central-line access
■ Stop/reverse anticoagulation if indicated
■ Treatment of underlying condition that may have caused the GI bleed

ALERT!

If the patient is experiencing a massive GI bleed with hemodynamic instability, Blakemore or Minnesota tube placements may be inserted. Surgery should be consulted, and the patient should be considered for transfer to a higher level of care.

Nursing Interventions

- Administer medications as ordered.
- Assess airway, breathing, and circulation.
- Assess hemodynamics and frequent vital signs (VS).
- Ensure two large-bore IVs are appropriately placed and patent.
- Maintain calm and therapeutic communication with the patient.
- Monitor emesis and administer antiemetic as needed.
- Monitor patient's stool for color and consistency. Perform a guaiac test if ordered.
- Perform serial CBCs to monitor H/H.
- Transfuse blood products as ordered (if consented by patient).

Patient Education

- Follow nutritional changes per provider recommendations.
- Follow up with resources for alcohol cessation, if indicated.
- Notify provider of any change in symptoms, pain, or sensation.
- Monitor for symptoms of bleeding, which include frank blood or black tarry stools.
- Self-assess for any changes or signs of worsening anemia including pallor, dizziness, fatigue, lightheadedness, palpitations, and shortness of breath.
- Stop anticoagulant medications if indicated by provider.
- Take medications as advised.

GASTROINTESTINAL INFECTIONS

Overview

- GI infections can be bacterial, viral, or parasitic. Bacterial infections include *Salmonella, Listeria monocytogenes, E. coli, Shigella*, and most notably *C. difficile* (with recent antibiotic intake). Parasitic infections include giardia. Viral infections include norovirus and rotavirus.

Signs and Symptoms

- Abdominal pain
- Diarrhea (watery or bloody, three or more loose stools/day)
- Fever
- Nausea
- Vomiting

Diagnosis

Labs

- Stool culture: May be positive for pathogenic bacteria.
- CBC: Will show elevated WBC.
- Blood cultures: May be positive if GI infection has spread.
- BMP: May show hypokalemia (K <3.5 mmol/L).

[🧠]   **COMPLICATIONS**

GI infection can result in dehydration and electrolyte abnormalities from vomiting and diarrhea that usually accompany infection. Infections can further progress to irritable bowel syndrome, chronic fatigue syndrome (giardia), sepsis, toxic megacolon, intestinal perforation, and necrotizing colitis.

Diagnostic Testing
- Abdominal x-ray
- CT scan of the abdomen
- Colonoscopy

Treatment

ALERT!

If a patient abruptly begins having watery diarrhea more than three times in 1 day, especially while receiving antibiotics, the patient should be tested for *C. difficile*.

- Symptom management
- Oral or IV fluid (Table A.3) and electrolyte supplementation (Table 8.3)
- Antiemetics
- Antibiotic therapy: ampicillin, azithromycin, fluoroquinolones, and tetracyclines
- *C. difficile:* Discontinue causative antibiotic; vancomycin, fidaxomicin, or metronidazole; and fecal transplant.

Nursing Interventions

- Administer medications and fluids as ordered/tolerated.
- Assess VS.
- Assess abdomen and GI tract frequently for changes.
- Assess I/Os to prevent dehydration.
- Draw and monitor serial labs as ordered.
- Monitor fever and provide cooling interventions if needed.
- Maintain skin integrity given increased stool output.
- Monitor stool output.

Patient Education

- Verbalize understanding of cause of GI infection and actions to prevent reinfection in the future. Cook meat thoroughly based on type and cut. Do not leave food out at room temperature. Obtain access to safe and clean drinking water.
- Take medications as ordered.
- Stay up to date about current status and plan of care.
- Stay up to date of any upcoming tests or procedures.

GASTROINTESTINAL SURGERIES

Overview

COMPLICATIONS

Complications of GI surgery include perforation, biliary leak, postsurgical or retroperitoneal bleeding, infection, sepsis, and death. Close postoperative monitoring is needed to identify changes and deterioration of condition.

- A GI surgery refers to an intervention performed on any organ or tissue housed within the abdominal space.
- Surgical interventions can be either open or laparoscopic and include adrenalectomy, appendectomy, bariatric surgery, cholecystectomy, colon and rectal surgery, hiatal hernia repair, Nissen fundoplication, nephrectomy, pancreatic surgery, retroperitoneal surgery, splenectomy, Roux-en-Y, and Whipple procedures.
- Many life-threatening or fatal complications can arise from GI surgery.

Signs and Symptoms

- Signs and symptoms of GI surgery complication: abdominal distention; abdominal pain; absent bowel sounds; changes in abdominal assessment: increased firmness, distention, rigidity, or pain; dyspnea; dull back pain; ecchymosis; fever; hemodynamic instability; and high volume of frank blood or output from drains, NG tube, surgical issues, or wound vac

Diagnosis

Labs

- Blood cultures
- BMP
- CBC
- Lactate

Diagnostic Testing

- Chest, abdomen, and pelvis CT scan
- Endoscopy
- MRI
- X-ray (chest and abdomen)

Treatment

- Ambulation per postoperative orders, moving out of bed to chair as ordered
- Incentive spirometer hourly
- Bowel rest as ordered with nasogastric tube (NGT) for gastric decompression, NPO, slow progression and advancement of enteral nutrition as ordered by surgeon and tolerated by patient
- Pain control
- Medications as ordered (Table 7.1)
- Treatment of surgical complications: for bleeding, blood product administration and continuous hemodynamic monitoring; for hemodynamic instability, IV fluids (Table A.3), continuous EKG monitoring, vasopressors (Table 2.3), and ionotropic agents as necessary for mean arterial pressure (MAP) goal >65; for infection, blood cultures, and antibiotics specific to disease process
- Possible transfer to higher level of care if hemodynamically unstable and condition deteriorating

Nursing Interventions

- Assess airway, breathing, and circulation.
- Administer postoperative medications as ordered.
- Apply abdominal binder and/or splinting pillow postoperatively as ordered.
- Change wound vac cannisters when filled and record output, color, and consistency.
- Continuously assess VS and notify provider of any changes.
- Draw and monitor serial postoperative labs as ordered.
- Encourage use of incentive spirometry postoperatively (instructions for use in Patient Education section).
- Monitor I/O, including volume and characteristics of gastric tube output.
- Monitor for postoperative DVT, pulmonary embolism (PE), or skin breakdown from positioning on the OR table. ▶

[⚙]   **ALERT!**

Postoperative complications resulting in severe hemodynamic instability may need immediate surgical consult with transfer back to the OR or to a higher level of care. Closely monitor changes to advocate for appropriate elevation in care as needed.

Nursing Interventions (*continued*)

■ Perform detailed assessment of drain output volume, color, and consistency. Empty drains as ordered by surgeon.

■ Perform detailed assessment of surgical incision site for drainage or oozing.

■ Perform dressing change daily or as frequently as ordered by provider.

■ Perform serial abdominal assessments for bleeding indications: dehiscence, evisceration, or rigidity.

■ Provide education to patient on patient-controlled analgesia (PCA) control. PCA is programmed to deliver a certain dose when the button is pressed. The button is on a timer based on the provider's order, and the PCA will only deliver one dose of pain medication per programmed time frame.

■ Take special precautions with bariatric patients. Monitor for signs of anastomotic leak or dumping syndrome, or signs of obstructive sleep apnea (OSA) and the need for NIPPV. Provide the opportunity for small, frequent meals and wait 30 minutes after meals to drink fluids; do not drink fluids with meals (to avoid dumping syndrome). Utilize reverse Trendelenburg to optimize breathing mechanics. Note that positioning the bed steeply upright may limit normal diaphragmatic excursion.

Patient Education

■ Brace the abdominal incision with a pillow when mobilizing to prevent pain and incision dehiscence.

■ Take medications as advised, including completing antibiotic regimen as prescribed.

■ Continue using incentive spirometry at home.

■ To use incentive spirometer, exhale deeply and then make a tight seal around the mouthpiece. Inhale as deeply as possible to the targeted volume. Repeat this 10 times every 1 to 2 hr.

■ In general, when caring for incisions after surgery: Clean hands prior to and after touching the surgical site. Assess the incision daily for any new redness, warmth around the site, foul or discolored drainage, edema, or bleeding. If bleeding occurs from the incision site, hold firm manual pressure over the incision and contact the provider immediately. Obtain necessary materials to perform dressing changes once discharged home. Change dressing daily as ordered by your provider, or if the dressing becomes soiled. After cleaning hands, remove the old dressing, clean and rinse the incision site, pat dry, and apply new dressing as directed. Avoid tight fitting clothes. Itchiness is expected as wounds heal. Do not scratch or pick at wounds.

POP QUIZ 7.3

A patient has been admitted to the PCU following an exploratory laparotomy for abdominal pain. During their admission assessment, they reported dull back and abdominal pain as a 2/10. An hr later, they are reporting the same back and abdominal pain as an 8/10. After completing a focused assessment, the nurse notes the surgical laparotomy sites are clean, dry, and intact; however, the abdomen is much firmer than when the patient was first admitted and is painful to palpation. VS: Heart rate (HR) 128, blood pressure (BP) 90/54, respiratory rate (RR) 20, T 98.2°F (36.8°C), and SpO_2 93% on 4 L of oxygen via nasal cannula. What should the nurse suspect?

■ For incisions with staples, stitches, or wound closure strip: Wait 24 hr following surgery to shower and wash unless otherwise directed by the provider. Clean the incision with mild soap and water. Do not scrub. Pat dry with a clean cloth once done bathing. Allow wound closure strips to fall off on their own; do not remove unless they do not fall off after 2 weeks.

■ For incisions with tissue glue closure: While skin glue is waterproof, avoid touching the glue for 24 hr and try to keep the wound dry for the first 5 days. Have showers rather than baths, to avoid soaking the wound. The glue will dry and fall away between 5 and 10 days. Do not pick or rub the glued area or put creams or lotions on the glue. Avoid direct sunlight.

HEPATIC DISORDERS
Overview

- Hepatic disorders include viral infections (hepatitis A, B, C), autoimmune hepatitis, cirrhosis, hemochromatosis, biliary atresia, nonalcoholic fatty liver disease, and nonalcoholic steatohepatitis (NASH).
- Some liver diseases can be reversed and treated, while others leave permanent scar tissue, resulting in cirrhosis or liver failure.

Signs and Symptoms

- Liver disease may present with no symptoms.
- If present, symptoms may include the following: altered mental status (AMS)/confusion, abdominal pain in the right upper quadrant, ascites, darker colored urine, edema, encephalopathy, ecchymosis, fatigue, itching, jaundice, nausea/vomiting, poor appetite, personality changes, and unexplained weight loss.

Diagnosis

Labs

- Albumin: May be <3.4 g/dL.
- Ammonia: May be >80 mcg/dL.
- Bilirubin may be >1.2 mg/dL.
- Blood and/or ascites fluid cultures
- CBC: May indicate elevated WBC in infection, decreased platelet count (<150,000/L).
- Comprehensive metabolic panel (CMP): Will show elevated AST/ALT (AST >40 u/L and ALT >56 u/L).
- PT/INR (PT >13.5 seconds, INR >1.1)
- PTT >35 seconds
- Lactate: May be elevated (<2 mmol/L)
- Serum copper levels: May be elevated in Wilson's disease.
- Toxicology screen: May be positive if illicit drugs are used.
- Viral: hepatitis A antibody, hepatitis B core antibody and surface antigen, hepatitis C antibody (and/or polymerase chain reaction [PCR]), and herpes simplex virus (HSV) PCR or serology tests

Diagnostic Testing

- Abdominal CT scan
- Abdominal ultrasound
- Chest x-ray
- Endoscopic retrograde cholangiopancreatography (ERCP)
- Head CT scan (if hepatic encephalopathy is suspected and to rule out other neurologic causes)
- Liver biopsy
- MRI
- Upper endoscopy (if varices suspected)

[🧠]   **COMPLICATIONS**

The major complication of liver disease is acute and/or chronic liver failure. There currently is no medical cure for liver failure. Liver transplant is available to those who meet eligibility criteria.

Treatment

- Acute hepatic failure: identify/reverse cause
- Alcohol cessation
- Coagulopathies possible: treatment is blood products such as fresh frozen plasma (FFP) and platelets
- Management of sequela of systemic effects of the disease
- Medication based on etiology (Table 7.1): lactulose, N-acetylcysteine and activated charcoal with acetaminophen toxicity, and rifaximin
- Lifestyle modifications: diet modifications, physical activity, and weight loss
- Surgery: liver resection, liver transplantation, and/or transjugular intrahepatic portosystemic shunt (TIPS) procedure

Nursing Interventions

- Administer medications as ordered.
- Assess abdomen frequently for changes.
- Assess airway, breathing, and circulation.
- Assess neurologic status for evidence of worsening disease or encephalopathy.
- Assess the need for noninvasive oxygen or intubation in severe situations.
- Assess VS and hemodynamic stability.
- Draw and monitor serial labs as ordered.
- Monitor and record bowel movement frequency, consistency, and volume for all hepatic disorders, particularly if taking lactulose.
- Monitor for signs and symptoms of bleeding.
- Monitor I/Os daily.
- If the patient receives a liver transplant, monitor the following postoperatively: Administer hemodynamic support with albumin, fluids, or vasopressors. Assess and monitor all lines, drains, and tubes. Assess VS. Draw and monitor serial labs, tacrolimus levels, and blood glucoses. Encourage working with physical and occupational therapy (PT/OT) to regain functional ability postsurgery. Transition to advanced diet as tolerated once extubated.

Patient Education

- Call the provider for any new signs of bleeding, including increased bruising.
- Follow up with alcohol cessation or mental health resources, if indicated.
- If liver transplantation is received, take antirejection and immunosuppressive medications as prescribed.
- Self-monitor for worsening symptoms of disease (see Signs and Symptoms).
- Strictly adhere to follow-up office visits and testing.
- Take medications as prescribed.

[⚡] **ALERT!**

While the United Network for Organ Sharing (UNOS) is the governing body for organ allocation in the United States, each hospital and health system is responsible for determining which patients meet eligibility criteria to be added to the solid organ transplant list. For alcoholic liver disease, some hospitals require 6 months of sobriety prior to being listed; however, others are moving away from this requirement. Check with your institution for the most current policy for liver transplantation eligibility.

 POP QUIZ 7.4

A patient with alcoholic liver disease and associated cirrhosis has been without alcohol for 3 months. He has consistently been compliant with his treatment plan and medications and is ready to be listed for transplant. He was admitted to the PCU with hepatic encephalopathy. His wife asks if he will be listed for transplant because of his deteriorating condition. What is the most appropriate response?

ILEUS

Overview

- An ileus is the inability to tolerate oral intake due to the lack of GI propulsion with no sign of mechanical obstruction. There is an inability of the intestine to contract normally and move waste out of the body.
- The most common causes of ileus include surgery, medication, trauma, peritonitis, or severe illness. However, an ileus is often unavoidable after abdominal or retroperitoneal surgery and critical illness.

Signs and Symptoms

- Abdominal distention
- Absent or hypoactive bowel sounds
- Bloating
- Diffuse pain
- Inability to tolerate oral by mouth (PO) intake or pass gas
- Nausea and vomiting
- Slow onset of symptoms

Diagnosis

Labs

There are no labs specific to diagnose an ileus. However, the following may be helpful for an initial workup:

- Blood cultures
- BMP
- CBC

Diagnostic Testing

- Abdominal CT scan
- Abdominal x-ray

Treatment

- Bowel rest
- HOB at 30° or higher to prevent risk of aspiration
- IV fluids (Table A.3)
- NG tube insertion to assist with bowel decompression
- NPO
- Monitoring for presence of flatus
- Noting for any occurrence of bowel movements
- Treatment of underlying condition
- Physical activity

Nursing Interventions

- Administer medications and fluid and electrolyte replacement as ordered/needed.
- Assess for other signs of underlying disease or medication contributing to ileus.

[🧠] **COMPLICATIONS**

Complications of an ileus include aspiration due to vomiting and can result in a prolonged hospital stay with additional interventions.

[🌐] **NURSING PEARL**

Early recovery after surgery protocols includes minimal fasting before surgery; returning to normal eating, drinking, and activities within 1 day of surgery; and using multimodal analgesia with appropriate opioid use if needed. If implemented, these protocols help increase speed of recovery, shorten hospital stays, and significantly reduce complications like postoperative ileus.

Nursing Interventions (*continued*)

- Assess for symptoms of hypovolemia.
- Assess patient for intolerance to PO intake and/or vomiting.
- Assess vitals continuously.
- Draw and monitor serial labs as ordered.
- Encourage physical activity. Assist patient out of bed to the chair daily.
- Provide a safe environment and engage in therapeutic communication.
- Monitor for return of bowel function (passing flatus, active bowel sounds).
- Monitor volume of NG tube output.

Patient Education

- Ambulate in room or in the hallways with therapy.
- Notify nurse of any return of bowel function (passing flatus, having a bowel movement).

POP QUIZ 7.5

What interventions and protocols decrease the risk of developing a postoperative ileus?

IRRITABLE BOWEL SYNDROME
Overview

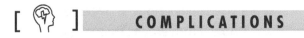

COMPLICATIONS

- Irritable bowel syndrome (IBS) is defined as abdominal pain/discomfort with altered bowel habits without a diagnosable cause.
- This can result from impaired motility, visceral sensation, brain–gut interactions, and psychosocial distress.

Complications of IBS can include hemorrhoids from chronic constipation or diarrhea, mood disorders (depression and/or anxiety), and overall poor quality of life. IBS has also been found to increase the risk of epilepsy, a more serious complication that can result in permanent brain damage.

Signs and Symptoms

- Abdominal pain or discomfort
- Altered bowel habits including constipation, diarrhea, or both
- Bloating
- Distention
- Pain location changes
- Stool changes
- Worsened symptoms with food intake

Diagnosis

Labs

There are no labs specific to diagnose IBS. However, the following are indicated if IBS is atypical, or if the patient complains of alarming symptoms (weight loss, hematochezia, iron deficiency):

- CBC
- CMP
- Fecal tests: Leukocytes, *C. difficile,* giardia, cryptosporidium
- Inflammatory markers: C-reactive protein (CRP), erythrocyte sedimentation rate (ESR)
- Thyroid-stimulating hormones (TSH)

Diagnostic Testing

There are no diagnostic tests specific to diagnose IBS. However, the following are indicated if IBS is atypical, or if patient complains of alarming symptoms (weight loss, hematochezia, iron deficiency):

- Intestinal biopsy via colonoscopy
- Abdominal x-ray

Treatment

- Symptom management: For constipation, use fiber supplements and laxatives; for diarrhea, use loperamide and probiotics.
- Increased physical activity, which increases colonic transit time to improve symptoms
- Diet modifications: avoidance of foods that fall under the FODMAP category, such as dairy, fruit, highly fermentable carbohydrates, onions, sorbitol, vegetables, and wheat
- Low-dose tricyclic antidepressant or selective serotonin reuptake inhibitor (SSRI; Table 11.1) if constant and chronic abdominal symptoms persist

Nursing Interventions

- Administer medications as ordered.
- Assess bowel movement frequency.
- Assess for changes in quality and sensation of pain.
- Assess for new or worsening symptoms of IBS.
- Assess quality and consistency of stool, if possible.
- Continuously assess VS.
- Perform frequent abdominal physical assessments.
- Provide safe space and engage in therapeutic communication to support the patient.

Patient Education

- Make note of any patterns in symptom presentation.
- Stay up to date on current status and plan of care.
- Work with a registered dietician or nutritionist to modify diet and avoid FODMAPs.
- Take medications as prescribed.

ISCHEMIC BOWEL

Overview

- Ischemic bowel occurs when there is a decrease in blood flow to the small or large intestine, resulting in cell and tissue death.
- The cause of decreased blood flow can be acute or chronic and result from atherosclerotic disease, mesenteric venous thrombosis, mesenteric arterial thrombosis, intestinal hypoperfusion during systemic shock, or mesenteric arterial embolism.

NURSING PEARL

FODMAP stands for fermentable oligosaccharides, disaccharides, monosaccharides, and polyols. It includes dairy, fruit, highly fermentable carbohydrates, onions, sorbitol, vegetables, and wheat. Adhering to a FODMAP-free diet may require additional assistance and support from a nutritionist or dietician.

POP QUIZ 7.6

A patient diagnosed with IBS is trying to order a breakfast tray while avoiding foods that fall under the FODMAP category. The patient asks if they are able to have scrambled eggs for breakfast. What should the nurse's response be?

COMPLICATIONS

Complications of bowel ischemia include bowel infarction and perforation, necrotic bowel, multiple organ dysfunction syndrome (MODS), toxic megacolon, fistula, colonic stricture, and sepsis. For severe bowel infarction, surgery may be indicated.

Signs and Symptoms

- Abdominal pain
- Bowel habit changes
- Guarding
- Rebound tenderness
- Sepsis: Chills or rigors, diaphoresis, elevated lactate and WBC counts, fever, hypotension, and tachycardia

Diagnosis

Labs

- Amylase >140 u/L
- BMP: May show hyperkalemia >5.0 mmol/L.
- CBC: May show elevated WBCs in infection (>11,000/mcL).
- Lactate: May be elevated >2 mmol/L.

Diagnostic Testing

- CT angiography
- Duplex ultrasound
- Invasive angiography
- MRI with angiography

Treatment

- Antibiotics
- Electrolyte replacement as needed
- Hemodynamics support: blood products and volume replacement
- Pain control
- Oxygen support
- Surgical intervention: endovascular and/or open surgery

Nursing Interventions

- Administer lactulose to ordered number of daily bowel movements or ammonia level as ordered.
- Administer medications as ordered.
- Assess airway, breathing, and circulation.
- Assess the need for noninvasive oxygen or intubation in severe situations.
- Assess neurologic status for evidence of worsening disease.
- Assess abdomen frequently for changes.
- Assess abdominal incisions each shift and monitor for signs of infection including redness, warmth to the touch, swelling or edema, bleeding, or foul-smelling or purulent drainage.
- Draw and monitor serial labs as ordered.
- Encourage pulmonary hygiene through ambulation, position changes, and incentive spirometry.
- Monitor for evidence of systemic infection including fever, hypotension, or tachycardia.
- Provide abdominal binder or splinting pillow.

Patient Education

- Continue using incentive spirometry at home. See Patient Education in Gastrointestinal Surgeries for instructions. ▶

[📝]   POP QUIZ 7.7

Laboratory tests are nonspecific for diagnosing bowel ischemia. What imaging is critical for diagnosis?

Patient Education (*continued*)

- Monitor for recurring symptoms of recurrent ischemia and/or infection, which include abdominal pain, changes in bowel habits, fatigue or malaise, fever, increased heart rate, and low blood pressure.
- Monitor for surgical site infection by assessing for new or worsening redness, warmth to the touch, swelling, foul-smelling or purulent drainage, or fever.
- Perform incision care until appropriately assessed by provider at follow-up appointment. See Patient Education in Gastrointestinal Surgeries instructions.
- Take medications as prescribed.

MALNUTRITION

Overview

- Malnutrition is defined as insufficient total calorie intake, which can be chronic or acute.
- There are a variety of causes for malnutrition, including chronic or acute disease, mental health disorders, or physical access to food.

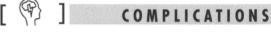

COMPLICATIONS

Malnutrition complications can result in electrolyte abnormalities and risk of developing refeeding syndrome, heart failure (HF) and/or dysrhythmia, impaired wound healing, urinary tract infection (UTI), sepsis, GI malabsorption, endocrinologic dysfunction, hypothermia, and death.

Signs and Symptoms

- Decreased muscle function and strength
- Decreased oral intake
- Dehydration
- Edema
- Electrolyte abnormalities: hypokalemia, hypomagnesemia, hypocalcemia, and hypoglycemia
- Frequent infections
- Mood changes: apathy, anxiety, depression, and self-neglect
- Poor wound healing
- Weight loss

Diagnosis

Labs

- Albumin <3.5 g/dL/prealbumin <10 mg/dL
- CBC is drawn to rule out anemia
- CMP
- Lactate
- Osmolality >295 mosm/kg
- Thiamine <2.5 mcg/dL
- Vitamin D <20 mg/mL

Diagnostic Testing

- EKG to detect electrolyte abnormalities

ALERT!

Thiamine plays a central role in carbohydrate metabolism. Thiamine deficiency can alter cellular energy production, especially in the brain, which requires glucose metabolism. Signs of thiamine deficiency include Wernicke's encephalopathy, cardiomyopathy, lactic acidosis, and peripheral neuropathy. Common etiologies of thiamine deficiency are alcoholism, hypermetabolic states, furosemide therapy, and magnesium depletion.

Treatment

- Appetite stimulants in patients with malignancies, those receiving chemotherapy, or those with poor oral intake
- Electrolyte replacement based on CMP results

Treatment (*continued*)

- Enteral/parenteral nutrition: enteral nutrition via temporary (or permanent) tube feeding: NG, orogastric (OG), gastrostomy, or jejunostomy; parenteral nutrition, if unable to tolerate enteral feeds
- IV fluid replacement (Table A.3)
- Medication management dependent on condition for patients with malnourishment
- Nutritional supplementation, including necessary vitamins and protein, if not contraindicated
- Psychiatric consult if needed
- PO intake if able
- Treatment of associated infections

ALERT!

In the first week of severe malnutrition, patients are most likely to develop refeeding syndrome. Patients should be slowly given between 60% and 80% of required calorie intake for age to prevent this complication.

Nursing Interventions

- Administer nutritional, electrolyte, and fluid replacement medications as ordered based on lab results.
- Assess VS for early indications of change in status.
- Consult dietary requirements and nutrition as needed.
- Consult a social worker to be sure patient has adequate resources for food.
- Draw and monitor serial labs as ordered.
- Minimize interruptions in enteral and parenteral nutrition.
- Monitor I/O and nutritional intake.
- Monitor for signs of malnutrition, including routine skin assessment for wounds.
- Monitor for signs of respiratory distress or aspiration following NG or OG tube placement.
- Monitor securement and site marking for NG and OG tubes.
- Provide protein supplementation as indicated.
- Provide safe therapeutic environment.

Patient Education

- Adhere to dietary recommendations made by provider. Choose high-protein, nutrient-dense foods if possible. Consult a dietician or nutritionist to help establish improved dietary choices. Consult a social worker to help get resources to obtain food.
- Follow up with alcohol or drug cessation resources if indicated.
- Self-monitor for status or symptom changes if possible.
- Take medications as ordered.

PANCREATITIS
Overview

- *Pancreatitis* is an inflammatory condition related to autodigestion of the pancreas by proteases.
- This process can range from mild edema to pancreatic necrosis and hemorrhage.
- Pancreatitis can be classified as acute or chronic. *Acute pancreatitis* is the result of pancreatic injury. *Chronic pancreatitis* occurs when permanent damage is sustained to the structure and endocrine and exocrine functions of the pancreatitis.
- Both acute and chronic pancreatitides are commonly caused by alcohol abuse.

COMPLICATIONS

Complications of acute pancreatitis include pancreatic pseudocyst, necrosis, peripancreatic fluid collection, acute respiratory distress syndrome (ARDS), compartment syndrome, acute kidney injury (AKI), disseminated intravascular coagulation (DIC), and death. Complications of chronic pancreatitis include pseudocysts and pseudoaneurysms, diabetes, and pancreatic cancer.

Signs and Symptoms

- AMS
- Dehydration
- Diaphoresis
- Diffuse visceral tenderness
- Distended abdomen
- Hemorrhagic signs: Cullen's sign, Grey Turner's sign
- Hypoactive or absent bowel sounds
- Low-grade fever
- Nausea/vomiting
- Rebound tenderness
- Steatorrhea
- Upper abdominal pain radiating to the back
- Weight loss

Diagnosis

Labs

- BMP: May show elevated BUN and creatinine.
- CBC: May show elevated WBC with pancreatic inflammation or infection.
- CRP: May be elevated with increased inflammation.
- Ionized calcium
- Lactate may be elevated >2.2 mmol/L.
- Serum amylase >140 u/L
- Serum lipase >140 u/L
- Triglycerides >10 mmol/L
- Urine amylase >21.2 IU/h

Diagnostic Testing

- Abdominal CT scan
- MRI
- X-ray
- Ultrasound

Treatment

- Electrolyte replacement
- ERCP if biliary tract occlusion suspected
- Medications: analgesics (Table A.2), antibiotics (Table A.1), antiemetics (Table 7.1), insulin (Table 4.1), IV fluids (Table A.3), pancreatic enzyme replacement (Table 7.1), and vasopressors (Table 2.3)
- Nutritional support: NPO initially, and enteral feeding below the duodenum
- Pain management
- Primary goals in the inpatient setting: blood sugar management, fluid resuscitation and blood pressure support, GI prophylaxis, and pain and nausea management

Nursing Interventions

- Administer nutritional, electrolyte, and fluid replacement medications as ordered.
- Assess for signs of retroperitoneal bleeding. ▶

Nursing Interventions (*continued*)

■ Assess respiratory status for early signs of atelectasis or effusions.
■ Complete detailed frequent head to toe assessment to assess for systemic change.
■ Continuously assess VS.
■ Draw and monitor serial labs as ordered.
■ Monitor and treat elevated blood glucose.
■ Monitor urine output for signs of hypoperfusion or adequate resuscitation.
■ Provide safe therapeutic environment.

Patient Education

■ Follow dietary and lifestyle modification recommendations.
■ Self-monitor for status or symptom changes if possible.
■ Take medications as ordered.
■ Participate in an alcohol cessation program.
■ Modify daily diet. If assistance is needed, consider working with a nutritionist or dietician to assist with lifestyle modifications.

RESOURCES

American Association of Critical-Care Nurses. (2018). The gastrointestinal system. In T. Hartjes (Ed.), *Core curriculum for high acuity, progressive care, and critical-care nursing* (7th ed., pp. 552–598). Elsevier.

Cleveland Clinic. (2019, March 20). *Small bowel obstruction*. https://my.clevelandclinic.org/health/diseases/15850-small-bowel-obstruction

Gupta, E. (n.d.). *GERD diet: Foods that help with acid reflux (heartburn)*. Johns Hopkins Medicine. https://www.hopkinsmedicine.org/health/wellness-and-prevention/gerd-diet-foods-that-help-with-acid-reflux-heartburn

Mayo Clinic. (2017, June 6). *Over-the-counter laxatives for constipation: Use with caution*. https://www.mayoclinic.org/diseases-conditions/constipation/in-depth/laxatives/art-20045906

Mayo Clinic. (2020, October 15). *Irritable bowel syndrome*. https://www.mayoclinic.org/diseases-conditions/irritable-bowel-syndrome/symptoms-causes/syc-20360016

National Institute of Diabetes and Digestive and Kidney Diseases. (n.d.-a). *Acid reflux (GER & GERD) in adults*. U.S. Department of Health and Human Services. https://www.niddk.nih.gov/health-information/digestive-diseases/acid-reflux-ger-gerd-adults

National Institute of Diabetes and Digestive and Kidney Diseases. (n.d.-b). *Liver disease*. U.S. Department of Health and Human Services. https://www.niddk.nih.gov/health-information/liver-disease

National Institute of Diabetes and Digestive and Kidney Diseases. (n.d.-c). *Treatment for gastroparesis*. U.S. Department of Health and Human Services. https://www.niddk.nih.gov/health-information/digestive-diseases/gastroparesis/treatment

Prescribers' Digital Reference. (n.d.-a). *Amitriptyline hydrochloride* [Drug information]. PDR Search. https://www.pdr.net/drug-summary/Amitriptyline-Hydrochloride-amitriptyline-hydrochloride-1001#11

Prescribers' Digital Reference. (n.d.-b). *Colace capsules (docusate sodium)*[Drug information]. PDR Search. https://www.pdr.net/drug-summary/Colace-Capsules-docusate-sodium-1023

Prescribers' Digital Reference. (n.d.-c). *Ledipasvir/Sofosbuvir* [Drug information]. PDR Search. https://www.pdr.net/drug-summary/Harvoni-ledipasvir-sofosbuvir-3630#11

Prescribers' Digital Reference. (n.d.-d). *Loperamide hydrochloride* [Drug information]. PDR Search. https://www.pdr.net/drug-summary/Loperamide-Hydrochloride-Capsules-loperamide-hydrochloride-2664#15

Prescribers' Digital Reference. (n.d.-e). *Metoclopramide* [Drug information]. PDR Search. https://www.pdr.net/drug-summary/Metoclopramide-Injection-metoclopramide-3898

Prescribers' Digital Reference. (n.d.-f). *Ondansetron hydrochloride* [Drug information]. PDR Search. https://www .pdr.net/drug-summary/Zofran-Injection-ondansetron-hydrochloride-243.2904

Prescribers' Digital Reference. (n.d.-g). *Pantoprazole sodium* [Drug information]. PDR Search. https://www.pdr.net/ drug-summary/Protonix-I-V--pantoprazole-sodium-2096.5821

Prescribers' Digital Reference. (n.d.-h). *Potassium chloride* [Drug information]. PDR Search. https://www.pdr.net/ drug-summary/Micro-K-10-potassium-chloride-770

Prescribers' Digital Reference. (n.d.-i). *Sennakot (Sennosides)* [Drug information]. PDR Search. https://www.pdr .net/drug-summary/Senokot-sennosides-3182#5

Saunders, J., & Smith, T. (2010). Malnutrition: Causes and consequences. *Clinical Medicine, 10*(6), 624–627. https:// www.ncbi.nlm.nih.gov/pmc/articles/PMC4951875

Weaver, K. R., Melkus, G. D. E., & Henderson, W. A. (2017). Irritable bowel syndrome. *The American Journal of Nursing, 117*, 48–55. https://www.ncbi.nlm.nih.gov/pmc/articles/PMC5453305/

8 RENAL SYSTEM

ACUTE KIDNEY INJURY

Overview

- Acute kidney injury (AKI) refers to the sudden decrease in kidney function, resulting in the retention of urea and other waste products and in the dysregulation of extracellular volume and electrolytes.
- While AKI can be associated with a high mortality rate, it can also be reversible in certain situations.
- Causes of AKI are divided into three categories: prerenal, intrarenal, and postrenal. Prerenal results from blood flow changes, including hypovolemia, hypotension, renal vasoconstriction, and glomerular efferent arteriolar vasodilation. Intrarenal causes include acute tubular necrosis secondary to major surgery, shock, sepsis, blood transfusion reaction, rhabdomyolysis related to trauma, prolonged hypotension, and nephrotoxic drug administration (Table 8.1). Postrenal causes result from mechanical obstruction in the outflow of urine including benign prostatic hyperplasia, prostate cancer, renal calculi, trauma, or extrarenal tumors.

COMPLICATIONS

Complications of AKI include electrolyte abnormalities (hyperkalemia, hyperphosphatemia, etc.), metabolic acidosis, pulmonary and peripheral edema, heart failure (HF) due to fluid overload, and central nervous system (CNS) effects (lethargy, altered mental status [AMS], and encephalopathy) due to uremia. These complications contribute to the increased mortality rate associated with AKI. Prompt identification and treatment is necessary to prevent these complications; transfer to a higher level of care may be indicated.

Signs and Symptoms

- Asterixis
- Edema and fluid retention
- Flank pain
- Hypovolemia
- Oliguria ▶

TABLE 8.1 Intrarenal Causes of AKI

ISCHEMIC CAUSES	NEPHROTOXIC CAUSES
Burns	Contrast dye
Cardiac surgery	Drug use
HF	Medications
Hemorrhage	Rhabdomyolysis
Sepsis	

AKI, acute kidney injury; HF, heart failure.

Signs and Symptoms (*continued*)

- Peaked T waves
- Metabolic acidosis
- Weakness
- Widening QRS complex

Diagnosis

Labs

- Arterial blood gas (ABG)
- Basic metabolic panel (BMP): Assess for an increased creatinine by ≥0.3 mg/dL (27 mcmol/L) relative to a known baseline value within 48 hr, or an increase to ≥1.5 times the known or presumed baseline value within 7 days.
- Complete blood count (CBC)
- Creatinine clearance
- Glomerular filtration rate (GFR)
- Urinalysis, protein, osmolality, albumin to creatinine ratios, electrolytes, and urine sediment examination
- Urine specific gravity

Diagnostic Testing

- Abdominal CT scan
- Chest x-ray
- Fluid challenge (to determine if AKI is prerenal unless contraindicated)
- Intravenous pyelography
- Kidneys, ureter, bladder (KUB)
- MRI
- Renal biopsy
- Renal ultrasound

[⚡]   **ALERT!**

In addition to lab findings, a decrease in urine volume to <0.5 mL/kg over 6 hr also indicates a possible AKI.

[⚡]   **ALERT!**

Medications are a common source of AKI. Dosages of drugs shown to cause nephrotoxicity may need to be adjusted or medications may need to be discontinued if AKI is suspected. Nephrotoxic agents that can cause kidney damage include heavy metals, certain medications, illicit drug use, rhabdomyolysis, and radiocontrast dye.

Treatment

- Identify cause/correct underlying problem.
- Nephrotoxic agents: Avoid if possible or administer renal dosage of certain medications.
- Dialysis if needed: Early initiation beneficial to prevent exacerbation of and currently manage acute and chronic renal failure, hemodialysis, peritoneal dialysis, and continuous renal replacement therapy (RRT) (may require transfer to higher level of care).
- Electrolyte level monitoring and replacement (Table 8.2).
- Fluid volume maintenance: Monitor for overload, fluid restriction, or IV hydration, depending on the patient's clinical status.
- Diuretics may be used to relieve hypervolemia among non-anuric patients with AKI (Table 8.3).
- Nutritional therapy if able to tolerate orally by mouth (PO): Offer high protein, and restrict potassium, phosphate, and sodium.

TABLE 8.2 Electrolyte Imbalances

ELECTROLYTE	CAUSES	SIGNS AND SYMPTOMS	TREATMENT
Calcium (normal value: 8.5–10.5 mmol/L)			
Hypercalcemia	• Cancer • Hyperparathyroidism	• Bone pain and fractures • Coma • Confusion • Depressed reflexes • Dehydration and polyuria • Dysrhythmias • EKG changes include shortened ST and QT segments/intervals • Fatigue • Heart blocks • Hypotonicity • Lethargy • Neurologic changes including confusion, psychosis, personality changes, memory issues, stupor, and coma • Nephrolithiasis • Seizures • Ventricular dysrhythmias • Weakness	• Furosemide to promote diuresis • Calcitonin • Hemodialysis if patient cannot tolerate additional fluids • High-rate IV fluids. (0.9% NS)
Hypocalcemia	• Fluoride poisoning • Hypomagnesemia • Hypoparathyroidism • Pancreatitis • Thyroid surgery • Toxic shock syndrome • Tumor lysis syndrome	• EKG changes include prolonged ST and QT segment, and ventricular tachycardia • Facial paralysis • Hyperreflexia • Laryngeal spasm • Muscle cramps • Neurologic changes including anxiety, depression, or confusion • Numbness and tingling of the extremities and around the mouth • Positive Chvostek and Trousseau signs • Seizures • Tetany	• Replacement with either calcium gluconate or calcium chloride • Magnesium replacement • Vitamin D supplementation

(continued)

TABLE 8.2 Electrolyte Imbalances (*continued*)

ELECTROLYTE	CAUSES	SIGNS AND SYMPTOMS	TREATMENT
Magnesium (normal value: 1.5–2.2 mg/dL)			
Hypermagnesemia	• Increased use of magnesium-containing medications such as laxatives and antacids • Renal failure	• Ataxia • Absent deep tendon reflexes • Bradydysrhythmia • Cardiac arrest • Confusion • Drowsiness • Fatigue • Flushing • Muscular weakness • Paralysis • Respiratory depression/arrest • Somnolence	• Calcium, which binds to and removes excessive magnesium • Dialysis • Diuresis with IVF 0.9% NS or furosemide
Magnesium (normal value: 1.5–2.2 mg/dL) (continued)			
Hypomagnesemia	• Alcoholism • DKA, HHS • GI abnormalities • Malnutrition • Thyroid dysfunction	• AMS • Cardiac dysrhythmias • Coma • Concurrent electrolyte/hormonal abnormalities (hypocalcemia, hypoparathyroidism, hypokalemia) • Delirium • EKG changes including widening QRS complex, peaked T wave, prolonged PR interval • Hyperreflexia • Muscle tremors • Ocular nystagmus • Positive Chvostek and Trousseau signs • Seizure • Tetany/tremors • Torsades de Pointes	• IV magnesium sulfate
Phosphate (normal value: 3–4.5 mg/dL)			
Hyperphosphatemia	• Renal failure	• Anxiety • Concurrent hypocalcemia • Deposition of calcium phosphate precipitates in skin, viscera, and blood vessels • Facial twitching • Irritability • Muscle dysfunction: Tetany	• Aluminum hydroxide • Correct hypocalcemia with treatments in hypocalcemia section

(continued)

TABLE 8.2 Electrolyte Imbalances (*continued*)			
ELECTROLYTE	**CAUSES**	**SIGNS AND SYMPTOMS**	**TREATMENT**
Hypophosphatemia	• Alcoholism • TPN	• CNS depression including confusion and coma • Dysrhythmias • Decreased stroke volume • Fatigue • Lethargy • Muscle weakness including decreased respiratory drive • Osteomalacia • Rhabdomyolysis	• Replace with PO or IV sodium or potassium phosphate
Potassium (normal value: 3.5–5 mmol/L)			
Hyperkalemia	• Adrenal cortical insufficiency • Blood administration • Crush injuries • DKA • Potassium sparing diuretic use • Renal failure • Rhabdomyolysis	• Bradycardia • Cardiac arrest • EKG abnormalities including flattening or missing P waves, widening QRS complex, shortened QT interval, peaked T waves • Leg cramps • Paralysis of skeletal muscle • Respiratory failure • Weakness	• Calcium chloride, sodium bicarbonate, insulin, and glucose administration • Correct acidosis • Dialysis • Eliminate drugs that may be the cause • Furosemide • Kayexalate
Hypokalemia	• GI loss • Malnutrition • Renal failure	• Dysrhythmias • Cardiac arrest • Decreased GI motility • EKG findings: Flattened T waves, emergence of the U wave, peaked P waves with increased amplitude • Fatigue • Hyperglycemia • Ileus • Muscle cramping • Paralysis • Respiratory failure • Weakness	• PO or IV potassium chloride replacement

(*continued*)

TABLE 8.2 Electrolyte Imbalances (*continued*)

ELECTROLYTE	CAUSES	SIGNS AND SYMPTOMS	TREATMENT
Sodium (normal value: 135–145 mEq/L)			
Hypernatremia	• Water loss • Cushing's syndrome • Hyperaldosteronism • GI loss • DI • DKA • Hyperosmolar hyperglycemic syndrome	• Agitation • AMS • Coma • Dehydration • Irritability • Lethargy • Weakness • Seizures	• Replacement with free water via PO or through NG tube • IV D5 or D5 1/2 if unable to tolerate enteral administration • Gradual correction to prevent cerebral edema or neurologic complications
Sodium (normal value: 135–145 mEq/L) (continued)			
Hyponatremia	• CHF • Cirrhosis with ascites • Excess water intake • Fluid overload • Hypothyroidism • Renal failure • SIADH • Thiazide diuretics	• Coma • Confusion • Nausea • Headache • Irritability • Lethargy • Seizures • Vomiting	• Sodium tablets and restrict free water • 3% NS intravenously • Gradual correction to prevent cerebral edema and osmotic demyelination

AMS, altered mental state; CHF, congestive heart failure; CNS, central nervous system; DI, diabetes insipidus; DKA, diabetic ketoacidosis; GI, gastrointestinal; HHS, hyperosmolar hyperglycemic syndrome; IV, intravenous; IVF, intravenous fluids; NG, nasogastric; NS, normal saline; PO, orally by mouth; SIADH, syndrome of inappropriate antidiuretic hormone; TPN, total parenteral nutrition.

TABLE 8.3 Renal Medications

INDICATIONS	MECHANISM OF ACTION	CONTRAINDICATIONS, PRECAUTIONS, AND ADVERSE EFFECTS
Alkalinizing agents (e.g., sodium bicarbonate)		
• Management of metabolic acidosis, adjunct treatment of life-threatening hyperkalemia	• Act as alkalinizing agent by releasing bicarbonate ions, thus correcting metabolic acidosis and shifting potassium intracellularly	• Contraindications include metabolic or respiratory acidosis, hypocalcemia, and hypernatremia. • Use caution in CHF, renal failure, or concurrent use with corticosteroids. • Adverse effects include edema, metabolic alkalosis, hypernatremia, hypocalcemia, hypokalemia, sodium and water retention, tetany, and cerebral hemorrhage.

(continued)

TABLE 8.3 Renal Medications (*continued*)

INDICATIONS	MECHANISM OF ACTION	CONTRAINDICATIONS, PRECAUTIONS, AND ADVERSE EFFECTS
Calcium supplementation (e.g., calcium gluconate, calcium chloride)		
• Treatment and prevention of hypocalcemia, emergency treatment of hyperkalemia, hypermagnesemia, and adjunct treatment in cardiac arrest	• Replaces calcium in deficiency and helps maintain cell membrane and capillary permeability • Assists with contractility of cardiac, skeletal, and smooth muscle	• Medication is contraindicated in hypercalcemia, renal calculi, and ventricular fibrillation. • Use caution in patients receiving digoxin, patients with severe respiratory compromise, and patients with renal or cardiac disease. • Adverse effects include cardiac arrest, syncope, dysrhythmias, phlebitis, and calculi.
Cation exchanger (e.g., patiromer, zirconium cyclosilicate)		
• Treatment of hyperkalemia	• Binds potassium in GI lumen to increase fecal potassium excretion, thus decreasing serum potassium	• Use caution in patients with constipation, fecal impaction, GI obstruction, or a history of hypomagnesemia. • Do not give with other medications. Administer either 3 hr before or after any other medication. • Adverse effects include hypomagnesemia, constipation, hypokalemia, edema, diarrhea, and abdominal pain.
Diuretics: Loop (furosemide)		
• Fluid overload • Renal dysfunction	• Secretion of electrolytes and water by preventing resorption and increasing urine output	• Contraindications include hypersensitivity and cross sensitivity with sulfonamides (thiazide diuretics). • Use caution in hypokalemia, digoxin therapy, cardiac disease, and dysrhythmia. • Adverse effects include hypokalemia, dehydration, hypomagnesemia, and hyponatremia.
Dextrose (D50)		
• Hypoglycemia related to regular IV insulin administration to treat hyperkalemia	• Glucose replacement and supplementation	• Contraindications include hyperglycemia. • Adverse effects include hyperglycemia.
Electrolytes (magnesium sulfate)		
• Hypomagnesemia	• Increase magnesium levels to maintain acid–base balance, electrolyte balance, and homeostasis	• Contraindications include hypermagnesemia, hypocalcemia, anuria, and heart block. • Use caution in renal insufficiency. • Adverse effects include decreased respiratory drive, dysrhythmia, hypotension, drowsiness, diarrhea, and muscle weakness.

(continued)

TABLE 8.3 Renal Medications (*continued*)

INDICATIONS	MECHANISM OF ACTION	CONTRAINDICATIONS, PRECAUTIONS, AND ADVERSE EFFECTS
Electrolytes, phosphorous supplements (e.g., sodium phosphate, potassium phosphate)		
• Hypophosphatemia	• Increase serum phosphorous levels to maintain electrolyte balance	• Contraindications include hyperkalemia, hyperphosphatemia, infected phosphate stones, and severe renal impairment. • Use caution in patients with HTN, CHF, severe hepatic disease, renal insufficiency, and dehydration. • Adverse effects include dysrhythmia, abdominal discomfort, nausea, vomiting, diarrhea, and arthralgia.
Electrolytes (potassium chloride)		
• Hypokalemia	• Maintain acid–base balance and homeostasis	• Contraindications include hyperkalemia, hypermagnesemia, and severe renal disease. • Use caution in cardiac disease and/or dysrhythmia, renal impairment, or patients using potassium-sparing diuretics. • Adverse effects include dysrhythmia, confusion, restlessness, abdominal pain, flatulence, and IV site pain/burning.
Mineral binding agents (e.g., sodium polystyrene)		
• Treatment of life-threatening hyperkalemia	• Exchange sodium ions for potassium ions in the intestines, allowing for excretion of excessive potassium from the GI tract	• Medication is only used in rare settings. • Medication may be used *only* in a patient who meets *all* the following criteria: (a) Potentially life-threatening hyperkalemia, (b) dialysis is not readily available, (c) new cation exchangers are not available, and (d) other therapies to remove potassium have failed or are not possible. • Do not give to the following patients due to the high risk for intestinal necrosis: Postoperative patients, patients with an ileus or who are receiving opiates, patients with a large or small bowel obstruction, or patients with underlying bowel disease. • Adverse effects include constipation, fecal impaction, nausea and vomiting, hypocalcemia, hypokalemia, sodium retention/hypernatremia, hypomagnesemia, and intestinal necrosis.
Polypeptide hormones (calcitonin)		
• Treatment of hypercalcemia	• Inhibit osteoclastic bone resorption and promote renal excretion of calcium-lowering serum calcium levels	• Contraindications include hypersensitivity to salmon protein or gelatin diluent. • Adverse effects include nausea and vomiting, facial flushing, and anaphylaxis.

(continued)

TABLE 8.3 Renal Medications (*continued*)

INDICATIONS	MECHANISM OF ACTION	CONTRAINDICATIONS, PRECAUTIONS, AND ADVERSE EFFECTS
Short-acting human insulin (regular insulin)		
• Hyperkalemia	• Forces potassium to move intracellularly	• Medication is given intravenously. • Contraindications include hypoglycemia. • Use caution in infection, stress, and changes in diet. • Adverse effects include hypoglycemia.
Vitamin D (vitamin D$_3$: calcitriol, cholecalciferol, etc.)		
• Management of hypocalcemia in chronic renal disease or hypoparathyroidism	• Activation in the liver to promote the absorption of calcium and decrease PTH concentration to improve calcium and phosphorous homeostasis in patients with deficiency with or without CKD	• Contraindications include hypercalcemia, vitamin D toxicity, and malabsorption problems. • Use caution in patients receiving concurrent digoxin therapy. • Adverse effects include dizziness, dyspnea, pancreatitis, dysrhythmias, and edema.

CHF, congestive heart failure; CKD, chronic kidney disease; GI, gastrointestinal; HTN, hypertension; IV, intravenous; PTH, parathyroid hormone.

Nursing Interventions

- Administer medications as ordered.
- Assess and maintain sterility of dialysis sites and lines.
- Assess atrioventricular (AV) fistula, if applicable: auscultate for bruit; palpate for thrill, and assess skin color, pulse, and capillary refill of distal extremity.
- Assess EKG tracings for signs of worsening condition, electrolyte imbalances, or respiratory compromise.
- Assess vital signs (VS) for signs of worsening condition or respiratory compromise.
- Maintain strict intake and outputs (I/O).
- Monitor and draw serial labs as ordered.
- Monitor fluid volume status: extra heart sounds (S3/S4, gallops, murmurs, and/or pericardial friction rubs), fluid intake from PO and/or intravenous (IV) fluids, jugular vein distention (JVD), lung sounds, mucous membranes, peripheral edema, skin turgor, and urine output.
- Monitor neurologic status. Assess for altered mental status and decreased level of consciousness.
- Perform bladder scan, if needed.
- Provide therapeutic communication and support.

[ ]   **NURSING PEARL**

Multiple medications have nephrotoxic properties. Antibiotics, drug classes such as aminoglycosides, beta-lactams, quinolones, and sulfonamides are commonly used nephrotoxic medications. Make sure to monitor the patient's creatinine and blood urea nitrogen (BUN) when administering these medications.

[⚙]   **ALERT!**

The National Kidney Foundation recommends that patients receiving dialysis avoid drinking more than 32 oz of fluid per day. When teaching both patients and family, provide education on the importance of this guideline and how exceeding this fluid intake may impact clinical status.

Patient Education

- Avoid nephrotoxic agents (certain antibiotics, diuretics, contrast dye, statins, antihypertensives, or benzodiazepines) unless directed by provider.
- Confirm understanding of renal diet modifications, including any diets with fluid restrictions, high protein, and low potassium, phosphate, and sodium.
- Follow up with scheduled outpatient appointments, dialysis appointments, and blood draws.
- Self-monitor for signs of fluid overload, worsening dyspnea, palpitations, or chest pain and call for help if indicated.

CHRONIC KIDNEY DISEASE

Overview

- Unlike AKI, chronic kidney disease (CKD) is the irreversible loss of kidney function that will progress to end-stage renal disease (ESRD).
- *CKD* is defined as the presence of kidney damage or decreased kidney function, as evidenced by an estimated GFR of <60 mL/min/1.73 m^2, for 3 or more months, irrespective of the cause.

Signs and Symptoms

CKD affects every body system and has many symptoms of varying degree and severity depending on the stage. Signs and symptoms include any of the following:

- Urine output changes: oliguria or anuria
- Cardiovascular abnormalities: coronary artery disease (CAD), HF, HTN, pericarditis, or peripheral arterial disease (PAD).
- Gastrointestinal (GI) disturbances: gastritis, GI bleed, nausea, and vomiting
- Endocrine disturbances: amenorrhea in women, erectile dysfunction in men, and thyroid abnormalities
- Hematologic abnormalities: anemia, bleeding, and infection
- Neurologic abnormalities: encephalopathy, peripheral neuropathy, restless leg syndrome, and sleep disturbances
- Pulmonary complications: pneumonia, pulmonary edema, and uremic pleuritis
- Integumentary changes: dry, scaly skin; ecchymosis; pruritus
- Musculoskeletal: *Calciphylaxis* is buildup of calcium in the blood vessels, skin, and visceral fat that causes painful ulcers and infection; soft tissue and vascular calcifications may also be a concern.

POP QUIZ 8.1

A patient with AKI is admitted to the progressive care unit (PCU) with a potassium value of 6.5 mmol/L. The patient has received calcium gluconate, regular insulin IV, and glucose with minimal improvement in potassium level. If this patient is unresponsive to medical therapy, what is the next step to lower potassium?

COMPLICATIONS

- Complications of CKD include electrolyte abnormalities (hyperkalemia, hyperphosphatemia), metabolic acidosis, hypertension (HTN), anemia, ESRD, and death.
- Complications of ESRD include electrolyte and acid–base abnormalities, mineral and bone disorders, anemia, HTN, dysrhythmia, and death. Careful monitoring and compliance with dialysis appointments is essential to managing ESRD.

ALERT!

Risk factors for CKD include diabetes type 1 and type 2, HTN, glomerulonephritis, chronic tubulointerstitial nephritis, hereditary or polycystic disease, vasculitis, plasma dyscrasia or cancer, and sickle cell nephropathy. Minority populations including African and Native Americans and Hispanic males are most likely to develop CKD. Dialysis and renal transplant are the only effective therapy options for ESRD.

Diagnosis

Labs

- ABG
- Albumin
- BMP
- GFR (see Nursing Pearl: Stages of CKD section for lab values of GFR)
- CBC
- Creatinine clearance
- Lipid profile
- Urinalysis

Diagnostic Testing

- Abdominal and pelvic CT scan
- MRI
- Renal biopsy
- Renal ultrasound

Treatment

- Dialysis: continuous RRT (requires transfer to higher level of care), hemodialysis
- Kidney transplant
- Medications to manage complications, including the following (Table 8.3): anemia (Table 5.4), dyslipidemia, HTN (Table 2.3), and metabolic/electrolyte disorders
- Nutritional therapy: fluid restriction; low-protein diet of 0.6 to 0.8 g/kg/d; sodium, potassium, and phosphate restriction

Nursing Interventions

- Refer to AKI, Nursing Interventions.

Patient Education

- Refer to AKI, Patient Education.

ELECTROLYTE IMBALANCE

Overview

- It is important to maintain normal electrolyte levels for the body to function appropriately.
- Renal disease often impairs the natural electrolyte balance within the body (Table 8.2).

NURSING PEARL

Stages of CKD:

- *Stage 1:* Kidney damage with normal or slightly increased GFR (>90 mL/min/1.73 m²)
- *Stage 2:* Mild loss in GFR (60–89 mL/min/1.73 m²)
- *Stage 3:* Moderate loss in GFR (30–59 mL/min/1.73 m²)
- *Stage 4:* Severe loss in GFR (15–29 mL/min/1.73 m²)
- *Stage 5:* Kidney failure (ESRD) requiring dialysis (GFR <15 mL/min/ 1.73 m²)

ALERT!

Consider consulting a dietician or nutritionist to assist with meal planning and food options when preparing for discharge.

POP QUIZ 8.2

A patient has been admitted to the PCU with the following lab values: creatinine of 3.4, estimated GFR <60, and potassium 5.8. Upon admission assessment, the patient reports that she typically eats a big bowl of fruit for breakfast. For lunch, she usually has milk with a peanut butter sandwich. For dinner, she has broccoli, beans, or potatoes with meat protein. What should the nurse's next action be?

COMPLICATIONS

While many electrolyte imbalances can be asymptomatic, it is essential that electrolytes be closely monitored in patients with renal disease to prevent dangerous complications, such as lethal dysrhythmias.

Diagnosis

Labs

- BMP
- Magnesium
- Parathyroid hormone
- Vitamin D levels

Diagnostic Testing

- EKG tracings help signal electrolyte abnormalities as evidenced by changes in cardiac conduction.

Nursing Interventions

- Administer medications to treat corresponding electrolyte imbalance as ordered (Tables 8.2 and 8.3).
- Assess musculoskeletal and neurologic status for changes or worsening condition.
- Draw and monitor serial labs as ordered.
- Ensure appropriate nutrition by adhering to fluid and electrolyte restrictions or supplementations.
- Monitor EKG tracings for electrolyte-related changes.

Patient Education

- Follow specific diet for corresponding electrolyte abnormality (Table 8.4).
- Follow up with lab draws to monitor levels of electrolytes.
- Self-monitor for worsening symptoms of corresponding electrolyte abnormality (Table 8.2), if possible.
- Take medications as prescribed to maintain regular electrolyte levels.

[⚡]   ALERT!

Chvostek sign is a twitching of the facial muscles when tapping on the facial anterior nerve.

Trousseau sign is a carpopedal spasm that occurs while inflating a blood pressure cuff on the arm. Both are abnormal and can indicate an electrolyte abnormality.

[📝]   POP QUIZ 8.3

A patient diagnosed with hypokalemia is not responding appropriately to potassium supplementation. What additional labs should be checked?

TABLE 8.4 Electrolyte-Rich Foods	
ELECTROLYTE	**FOODS**
High-potassium foods	• Vegetables: ◦ Broccoli ◦ Mushrooms ◦ Leafy greens ◦ Peas ◦ Potatoes ◦ Spinach ◦ Sweet potatoes • Dairy products: Milk, yogurt • Fish: Tuna, cod, or halibut • Beans or legumes

(continued)

TABLE 8.4 Electrolyte-Rich Foods (*continued*)

ELECTROLYTE	FOODS
High-sodium foods	• Boxed or frozen meals • Canned foods • Cottage cheese • Deli meat • Ham • Hot dogs • Jerky or dried meats • Pickles • Pizza • Pork rinds • Shrimp • Salad dressing • Soups • Tortillas • Vegetable juice

RESOURCES

American Heart Association. (2005). Part 10.1: Life-threatening electrolyte abnormalities. *Circulation*, *112*(24), IV-121–IV-125. https://doi.org/10.1161/CIRCULATIONAHA.105.166563

Griffin, B. R., Liu, K. D., & Teixeira, J. P. (2020, March). Critical care nephrology: Core curriculum 2020. *American Journal of Kidney Diseases*, *75*, 435–452. https://www.ncbi.nlm.nih.gov/pmc/articles/PMC7333544

National Kidney Foundation. (2019, May 31). *Sodium and your CKD diet: How to spice up your cooking*. https://www.kidney.org/atoz/content/sodiumckd

National Kidney Foundation. (2020, June 15). *Potassium and your CKD diet*. https://www.kidney.org/atoz/content/potassium

Prescribers' Digital Reference. (n.d.-a). *Calcitonin-salmon rDNA origin* [Drug information]. PDR Search. https://www.pdr.net/drug-summary/Fortical-calcitonin-salmon--rDNA-origin--1939

Prescribers' Digital Reference. (n.d.-b). *Calcium chloride* [Drug information]. PDR Search. https://www.pdr.net/drug-summary/10--Calcium-Chloride-calcium-chloride-3148

Prescribers' Digital Reference. (n.d.-c). *Potassium chloride* [Drug information]. PDR Search. https://www.pdr.net/drug-summary/K-Tab-potassium-chloride-1073

Prescribers' Digital Reference. (n.d.-d). *Regular, human insulin rDNA origin* [Drug information]. PDR Search. https://www.pdr.net/drug-summary/Humulin-R-regular--human-insulin--rDNA-origin--2912.3423

Prescribers' Digital Reference. (n.d.-e). *Sodium polystyrene sulfonate* [Drug information]. PDR Search. https://www.pdr.net/drug-summary/Kayexalate-sodium-polystyrene-sulfonate-2925.1687#14

Prescribers' Digital Reference. (n.d.-f). *Veltassa (patiromer)* [Drug information]. PDR Search. https://www.pdr.net/drug-summary/Veltassa-patiromer-3812

9 MUSCULOSKELETAL SYSTEM

FALLS

Overview

- A *fall* can result from a multitude of physical or environmental factors (Table 9.1).
- Patients can experience falls inside or outside of the hospital due to acute illness, medications, delirium, or overestimation of one's strength or functional ability.
- Falls increase morbidity and mortality and can lead to decreased functioning in all patients.

[ ]   **COMPLICATIONS**

Falls can result in an acute fracture, traumatic brain injury (TBI), subdural hematoma, pain, surgical intervention, decreased functioning ability, fear of additional falls, decreased quality of life, and/or transfer to an assisted living facility.

TABLE 9.1 Physical and Environmental Fall Risk Factors

Cognitive risk factors	• Acute or chronic memory impairments related to intellectual disabilities, dementia, or TBIs
Environmental risk factors	• Patients who live alone • Poor lighting in residence • Slippery floors • Tripping hazards (rugs, small animals, poor footwear, etc.) • Uneven surfaces
Psychological risk factors	• Fear of falling
Physical risk factors	• Female gender • History of previous falls • Increased age • Patients with comorbidities including electrolyte or metabolic abnormalities, dysrhythmias or syncopal episodes, MI, stroke, infection, arthritis, vascular disease, thyroid dysfunction, diabetes, depression, COPD, incontinence, vertigo, and orthostatic hypotension or AMS • Patients with immobility, deconditioning, and/or gait impairments • Polypharmacy (benzodiazepines, antiarrhythmics, digoxin, diuretics, sedatives, and psychotropics) • Poor nutrition
Sensory risk factors	• Hearing impairments • Patients with neuropathy or poor circulation to the lower extremities • Vision impairment

AMS, altered mental status; COPD, chronic obstructive pulmonary disease; MI, myocardial infarction; TBI, traumatic brain injury.

Signs and Symptoms

Patients who have fallen may present with any of the following:

- Altered mental status (AMS)
- Bruising
- Confusion
- Cuts or scrapes
- Fractures
- Head or facial trauma
- Lacerations
- Memory loss

Diagnosis

Labs

There are no labs specific to diagnose falls. However, the following may be helpful to clarify the etiology, cause, and extent of sustained injury:

- Basic metabolic panel (BMP): Assess electrolyte abnormalities to rule out anemia
- Complete blood count (CBC): Determine if fall is related to infectious process (white blood cell [WBC] count may be elevated) or anemia (low hemoglobin [Hgb] and hematocrit [Hct])
- Coagulation panel: Determine coagulation status if patient on blood thinners (may be elevated)
- Glucose point of care: Assess for hyper- or hypoglycemia or autonomic neuropathy related to diabetes
- Serum 25-hydroxyvitamin D levels: Identify individuals with vitamin D deficiency who may benefit from vitamin D supplementation

Diagnostic Testing

There are no diagnostic tests specific to diagnose falls. However, the following may be helpful to clarify the etiology, cause, and extent of sustained injury:

- CT scan of the head, chest, and/or abdomen
- MRI
- Transthoracic echocardiogram (TTE)
- Ultrasound
- X-rays of the chest, pelvis, spine, or extremities

Treatment

- Address/treat secondary injuries resulting from the fall. If a fracture was sustained, consult ortho/trauma for evaluation and possible surgery. If a neurologic injury was sustained, see Chapter 6.
- Perform an extremity examination to uncover possible deformities of the feet contributing to risk of falling (bunions, callouses, and arthritic deformities).
- Perform a full workup to determine any underlying causes; for example, a syncopal episode may require a full cardiac workup (Chapter 2).
- Order a physical therapy/occupational therapy (PT/OT) consult.
- Review/discontinue unnecessary medications contributing to polypharmacy.
- Assess visual acuity, hearing, and muscle function.
- Provide vitamin D supplements as needed (Table 9.2).

 [🌐] **NURSING PEARL**

Patients who take certain medications such as benzodiazepines, antiarrhythmics, digoxin, diuretics, sedatives, and psychotropics have been found to be at higher risk for falls.

 [⚡] **ALERT!**

Be alert to older adult patients taking anticoagulants who have experienced a fall with head trauma, as they are at increased risk for intracranial bleeding.

TABLE 9.2 Musculoskeletal Medications

INDICATIONS	MECHANISM OF ACTION	CONTRAINDICATIONS, PRECAUTIONS, AND ADVERSE EFFECTS
Antiparkinson agents (levodopa/carbidopa)		
• Treatment of motor fluctuations in patients with advanced Parkinson disease	• Cross the blood-brain barrier to increase dopamine levels within the corpus striatum to improve nerve impulse and decrease motor symptoms	• Contraindications include concurrent use with MAOIs. • Do not abruptly discontinue. • Use caution with cardiac disease; MI; hypotension; behavioral changes; depression; psychosis; coadministration with other CNS depressants; GI disease; diabetes mellitus; melanoma; pheochromocytoma; pulmonary, hepatic, and renal disease; peripheral neuropathy; HF; and electrolyte imbalances. • Adverse effects include akinesia, seizures, GI bleeding, GI obstruction, MI, new primary malignancy, angioedema, hypotension, depression, confusion, hallucinations, increased hepatic enzymes, urinary incontinence, edema, blurred vision, nausea, anxiety, and vomiting.
Vitamin D supplement (ergocalciferol)		
• Vitamin D deficiency	• Metabolize vitamin D into calcitriol, which promotes renal reabsorption of calcium, increases intestinal absorption of calcium and phosphorus, and increases calcium mobilization from bone to plasma, which promotes skeletal strength and increases muscle fiber growth to help with balance	• Vitamin D supplements are contraindicated in hypercalcemia and malabsorption syndrome. • Use caution in renal failure, renal disease, and pregnancy. • Adverse effects include fatigue, headache, nausea, increased thirst, and increased urinary frequency.
Vitamin B$_{12}$ supplements (cyanocobalamin)		
• Vitamin B$_{12}$ deficiency	• Assist in metabolic processes, such as fat and carbohydrate metabolism, protein synthesis, cell production, and hematopoiesis	• Vitamin B$_{12}$ is contraindicated in cobalt hypersensitivity. • Use caution in renal impairment, myelosuppression, uremia, infection, iron or folate deficiency, and polycythemia. • Adverse effects include headache, nausea, anxiety, ataxia, diarrhea, itching, swelling, infection, thrombocytosis, or hypokalemia.

CNS, central nervous system; GI, gastrointestinal; HF, heart failure; MAOIs, monoamine oxidase inhibitors; MI, myocardial infarction.

Nursing Interventions

- Assist the patient to the bathroom if not using a Foley catheter/bedpan.
- Consult social work to perform in-home assessment.
- Discuss mobility orders with the patient (bedrest, with assistance, with assistive device, etc.).
- Instruct patient on fall risk precautions.
- Maintain fall precautions as ordered: Adjust bed rails as ordered, keep call bell and personal belongings within reach, lower bed to lowest setting, place appropriate signage on door, place appropriate falls wrist band on patient, and use antislip socks in the fall color corresponding to hospital policy (e.g., yellow).
- Obtain postural vital signs (VS) to rule out orthostatic hypotension.
- Perform serial neurologic assessments if patient sustained a head bleed from the fall or shows any signs of deterioration in neurologic status.
- Provide assistive devices (walker, cane) and personal support (gait belt) to maintain patient safety while ambulating.
- Provide a safe environment free of tripping hazards if patient is ambulatory. Remove or secure clutter on the floor, IV lines/tubes, medical devices, and sequential compression devices (SCDs).
- Provide therapeutic communication.

Patient Education

- Engage in exercise programs that encourage balance, endurance, flexibility, and resistance, such as tai chi and yoga.
- Collaborate with caregivers on home modifications to decrease environmental risk for falls.
- Encourage proper nutrition.
- Use call bell for needs outside of reach (e.g., lunch tray, book, and personal belongings).
- Home assessment: Add nonslip surfaces/mats; add rails; use fall alert system, if appropriate; flatten uneven surfaces; place ramps over steps; remove rugs; and utilize shower chairs.

POP QUIZ 9.1

A patient is admitted to the progressive care unit (PCU) after an unwitnessed fall at home. During your intake assessment, you learn that the patient has a past medical history of diabetes, atrial fibrillation (A-fib), and gastroesophageal reflux disease (GERD). The patient also wears glasses. He lives alone, but his daughter visits daily. She is currently working to fall proof his house by removing loose rugs and installing handrails on the stairwells. Which of the five types of risk factors for falls does this patient currently present with?

GAIT DISTURBANCES

Overview

- A *gait disturbance* is any deviation from a normal walking pattern that results in an increased risk for an injury or fall.
- Gait disturbances can occur due to a multitude of conditions, including degenerative disk or bone disease, Parkinson disease, multiple sclerosis, kyphosis, muscle atrophy, or any condition that causes exercise intolerance and decreased mobility.
- Neurologic and musculoskeletal abnormalities are the most common cause of gait abnormalities and disturbances.

COMPLICATIONS

Patients with gait abnormalities are at increased risk for falls, paralysis, syncope, skeletal fractures, epidural/subdural trauma, and psychosocial stigma. Those who do experience a fall are at increased risk for morbidity, mortality, and reduced functioning.

Signs and Symptoms

- Symptoms of gait disturbances may include abnormalities in any of the following: arm swing, posture, running pattern, speed, stance, standing, step length, and walking pattern.
- Additionally, gait disturbances may manifest as freezing, heels walking, positive Romberg's test, tandem gait, toes walking, and turning.

Diagnosis

Labs

There are no labs specific to diagnose gait disturbances.

Diagnostic Testing

Imaging is dependent on findings obtained during history and physical:

- CT scan
- MRI
- X-rays

Treatment

Treatment is dependent on etiology of the gait disturbance:

- Aerobic exercise
- Electrical stimulator
- Low resistance strength training
- Medications (Table 9.2): Dopamine agonist/ antiparkinson agents and vitamin B_{12}
- Muscle strengthening
- Shoe lifts
- Solid or hinged ankle foot orthosis
- Surgery

ALERT!

Gait abnormalities resulting from Parkinson disease are best treated with a combination of medication therapy, deep brain stimulation, and allied health support including treadmill walking, cognitive training, and home-based exercise programs.

Nursing Interventions

Maintain fall precautions as ordered (see Falls section for additional details).

Patient Education

- Follow treatment guidelines for specific etiology causing gait disturbances.
- Use assistive devices as ordered.
- See the Falls section for additional patient education.

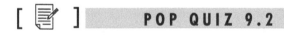

POP QUIZ 9.2

Patients with gait abnormalities resulting from Parkinson disease would benefit from which therapies to improve stability?

IMMOBILITY

Overview

- Immobility can result from critical illness, lack of motivation, or a combination of both.
- For patients admitted to the PCU, immobility may complicate primary illness and result in an increased length of stay due to a range of both short- and long-term effects.

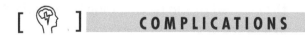

COMPLICATIONS

Immobility can result in pressure ulcers, deformities, joint pain, loss of muscle and bone mass, deep vein thrombosis (DVT), pulmonary embolism (PE), atelectasis, pneumonia, and decreased functioning in cardiovascular, endocrine, immune, gastrointestinal (GI), excretory, vestibular, cognitive, and psychologic systems. These can impact morbidity and mortality rates.

Signs and Symptoms

- Flaccid extremities
- Lack of motivation
- Lack of movement/inability to mobilize any part of the body
- Muscle atrophy

Diagnosis

Labs

There are no labs specific to diagnose immobility. However, the following may be helpful in the initial workup to understand causes for immobility.

- BMP
- CBC
- Coagulation panel

Diagnostic Testing

- Imaging to rule out underlying etiology: CT scans, MRI, and x-ray
- Musculoskeletal assessment (e.g., the timed up and go test)
- Neurologic assessment: cognitive functioning, gait assessment, and motor strength

Treatment

- Identification and correction of underlying cause of functional disability as possible
- Participation in PT and OT sessions: scheduled activity sessions to encourage mobility; repetition of skills practiced with PT, which may include sitting at the side of the bed, standing, pivoting to a chair, and ambulating; activity as often as safely possible, being mindful of potential removal of drains, lines, or tubes; and can be completed in a bed or chair (e.g., arm raises, calf pumps, and leg raises)
- Administration of corresponding treatments and medications to assist in correcting underlying cause of functional disability
- Identification and treatment of any complications of prolonged immobility if present: Clot prevention, pneumonia, and pressure ulcer prevention

Nursing Interventions

- Administer anticoagulation medications as ordered.
- Coordinate mobilization or ambulation attempts with additional support staff as needed (e.g., respiratory therapy and PT).
- Communicate directions and plan for mobilization effectively; secure all devices, drains, lines, and tubes prior to mobilization or ambulation and place the call bell within reach if mobilizing patient out of bed to the chair.
- Encourage the patient to perform daily care as much as independently possible (e.g., brushing teeth, washing face, and brushing hair).
- Monitor VS changes during activity. ▶

[🌐]   NURSING PEARL

While immobility may be due to critical illness, sometimes it may be due to a lack of personal patient motivation. To help encourage and motivate the patient, develop a therapeutic relationship and seek to understand motivations. Motivating factors could be family (kids, grandkids, spouse), pets, work, or hobbies. Encourage the patient and establish achievable goals both in and out of the hospital.

Nursing Interventions (*continued*)

■ Prevent pressure ulcers: Change pads, dressings, diapers, or sheets if wet or soiled; keep skin clean and dry; offload pressure on bony prominences by turning patient with pillows and elevating heels; reposition frequently to alleviate pressure on bony prominences and redistribute weight; monitor for new areas of skin breakdown; pad bony prominences and skin that comes into contact with lines, drains, or tubes to prevent skin breakdown; perform skin assessment each shift and document changes as noted; turn every 2 hr as ordered; elevate heels to prevent skin breakdown; and encourage appropriate nutrition to decrease risk of pressure ulcers.

■ Provide emotional and therapeutic support for patients engaging in physical activity during or shortly following critical illness: Create and encourage attainable goals; celebrate accomplishments and improvements; and encourage and motivate patient, if possible, to perform physical activity and regain mobility to achieve postdischarge goal.

Patient Education

■ Identify personal motivating factors; create future goals to help motivate the patient to remain as active as possible; and perform physical activity with others at a gym, with family members, or with support groups.

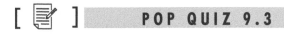

POP QUIZ 9.3

Promoting physical activity and preventing immobility are essential to prevent which three major pulmonary, integumentary, and circulatory complications?

■ If the patient is completely immobile or requires total care, the family might consider obtaining a home lift to assist with mobility and turning or consult home healthcare assistance.

■ Offload pressure on bony prominences at home by elevating extremities, turning, and repositioning.

■ Perform as much activity as physically able to prevent additional loss of mobility: Start slow and increase pace as able and indicated by provider, and set appropriate and attainable goals.

RESOURCES

Agency for Healthcare Research and Quality. (2021). *Tool 3H: Morse fall scale for identifying fall risk factors*. https://www.ahrq.gov/patient-safety/settings/hospital/fall-prevention/toolkit/morse-fall-scale.html

Alaparthi, G. K., Gatty, A., Samuel, S. R., & Amaravadi, S. K. (2020, November 26). Effectiveness, safety, and barriers to early mobilization in the intensive care unit. *Critical Care Research and Practice*. https://www.ncbi.nlm.nih.gov/pmc/articles/PMC7714600

Deglin, J. H., Vallerand, A. H., & Sanoski, C. A. (2011). *Davis's drug guide for nurses*. F.A. Davis.

Epocrates. (n.d). *Cyanocobalamin (vitamin B12) adult dosing* [Drug information]. Epocrates Web. https://online.epocrates.com/drugs/1877/cyanocobalamin-vitamin-B12?MultiBrandAlert=true

Huether, S. E., & McCance, K. L. (2012). *Understanding pathophysiology*. Elsevier/Mosby.

InformedHealth.org. (2018, November 15). *Pressure ulcers: Overview*. Institute for Quality and Efficiency in Health Care. https://www.ncbi.nlm.nih.gov/books/NBK326428

Lewis, S. M. (2011). *Medical-surgical nursing: Assessment and management of clinical problems*. Mosby.

Lupescu, O., Nagea, M., Patru, C., Vasilache, C., & Popescu, G. I. (2015, June). Treatment options for distal femoral fractures. *Maedica, 10*(2), 117–122. https://www.ncbi.nlm.nih.gov/pmc/articles/PMC5327816

National Institute on Aging. (n.d.). *Prevent falls and fractures*. U.S. Department of Health and Human Services. https://www.nia.nih.gov/health/prevent-falls-and-fractures

Parida, S., & Mishra, S. K. (2013, November). Urinary tract infections in the critical care unit: A brief review. *Indian Journal of Critical Care Medicine, 17*(6), 370–374. https://www.ncbi.nlm.nih.gov/pmc/articles/PMC3902573/

Prescribers' Digital Reference. (n.d.-a). *Ergocalciferol* [Drug information]. PDR Search. https://www.pdr.net/drug-summary/Ergocalciferol-ergocalciferol-24306#10

Prescribers' Digital Reference. (n.d.-b). *Sinemet* [Drug information]. PDR Search. https://www.pdr.net/drug-summary/Sinemet-carbidopa-levodopa-388#11

Wu, X., Li, Z., Cao, J., Jiao, J., Wang, Y., Liu, G., Liu, Y., Li, F., Song, B., Jin, J., Liu, Y., Wen, X., Cheng, S., & Wan, X. (2018). The association between major complications of immobility during hospitalization and quality of life among bedridden patients: A 3 month prospective multi-center study. *PLoS One, 13*(10), Article e0205729. https://www.ncbi.nlm.nih.gov/pmc/articles/PMC6185860/#:~:text=Immobility%20is%20independently%20associated%20with,(UTI)%20%5B4%5D

ACUTE AND CHRONIC PAIN

Overview

- Acute and/or chronic pain exacerbations are common causes for hospital admissions. *Acute pain* is sudden, often resulting from acute injury, trauma, or disease process. *Chronic pain*, in contrast, persists for 6 or more months.

- In the hospital setting, pain can be caused by devices such as drains, endotracheal tubes, Foley catheters, or invasive monitoring lines; immobility; invasive procedures; suctioning; surgical incisions; trauma; and wound care.

- It is important to identify the cause of pain to appropriately treat the pain. The pain or discomfort can often be relieved by nonpharmacologic intervention and assessing for and treating complications from the previously noted causes.

[🧠] COMPLICATIONS

If pain is not treated, delayed wound healing, hyperglycemia, atelectasis, delirium, depression, and posttraumatic stress disorder (PTSD) may occur.

[🤲] NURSING PEARL

Physiologic reactions to pain such as tachycardia should be monitored, as this can exacerbate or worsen the clinical condition.

Signs and Symptoms

- Agitation
- Anxiety
- Crying
- Dependence/substance abuse (chronic pain)
- Depression (chronic pain)
- Facial grimacing
- Feelings of discomfort that can be described as burning, dull, pressure, ripping, sharp, stabbing, tearing, and tingling
- Hypertension (HTN)
- Muscle tension
- Tachycardia
- Vocalization of distress: Yelling or screaming

Diagnosis

Labs

There are no labs specific to the diagnosis of acute and chronic pain. However, the following may be indicated based on the patient's clinical status:

- Arterial blood gas (ABG)
- Complete blood count (CBC)
- Comprehensive metabolic panel (CMP)

Diagnostic Testing

Further workup may be indicated if pain is suspected in a specific area on the body:

- CT scan
- MRI
- Ultrasound
- X-ray

Treatment

- Analgesics (Table A.2)
- Identification and treatment of the cause of the pain
- Methods to prevent pain from occurring, such as avoidance of triggers (if known), frequent assessment, and timely medication administration
- Nerve blocks, if appropriate
- Nonpharmacologic intervention, including elevation of affected extremity, hot/cold compress, and rest
- Possible need for sedation if analgesics alone cannot treat pain; may require transfer to a higher level of care

Nursing Interventions

- Assess pain as the sixth vital sign (VS). Use the appropriate pain scale for the patient (e.g., 0–10, Faces, and pain assessment in advanced dementia scale).
- Collaborate with interdisciplinary team for a pain management plan.
- Ensure analgesic reversal medications are easily available in the event of accidental oversedation.
- Ensure pain assessment accuracy by utilizing the appropriate pain scale for the patient.
- Provide nonpharmacologic methods to reduce pain, such as repositioning, cold or heat, range of motion, relaxation techniques, and providing a calm environment.

Patient Education

- Avoid self-medicating with illicit drugs, unprescribed medications, or alcohol.
- Consult with a pain clinic for outpatient follow-up and maintenance of medication regimens.
- Ensure family or caregiver is involved in pain management plan.
- Ensure realistic pain score goals.
- Ensure understanding of pain management plan at discharge.
- Follow up with outpatient appointments as scheduled.
- If applicable, seek extra support through or continue to attend Alcoholics Anonymous (AA) and/or Narcotics Anonymous (NA) meetings.
- If pain is worsening or the prescribed regimen is no longer working, contact the provider, pain management service, or clinic for further workup.
- Take prescribed medications as ordered. ▶

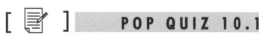

POP QUIZ 10.1

A patient returns from surgery, where they had a laparoscopic hysterectomy. They received pain medication in the post-anesthesia care unit (PACU) and were returned to the progressive care unit (PCU). On first assessment, the patient's abdomen is soft to palpitation and lap sites are clean, dry, and intact. The patient, however, reports pain of 6/10 in the lower abdomen that she describes as stabbing or cramping. The patient is only verbally responsive to touch and can keep her eyes open only for a few seconds. VS are as follows: Heart rate (HR) 91, blood pressure (BP) 105/74, respiratory rate (RR) 8, SPO$_2$ 92% on 4 LNC, and temperature 97.8°F (36.6°C). Given the patient's clinical presentation and pain rating, what should the nurse's next action be?

Patient Education (*continued*)

- Utilize nonpharmacologic interventions to manage pain.
- Utilize pain prevention methods.
- Utilize the minimum dosage of analgesics necessary to relieve pain.
- Wean pain medications as indicated per physician order.

END-OF-LIFE CARE

Overview

- Goals of care at the transition of end-of-life range from curing disease to improving comfort and quality of life.
- Care at the end-of-life requires collaboration between healthcare providers, patients, and families to provide care that focuses on comfort and minimal pain or suffering.

Signs and Symptoms

- Alterations in breathing: apnea, Cheyne–Stokes breathing, "death rattle"
- Cognitive changes
- Delirium
- Fatigue
- Lethargy
- Increased oral secretions
- Immobility
- Loss of interest in food or drink

Treatment

- Palliative care/hospice (see Palliative Care section for additional information).
- Medications to relieve pain and suffering: Antiemetics (Table 7.1), anxiolytics (Table 11.1), and opioid analgesics (Table A.2)
- Psychosocial and spiritual support

Nursing Interventions

- Administer medications as ordered for pain relief and symptom management.
- Assess for respiratory distress.
- Collaborate with patient, family, and all members of interdisciplinary care.
- Consider consult to spiritual care, palliative care, and/or hospice.
- Encourage nutrition as possible.
- Establish relationship and rapport with patient and family.
- Identify any cultural considerations the patient and family may have.
- Mobilize patient per patient request.
- Monitor family and patient behavior for signs of physical or emotional distress.
- Monitor lung sounds.
- Monitor sleep patterns.
- Provide oxygen if necessary (as determined by plan of care).
- Provide nonpharmacologic interventions to promote a calm and comfortable environment.

Patient Education

- Family: Learn what to expect in the final stages of death, and understand interventions to alleviate and reduce pain or suffering.
- Learn the importance of legal documents such as advanced directives and power of attorney and share them with the family.

HEALTHCARE-ACQUIRED INFECTIONS

Overview

- *Healthcare-acquired infections* are infections that were not present on admission but are acquired through the course of a hospital stay.
- Common health-acquired infections are catheter-associated urinary tract infections (CAUTIs), central line-associated bloodstream infections (CLABSIs), and surgical site infection

COMPLICATIONS

Healthcare-acquired infections can complicate a patient's condition, lead to prolonged hospitalization, and cause bacteremia, sepsis, septic shock, and death. Infection protocols should be enforced in all areas of the hospital to prevent these complications.

(SSIs) (see Surgical Wound section). *CAUTIs* are urinary tract infections (UTIs) that result from a bladder catheter. *CLABSIs* are bloodstream infections that result from any type of central line insertion. Both CLABSIs and CAUTIs are preventable infections that can lead to severe complications in the acutely ill patient population.
- Healthcare staff should maintain a high standard for infection control and be vigilant in assessing for these infections to protect their patients.

Signs and Symptoms

- CAUTI: abdominal, flank, or suprapubic pain; altered mental status (AMS) or delirium; burning with urination; fever or chills; foul-smelling urine; positive urinary culture; pus or drainage around insertion site; and urine color or consistency changes (cloudy, dark, etc.)
- CLABSI: AMS or delirium, central line insertion site, and fever or chills
- SSI: Fever or chills, or the surgical incision site may feature pain, poor wound healing, pus or foul-smelling drainage, redness or warm to the touch, and swollen.

Diagnosis

Labs

- Basic metabolic panel (BMP)
- CBC: White blood cell (WBC) count likely elevated with an infectious process
- Cultures: Blood culture likely positive in patients with CLABSI, and urine culture likely positive in patients with CAUTI
- Lactate: Likely elevated in septic patients

Diagnostic Testing

- CT scan
- Ultrasound
- X-ray

Treatment

- Antibiotics (Table A.1)
- Fluid resuscitation
- Removal of infected line or tube; possible replacement of central line in new location as indicated per institutional protocol and patient clinical status
- Possible for SSI: drains, exploration and debridement, negative pressure wound therapy; see Wounds: Surgical Wounds section

Nursing Interventions

- Administer medications as ordered.
- Assess airway, breathing, and circulation.
- Assess lines, drains, tubes, and wounds for signs of infection.
- Assess VS for symptoms of infection: Fever, hypotension, and tachycardia.
- CAUTI prevention: Assess urinary output for color, consistency, and odor as frequently as recommended per institutional protocol; perform peri-care and Foley care every shift with institutionally recommended hygiene solutions; remove or exchange Foley as recommended per institutional protocol.
- CLABSI prevention: Assess central line site every shift, assess each port for patency each shift, change central line dressing per institutional protocol or if dirty/soiled, change intravenous (IV) tubing for all medications per institutional protocol, make sure dressing remains occlusive, and scrub the central line hubs for at least 15 seconds before use.
- SSI prevention: Assess the surgical site each shift; keep the surgical site clean and change dressing, as ordered; see the Surgical Wounds section for more information.
- Initiate appropriate isolation precautions.
- Provide medication management.
- Remove lines when no longer necessary.
- Perform frequent hand hygiene and don gloves. If a patient is on contact precautions, wear gown before entering room.

Patient Education

- If going home with a chronic indwelling urinary catheter, make sure to clean around the catheter at least daily and when soiled.
- Notify the nurse or healthcare team for any changes at the catheter, central line, or surgical site.
- Practice good infection prevention practices and frequent hand hygiene.

[⚡] **ALERT!**

Closely monitor wound drainage on either the dressing or surgically placed drain for changes in output, color, volume, or consistency. This may indicate postsurgical infection and require prompt assessment and intervention.

[📝] **POP QUIZ 10.2**

A 55-year-old female is admitted to the PCU with a suspected CAUTI. The provider ordered broad-spectrum antibiotics to be given now and every 8 hr for the next week. The nurse removes the antibiotics from the medication dispensing system but, before administering, notices that blood cultures were never collected in the emergency department. What should the nurse's next action be?

[🧠] **COMPLICATIONS**

Complications of influenza include secondary bacterial pneumonia, acute respiratory distress syndrome (ARDS), myositis, myocarditis, respiratory and multiorgan failure, and death. Prevention, early identification, and treatment are key to preventing these dangerous complications.

INFLUENZA

Overview

- *Influenza* (commonly called the flu) is a contagious viral disease that affects the upper and lower respiratory tract.
- While influenza can affect people of all ages, it is especially dangerous for young children, pregnant women, or patients who are older adults or immunocompromised.

Signs and Symptoms

- Congestion
- Cough
- Cyanosis
- Dyspnea
- Fever
- Fatigue
- Headache
- Hypotension
- Myalgia
- Respiratory distress
- Rhinorrhea
- Sore throat
- Tachycardia
- Weakness

Diagnosis

Labs

- ABG
- CBC
- Influenza swab for antigen or polymerase chain reaction (PCR) testing
- Respiratory viral panel
- Sputum cultures

Diagnostic Testing

- Chest x-ray

Treatment

- Antiviral therapy (e.g., oseltamivir; Table 10.1)
- Symptom management: acetaminophen for fever, and cough suppressants
- Support oxygenation: oxygen therapy as needed; respiratory therapy consult as needed; acid–base balance and CO_2 monitoring to avoid complications; and regular chest x-rays to monitor for worsening infection, new infection, or lung damage

Nursing Interventions

- Administer fluids to prevent dehydration.
- Assess airway, breathing, and circulation.
- Assess respiratory status and VS: Administer oxygen if needed, and administer antipyretics as needed.
- Initiate droplet precautions. ▶

TABLE 10.1 Multisystem Medications

INDICATIONS	MECHANISM OF ACTION	CONTRAINDICATIONS, PRECAUTIONS, AND ADVERSE EFFECTS
Antidote, other (activated charcoal)		
• Emergency use following toxic ingestion/poisoning	• Absorb ingested toxin, preventing it from being systemically absorbed in the stomach	• Use cautiously in intestinal bleeding, blockage or perforation, decreased level of consciousness, dehydration, slow digestion, and recent surgery. • Adverse effects include diarrhea, black stools, or vomiting.
Benzodiazepine antagonist, systemic antidotes (flumazenil)		
• Antidote for benzodiazepines • Overdose or toxicity	• Bind to GABA receptors to reverse the effects of benzodiazepine on the body	• Medication is contraindicated in patients who have received benzodiazepines to correct life-threatening conditions such as status epilepticus or increased ICP, or cyclic antidepressant overdose. • Monitor patient's level of consciousness, as re-sedation may occur following administration due to short half-life of drug. • Adverse effects include anxiety, vomiting, nausea, shivering, tremors, insomnia, headache, and agitation.
Mucolytics, systemic antidotes (N-acetylcysteine)		
• Antidote for acetaminophen	• Bind to oxygen free radicals to excrete them out of the body without causing cellular and organ damage	• Use cautiously in patients with history of asthma or bronchospasm. • Use cautiously in patients with esophageal ulcers, as it may induce vomiting and potentiates risk for GI bleed. • Adverse effects include flushing, rash, itching, nausea, and vomiting.
Neuraminidase inhibitor antivirals (oseltamivir)		
• Management of influenza A	• Competitively inhibit enzyme from influenza virus	• Medication is contraindicated in bacterial infections and immunosuppression. • Use cautiously in cardiac and pulmonary diseases, hepatic disease, renal failure, and psychosis. • Adverse effects include seizures, angioedema, hallucinations and confusion, headache, rash, emotional lability, anxiety, and agitation.
Opiate antagonist (naloxone)		
• Antidote for opioid toxicity or overdose	• Antagonizes pain receptors in the body to inhibit the effects of opioids on the body	• Monitor patient frequently, as respiratory depression may occur after initial improvement of symptoms. • Use cautiously in patients with cardiovascular conditions, as it may cause hypotension or ventricular dysrhythmias. • Adverse reactions include tremor, agitation, pain, headache, and vomiting.
Topical sulfonamides (silver sulfadiazine)		
• Gram positive and negative bacterial infection (topical)	• Disrupt bacteria and break down cell membrane to fight infection	• Do not give to patients with sulfa hypersensitivity. • Use cautiously in patients with hepatic and renal impairment or hematologic disease.

GABA, gamma-aminobutyric acid; GI, gastrointestinal; ICP, intracranial pressure.

Nursing Interventions (*continued*)

- Encourage pulmonary hygiene (turn cough and deep breath).
- Encourage use of incentive spirometry.
- If status continues to worsen despite escalation of oxygenation therapy, notify the provider and prepare for transport to a higher level of care. Patient may require pressors, ventilation, and/or extracorporeal membrane oxygenation (ECMO) support depending on clinical status.
- Update patient on current status, such as improving labs or VS.

Patient Education

- Get seasonal influenza vaccine in future influenza seasons.
- Infection control: Stay home until fever free for at least 24 hr (without the use of antipyretics) before returning to normal activities.
- Take over-the-counter (OTC) medications to manage symptoms.

MULTIDRUG-RESISTANT ORGANISMS

Overview

- Multidrug resistance develops when bacteria evolve and become resistant to certain antibiotics.
- Multidrug resistant organisms (MDROs) render many pharmacologic treatments ineffective, as these antibiotics can no longer be used to control or kill the bacteria.

COMPLICATIONS

Organisms resistant to pharmacologic treatment can result in deterioration of condition, sepsis, and death, especially in acutely ill or immunocompromised patients.

Signs and Symptoms

- Bacterial infections and organisms that are unresponsive to standard antibiotic therapy
- Deteriorating condition despite treatment: acid–base imbalances, altered mental status, cyanosis/hypoxia, fever or hypothermia, hypotension, irritability, lethargy, normal or decreased BP, oliguria, pallor, shortness of breath, skin warmth, tachycardia, and tachypnea

Diagnosis

Labs

- Positive cultures from any of the following, based on suspected location or type of infection: blood, fecal, sputum, and urine
- Sensitivity studies to determine medications to which MDROs are susceptible

NURSING PEARL

When treating an MDRO, collaboration between nursing, pharmacy, and medicine is necessary to implement an effective course of treatment.

Treatment

- Collaboration with pharmacy to devise appropriate pharmacologic combination therapy based on cultures
- Appropriate antimicrobial therapy based on susceptibilities from culture results

ALERT!

Patients with MDRO infections should be placed on the appropriate contact, respiratory, or airborne precautions to prevent further spread to other patients on the unit.

Nursing Interventions

- Administer medications as ordered.
- Assess airway, breathing, and circulation.
- Draw and monitor labs as ordered.
- Don institutionally required personal protective equipment (PPE) to enter the contact precaution room. This may include a disposable gown and gloves to reduce transmission to other patients and reduce contact with bodily fluids.
- Perform a complete head-to-toe assessment.
- Perform hand hygiene before entering and after leaving the room.

Patient Education

- Finish all the antimicrobial therapy prescribed as indicated, even if feeling better.
- Notify future providers of history of MDRO infection.
- Once discharged from the hospital, frequently wash hands, towels, bed sheets, kitchen, and bathroom countertops to prevent transmission to others.
- Stay up-to-date on infection status.
- Understand contact precautions if infected with MDRO.
- Understand and stay up-to-date on plan of care.

PALLIATIVE CARE

Overview

- Palliative care prioritizes quality of life by anticipating, treating, and preventing suffering for patients with terminal or serious illness.
- In addition to the physical and psychosocial aspects of care, palliative care also focuses on the emotional and spiritual needs of the patient.

Signs and Symptoms

Patients progressing toward palliative care may exhibit any of the following symptoms:

- Bowel habit changes
- Cognitive changes
- Delirium
- Difficulty sleeping/changes to sleep–wake cycles
- Fatigue
- Lethargy
- Increased oral secretions
- Immobility
- Loss of interest in food or drink

Treatment

- Consult to palliative care/hospice services
- Medications to relieve pain and suffering: antiemetics (Table 7.1), anxiolytics (Table 11.1), and opioid analgesics (Table A.2)
- Psychosocial and spiritual support
- Transfer to home or an outpatient hospice facility if applicable

Nursing Interventions

- Assess for acute changes in breathing and respiration.
- Assist frequently with peri-care and anticipate an increasing loss of bowel/bladder control.
- Collaborate with patient, family, and all members of the interdisciplinary team.
- Consider consult to spiritual care, social work, home care, and/or hospice.
- Provide small, frequent meals with foods the patient enjoys, as tolerated.
- Provide nonpharmacologic interventions to promote a calm and comfortable environment.
- Provide oxygen and IV hydration, if necessary, as determined by plan of care.

Patient Education

- Consult social work to provide information on how to set up legal documents such as an advance directive and power of attorney.
- Learn what to expect in the stages of death and ensure family understands.
- Understand and ensure family understands what to expect moving into palliative care. Palliative care, unlike hospice care, has no deadline/timeline. Quality of life is emphasized over duration of life.

RHABDOMYOLYSIS

Overview

- *Rhabdomyolysis* is the rapid breakdown of muscle and release of intracellular muscle constituents into the bloodstream.
- Rhabdomyolysis has many causes including trauma, drugs, infection, excessive muscular contraction, diabetic ketoacidosis (DKA), heatstroke, and severe electrolyte disorders.

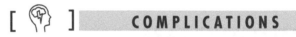

COMPLICATIONS

Rhabdomyolysis can result in acute kidney injury (AKI), chronic renal failure, electrolyte abnormalities (potassium, phosphate, calcium), and disseminated intravascular coagulation (DIC). It is essential to identify and treat rhabdomyolysis before the kidneys become compromised.

Signs and Symptoms

- Abdominal pain
- Dark-colored urine (cola/coffee colored)
- Fever
- Malaise
- Muscle pain
- Nausea and vomiting
- Tachycardia
- Weakness

Diagnosis

Labs

- BMP: elevated blood urea nitrogen (BUN) and creatinine; hyperkalemia; hyperphosphatemia; hypocalcemia; metabolic acidosis common, and increased anion gap possible; severe hyperuricemia.
- CBC: May indicate elevated WBC with infection and crush injuries.
- Elevated serum creatine kinase (CK) levels: At presentation, they are usually at least five times the upper limit of normal, but range from approximately 1,500 to over 100,000 international units/L; begins to rise within 2 to 12 hr following onset of muscle injury and reaches maximum within 24 to 72 hr. ▶

Labs (continued)

- Erythrocyte sedimentation rate (ESR) and C-reactive protein (CRP): Likely elevated with infection and crush injuries.
- Toxicology screen: May be positive.
- Urinalysis: Possible evidence of myoglobinuria from urine sample.

Diagnostic Testing

There are no diagnostic tests specific to diagnose rhabdomyolysis. However, the following may be helpful in the overall workup:

- CT scan
- Electromyography (EMG)
- MRI
- Muscle biopsy

Treatment

- Major therapy: Early and aggressive fluid resuscitation (Table A.3), no formal treatment guideline or protocol available, follow institutional guidelines.
- Dialysis: Management of hyperkalemia, correction of acidosis, or for the treatment of volume overload.
- Possible fasciotomy if complicated by compartment syndrome; pressure relief in compartment to increase muscle perfusion and prevent muscle breakdown and death.
- Treatment of metabolic abnormalities possibly required, including hypocalcemia (treated with calcium gluconate), hyperkalemia (treated with regular insulin, dextrose, nebulized beta 2 agonists, furosemide, sodium polystyrene, and so forth), and hyperuricemia (treated with allopurinol). In patients with DIC, fresh frozen plasma (FFP) may be used.

[⚡]   **ALERT!**

Hyperkalemia can develop in patients with rhabdomyolysis as a result from decreased renal clearance from AKI and additionally from potassium release from damaged muscle. Standard hyperkalemia treatments can help manage this complication.

Nursing Interventions

- Administer IV fluids as ordered. Ensure peripheral IV access site is patent or deliver high volume fluid resuscitation through central line if available.
- Assess and draw CK and BMPs as ordered to treat renal function, electrolyte changes, and assess whether patient is responding to fluid resuscitation.
- Maintain plasma pH <7.5.
- Monitor hourly urine output and labs for the following: urine output goal of 200 mL/hr, and urine pH >6.5.
- Monitor VS for EKG changes related to electrolyte abnormalities.
- Perform neurovascular checks if there is a concern for compartment syndrome.
- Treat electrolyte abnormalities as ordered.

Patient Education

- Stay up to date on current status, changes to condition, and/or plan of care (e.g., initiation of dialysis).
- Notify the nurse of status changes: Dizziness, new or worsening tremor, palpitations, worsening weakness, and worsening pain.
- Pursue drug and alcohol cessation as appropriate based on presenting condition.

[📝]   **POP QUIZ 10.3**

A patient with rhabdomyolysis is admitted to the PCU. They have received medical treatment for the resulting hyperkalemia; however, the most recent potassium on the BMP was 6.2. Urine output was 15 mL/hr over the last 2 hr. What should the next intervention be?

SEPSIS

Overview

- *Sepsis* refers to systemic inflammatory response syndrome with an accompanying infectious source.
- Sepsis has a high morbidity and mortality rate; early identification and treatment are essential to prevent complications.

Signs and Symptoms

- Changes in mentation: AMS, confusion, and delirium
- Cyanosis
- Dyspnea
- Pain
- Skin changes: cold and clammy, and warm and flushed
- VS changes: fever or hypothermia (>100.4°F (38°C) or <96.8°F (36°C), hypotension, tachycardia, and tachypnea

Diagnosis

Labs

- ABG: May indicate acidosis, hypoxemia, or hypercarbia.
- Blood cultures: Likely positive.
- Blood glucose
- CBC: Elevated WBC.
- CMP
- Coagulation panel
- CRP: Likely elevated.
- Lactate level: Likely >2 mmol/L if septic shock.
- Mixed venous $ScvO_2$
- Troponins
- Urinalysis
- Urine cultures

Diagnostic Testing

- Chest x-ray
- CT scan
- Ultrasound

Treatment

- Antibiotics (Table A.1)
- Corticosteroids (Table A.4)
- Fever control
- Identification and treatment of cause of infection
- If possible, removal of infectious source

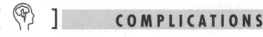

COMPLICATIONS

Complications of sepsis include septic shock, multiorgan failure, and death.

NURSING PEARL

Use the following criteria for grading sepsis and septic shock:

- *Systemic inflammatory response syndrome* is a systemic response to infection with at least two of the following symptoms:
  - Temperature outside of range 96.8°F–100.4°F (36°C–38°C)
  - HR >90
  - RR >20
  - $PaCO_2$ >32 mmHg
  - WBC outside of range 4,000 to 12,000
- *Sepsis* is an identified infection in combination with at least two criteria for systemic inflammatory response syndrome.
- *Severe sepsis* is sepsis with evidence of end organ dysfunction.
- *Septic shock* is severe sepsis with both of the following:
  - Persisting hypotension with vasopressor use to maintain mean arterial pressure (MAP) ≥65 mmHg
  - Lactate >2 mmol/L despite fluid resuscitation

NURSING PEARL

Positive blood cultures are helpful for individualized treatment; however, they are not a prerequisite for diagnosis. Up to 33% of sepsis patients have negative blood cultures due to intermittent bacteremia.

Treatment (*continued*)

- IV fluid resuscitation (Table A.3)
- Organ support: dialysis, ventilation
- Vasopressors—patient may require higher level of care (Table 2.3)

Nursing Interventions

- Administer medications as prescribed.
- Assess mental status.
- Collect and monitor serial labs and blood cultures.
- Follow infection prevention procedures: Assess bladder catheters for signs of infection; assess central line and IV insertion areas for signs of infection; change IV tubing and IV/central line dressings per institutional protocol; don gloves; perform frequent peri-care, at least once a shift; scrub IV hubs with alcohol for 15 seconds before use; and wash hands.
- Increase nutrition as possible.
- Monitor urine output.
- Monitor VS hourly.
- Perform head-to-toe assessment frequently to assess for changes.
- Provide nutritional support.
- Transfer to higher level of care if condition continues to deteriorate.
- Utilize cooling devices as allowed per institution/unit to control fever.

Patient Education

- Ensure blood glucose control if diabetic.
- Ensure early mobilization; ambulate as often as possible.
- Ensure pulmonary hygiene using incentive spirometry.
- Follow infection precaution practices while at home: Avoid others who are sick; avoid touching eyes, face, and mouth; if diabetic, be especially cautious of infection development, and assess feet daily; if performing other wound care, dress wound as ordered and monitor for signs or symptoms of infection; wash cuts or abrasions with antimicrobial soap and dress with clean dressing; and wash hands frequently.
- Maintain infection prevention strategies.
- Take medications, especially antibiotics, as prescribed.

SHOCK STATES

Overview

- *Shock* occurs when the body is unable to function properly as a result of inadequate oxygenation. This can be due to either decreased perfusion in the body or the cells being unable to utilize the oxygen delivered.
- Shock can be broken down into three stages. *Compensatory stage:* The sympathetic nervous system produces adrenalin to compensate for the body's loss of oxygen, resulting in tachycardia, peripheral vasoconstriction, and normalized BP. *Progressive stage:* The compensatory mechanisms are no longer sufficient enough to maintain hemodynamic stability and early organ dysfunction is starting. *Refractory stage:* The final stage of shock, leading to end or multiorgan damage and patient no longer responding to intervention. ▶

[🧠]   **COMPLICATIONS**

Shock states can progress rapidly and result in multiorgan failure and death. Early identification and treatment are needed to prevent further decompensation.

Overview (*continued*)

■ There are several different types of shock. The examination focuses on distributive and hypovolemic shock. *Distributive shock* occurs from profound peripheral vasodilation. Septic, anaphylactic, and neurogenic shock are classified as distributive shock. *Hypovolemic shock* occurs when there is decreased intravascular volume and perfusion to the body. It can be classified as either hemorrhagic or nonhemorrhagic.

Signs and Symptoms

■ Anaphylactic shock: hypotension, hypotonial, incontinence, syncope, and respiratory symptoms
■ Hypovolemic shock: agitation, confusion, dry mucous membranes, hypotension, lethargy, muscle cramps, orthostatic hypotension, tachycardia, and thirst

Diagnosis

Labs

Possible workup for a patient presenting with shock:

■ ABG
■ BMP
■ Blood cultures
■ Cardiac biomarkers
■ CBC
■ CMP
■ Coagulation panel
■ Lactate level
■ Plasma histamine
■ Serum or plasma total tryptase
■ Type and screen
■ Urinalysis

Diagnostic Testing

Imaging as indicated per patient status:

■ Chest x-ray
■ CT scan
■ Transthoracic echocardiogram
■ Ultrasound

Treatment

■ Anaphylactic shock: airway management; antihistamines (Table 5.4); bronchodilators (Table 3.1); causative agent removal, if known; corticosteroids (Table A.4); epinephrine (Table 2.3); IV fluids (Table A.3); and vasopressors (Table 2.3)
■ Hypovolemic shock: administration of blood products if severe blood loss and hemoglobin <7 g/dL; IV fluids if volume down and underresuscitated; stop/control bleeding; and surgery consult if hypovolemia due to rapid blood loss or suspected trauma

Nursing Interventions

■ Administer antibiotics, fluids, blood products, and other medications as needed.
■ Collect and monitor serial labs and blood cultures.
■ Educate patient on plan of care and possible OR procedures as needed. ▶

Nursing Interventions (*continued*)

- Monitor airway and breathing; administer oxygen as needed. Communicate as needed with respiratory therapy for additional respiratory support.
- Monitor intake and output (I/O) hourly and labs as ordered.
- Monitor VS hourly.
- Perform head-to-toe assessment frequently to assess for changes.
- Transfer to higher level of care if condition continues to deteriorate.

Patient Education

- Ensure infection prevention.
- Ensure pulmonary hygiene
- Identify and have rescue medications on hand for anaphylactic triggers.
- Once discharged after an anaphylactic reaction, carry an epinephrine auto-injector as needed. Consider wearing a medical alert bracelet or necklace. Drink adequate fluids, follow up with allergist for thorough allergy testing, and notify all other healthcare providers of history of anaphylaxis. Once possible allergy is identified, avoid as best as possible.
- Take medications, especially antibiotics, as prescribed.

TOXICITY

Overview

- Medication toxicity from both prescribed and non-prescribed medications is a common reason for admission to the PCU.
- The ingestion of toxins may be intentional or accidental.
- It is important to identify the ingested toxin and administer the antidote as soon as possible (Table 10.2).
- Toxins that can cause complications when ingested include illicit drugs, prescription medications, alcohol, chemicals, or illegally obtained analgesics or benzodiazepines.

[🧠]   **COMPLICATIONS**

Complications of toxicity or overdose include electrolyte abnormalities, cardiac dysrhythmia, AMS, seizures, respiratory depression, renal or hepatic failure, cardiac or respiratory arrest, and death.

Signs and Symptoms

- AMS
- Bradycardia
- Bradypnea
- Confusion ▶

TABLE 10.2 Toxins and Antidotes	
TOXIN	**ANTIDOTE**
Acetaminophen	*N*-Acetylcysteine
Benzodiazepine	Flumazenil
Opioid	Naloxone

Signs and Symptoms (*continued*)

- Hallucinations
- Hypotension
- Lethargy
- Respiratory depression
- Seizure
- Sweating
- Vomiting

Diagnosis

Labs

- Acetaminophen overdose: increased acetaminophen level >200 mcg/mL 4 hr or more after ingestion
- CMP may indicate electrolyte abnormalities, elevated aspartate aminotransferase/alanine aminotransferase (AST/ALT), and elevated creatinine and BUN
- Ethanol (ETOH) level
- Salicylate level: elevated with aspirin overdose ≥50 mg/dL
- Urine drug screen

Diagnostic Testing

There are no diagnostic tests specific to diagnose toxicity. However, the following may confirm complications:

- Chest x-ray to identify aspiration
- ECG to identify potential arrythmias
- Head CT to identify head trauma

Treatment

- Antidote if applicable (Table 10.2)
- Activated charcoal if within 4 hr of a known or suspected acetaminophen ingestion
- Hemodialysis
- IV fluid resuscitation (Table A.3)
- Respiratory support with continuous positive airway pressure (CPAP), bilevel positive airway pressure (BiPAP), or intubation (requiring transfer to higher level of care)

Nursing Interventions

- Assess psychologic status: Ask the patient about any suicidal ideations; initiate suicide or psychologic precautions if intentional, per institutional protocol; and maintain a sitter with 1:1 observation if indicated.
- Consult social worker for support resources at discharge.
- If naloxone given, prepare to address pain, discomfort, or aggressive behaviors.
- Insert nasogastric/orogastric (NG/OG) tube for gastric lavage.
- Maintain patent airway.
- Monitor for arrythmias.
- Monitor I/O.
- Monitor VS. Depending on agent ingested, VS may show tachypnea or bradypnea, hypotension or HTN, or tachycardia or bradycardia.
- Notify poison control.
- Provide supplemental oxygen, if indicated.

Patient Education

- Do not abruptly stop taking benzodiazepine or opioid medications, as it may cause withdrawal.
- Ensure effective pain management strategies.
- Follow appropriate guidelines for OTC medications: Acetaminophen can be taken every 4 to 6 hr, up to four times in a 24-hr period. Do not exceed more than 4,000 mg of acetaminophen in a 24-hr period. Aspirin should be taken at the recommended dose and time. For example, 81 mg of aspirin should be taken once daily. If taken for pain, one to two tablets of 325 mg can be taken every 4 to 6 hr with a daily limit of no more than 12 tablets in 24 hr. Extra strength aspirin (500 mg) can be taken every 4 to 6 hr with a daily limit of eight tablets in 24 hr.

WOUNDS

- Wounds in the PCU frequently occur from surgery, traumatic events, pressure injuries, or infectious sources.
- See Table 10.3 for the stages of wound healing.

PRESSURE INJURY
Overview

- *Pressure injuries*, also referred to as pressure ulcers, decubitus ulcers, or bed sores, are injuries to the skin and underlying tissue from prolonged pressure on the body's bony prominences.

[🧠]　　**COMPLICATIONS**

Pressure injuries can lead to the development of infection, osteomyelitis, bacteremia, sepsis, septic shock, and death. Frequent skin assessment and treatment are needed to prevent these complications.

- The most common site is the sacrum; however, pressure injuries can occur on the heels, hips, back of the head, shoulder blades, and elbows.
- Older adult and bed-bound patients are more prone to pressure injuries.
- Pressure injuries can also be device-related and can occur in relation to a nasal cannula, urinary catheter, endotracheal tube, or NG tube.
- Fragile skin, decreased blood flow, muscle volume loss, increased moisture, and nutritional deficits can contribute to increased risk of pressure injury.

TABLE 10.3 Stages of Wound Healing	
Inflammatory phase	• Occurs between days 0 and 3 • Hemostasis is achieved • Inflammation and phagocytosis occur
Proliferation phase	• Occurs between days 3 and 21 • Angiogenesis and collagen synthesis occurs • Granulation and epithelization occur
Maturation phase	• 21 days to 2 years • Reorganization of collagen

Source: Data from Hopkins Medicine.

Signs and Symptoms

- Changes in skin color (nonblanchable redness)
- Drainage from an open wound
- Erythema
- Open wound on a bony prominence area
- Pain or tenderness
- Skin loss, exposing deeper layers of skin
- Skin swelling

Diagnosis

Labs

There are no labs specific to diagnose pressure injuries.

However, the following may be included as workup for a wound infection:

- Blood or wound culture: Likely to indicate an organism.
- BMP
- CBC: May indicate elevated WBC.
- Lactate: May be elevated with severe infection.

Diagnostic Testing

There are no diagnostic tests specific to diagnose pressure injuries. However, the following may confirm the depth of injury and infection of bone/surrounding tissue:

- CT scan
- X-ray

Treatment

- Antibiotics if an infected ulcer has caused a serious infection (Table A.1)
- Changing position
- Consult to wound therapy, as needed
- Mepilex/padded sacral dressing
- Surgical debridement to remove dead tissue, if necessary
- Topical barrier creams or ointments
- Topical medications (Table 10.1)
- Wound care

Nursing Interventions

- Administer nutritional support: Administer liquid dietary supplements and increase protein intake. An NG tube may be needed to provide additional nutritional support for wound healing; obtain a nutrition consult.
- Change pads as soon as soiling is noted.
- Clean wounds with gentle cleanser and pat dry; do not scrub.
- Deeper wounds may require wet-to-dry dressings with normal saline-dampened gauze.
- Elevate heels off bed or utilize heel protector boots.
- Establish turning schedule: Perform Q2H turns to relieve pressure on bony prominences and utilize positioning wedge and pillows.
- Perform frequent perineal hygiene. ▶

[ ] **NURSING PEARL**

Pressure injuries can be staged according to severity.

- *Stage 1:* Nonblanchable erythema of the skin
- *Stage 2:* Erythema with partial-thickness skin loss
- *Stage 3:* Full-thickness ulcer involving subcutaneous fat
- *Stage 4:* Full-thickness ulcer with muscle or bone involvement
- *Unstageable:* Unable to visualize wound bed due to eschar or tissue covering the wound bed

Nursing Interventions (*continued*)

- Perform frequent wound assessments: Apply moisture barrier product, as well as protective foam/ adhesive dressing.
- Place on a pressure redistribution surface, such as a low air loss mattress or pressure relief overlay.
- Premedicate prior to wound changes as needed.
- Provide support surfaces and special cushions when sitting in the chair. Reposition at regular intervals while in the chair.
- Reposition movable devices.
- Utilize specialty pillows to prevent breakdown on the back of the patient's head.

Patient Education

- Learn and understand the importance of the following: Change pads, dressings, diapers, or sheets if wet or soiled; keep skin clean and dry; maintain incontinence care at home; consider using wicking materials to help reduce moisture or assistive devices like bedside urinals or female external suction catheters; and reposition frequently to alleviate pressure on bony prominences and redistribute weight. If completely immobile or requiring total care, consider obtaining a home lift to assist with mobility and turning or consult home healthcare assistance.
- Perform wound care as needed: For patient with diabetes, this includes daily skin checks, especially to the feet and heels. Diabetic neuropathy decreases the feelings and sensations to the feet, thus increasing the risk for pressure ulcer or wound development. In general, when caring for pressure ulcers, assess incision daily for any new redness, warmth around the site, foul or discolored drainage, edema, or bleeding; avoid tight-fitting clothes; and change dressing daily as ordered by provider, or if the dressing becomes soiled. After cleaning hands, remove the old dressing, clean and rinse the incision site, pat dry, and apply new dressing as directed. Clean hands prior to and after touching the wound. If possible, measure the wound to assess for any growth in width or depth. Itchiness is expected as wounds heal. Do not scratch or pick at wounds. Obtain necessary materials, if needed, to perform dressing changes once discharged home.

SURGICAL WOUNDS

Overview

- Surgical wounds result from a surgical incision, which may be superficial or involve all of the layers of the skin.
- Wound size can also vary greatly depending on the type of procedure and may be closed completely with sutures, staples, or glue, or left open to heal with wet-to-dry dressings or negative pressure wound therapy.

Signs and Symptoms

- Erythema around incision site
- Mild swelling
- Pain
- Possible signs of infection: Discharge, drainage, foul odor, pain, and redness
- Serous, serosanguineous, or sanguineous bloody drainage

[🧠]   **COMPLICATIONS**

Surgical wounds are at increased risk for developing infection. Signs of infection include worsening swelling or edema, redness, warmth to touch, purulent or foul-smelling drainage, increased pain, fever, chills, or diaphoresis. This infection can progress to sepsis, septic shock, and even death. Frequent assessment and monitoring are required to identify potential infection early to decrease the risk for developing further complications.

Diagnosis

Labs

There are no labs specific to diagnose surgical wounds. However, the following may be helpful as workup for a wound infection:

- Blood or wound culture: Likely indicates an organism.
- BMP
- CBC: May indicate an elevated WBC.
- Lactate: May be elevated with severe infection.

Diagnostic Testing

- CT scan
- Ultrasound
- X-ray

Treatment

- Additional surgical debridement if needed
- Antibiotics (Table A.1)
- Surgical drains: Drainage via suction or gravity to remove excess fluid
- Negative pressure wound therapy provides increased negative pressure to promote epithelization, increase blood flow, and continuously remove drainage
- Wound therapy consult as needed

Nursing Interventions

- Administer nutritional support with increased protein to promote wound healing.
- Apply abdominal binder as ordered.
- Empty and perform drain care as ordered: Ensure drain tubing is free of clots or obstructions and remains patent; monitor surgical drains for increasing output, frank bleeding, or purulent drainage.
- Monitor site for signs of infection which include new or worsening swelling or edema, redness, warmth to the touch, pain, and foul-smelling or purulent drainage.
- Monitor VS for additional signs/symptoms of infection including new or worsening fever, tachycardia, and hypotension.
- Perform dressing changes as ordered and if soiled. Ordered dressing changes may be daily, every shift, or more frequently depending on situation.
- Perform frequent neurologic assessments to identify AMS or confusion, which may indicate infection.
- Perform wound care as ordered. For wet-to-dry dressing, apply gauze moistened with sterile water. Support with abdominal (ABD) pad and tape, and manage wound vacuum-assisted closure (VAC) if applied to wound.
- Provide splinting pillow or support to brace when coughing, bearing down, or repositioning in bed.

Patient Education

- Follow up as scheduled with all outpatient appointments.
- Include family and caregiver in education for at home management if assistance in changing dressing is needed.
- Maintain a healthy, high-protein diet to promote wound healing.
- Monitor for new or worsening systemic infection including fever, tachycardia, hypotension, or confusion. ▶

Patient Education (*continued*)

- Perform dressing changes as needed. In general, when caring for wounds after discharge, assess incision daily for any new redness, warmth around the site, foul or discolored drainage, edema, or bleeding. Change dressing daily as ordered by provider, or if the dressing becomes soiled. After washing hands, remove the old dressing, clean and rinse the incision site, pat dry, and apply new dressing as directed. Itchiness is expected as wounds heal. Do not scratch or pick at wounds. Obtain necessary materials, if needed, to perform dressing changes once discharged home. Wash hands prior to and after touching the surgical site.
- Pursue smoking cessation as needed.
- Perform site inspection daily, assessing for new or worsening redness, swelling, warmth to touch, or purulent, foul-smelling drainage.
- Immunocompromised patients and those with diabetes or peripheral vascular disease (PVD) may have impaired wound healing due to these comorbid conditions. Diligently monitor wound healing.
- Take medications as prescribed, especially the full dose of antibiotics.

TRAUMATIC WOUNDS

Overview

- Traumatic wounds result from a sudden, unplanned injury.
- The size and damage sustained can also vary greatly but generally depends on the velocity, force, and item that caused the damage.
- Anatomical location of the traumatic wound injury also impacts the severity of the wound.
- Traumatic wounds, if involving an artery or major organ, can quickly progress to a medical emergency and require prompt treatment and intervention.

Signs and Symptoms

- Entry or exit wound
- Lacerations caused by blunt or sharp mechanism
- Sanguineous, serosanguinous, or sanguineous drainage
- Swelling or edema
- Pain
- Possible signs of infection: discharge, drainage, foul odor, pain, and redness

Diagnosis

Labs

Lab workup for a trauma patient may include:

- ABG
- CBC: May indicate a low hemoglobin and hematocrit if traumatic wound.
- CMP
- Coagulation panel
- Type and screen

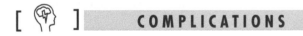

COMPLICATIONS

Complications of traumatic wounds include bleeding, hemorrhage, secondary injury to surrounding tissue, vasculature and organs, and infection. Depending on the type of secondary injury, a wide variety of complications can result. Most commonly, widespread traumatic wounds like those experienced in a crush injury can result in rhabdomyolysis and AKI. Other complications include infection which can progress to sepsis, septic shock, or death. Diligent monitoring is required to identify and treat wound complications early.

Diagnostic Testing
- CT scan
- Ultrasound
- X-rays

Treatment

- Utilize antibiotics (Table A.1).
- Consult with involved services (e.g., ears, nose, and throat [ENT] or neurosurgery for head/facial trauma; orthopedics for injuries involving bones).
- Manual or surgical removal of objects is conducted if fully or partially retained (bullet[s], shrapnel, or other debris).
- Surgical intervention may involve debridement (burns, retained gravel, etc.) or closure of traumatic wound; surgical drains utilize suction or gravity to remove drainage.
- Negative pressure wound therapy provides increased negative pressure to promote epithelization, increase blood flow, and continuously remove drainage.

Nursing Interventions

See Surgical Wounds, Nursing Interventions.

Patient Education

See Surgical Wounds, Patient Education.

RESOURCES

Centers for Disease Control and Prevention. (2021, August 20). *Get ahead of sepsis – Know the risks. Spot the signs. Act fast*. U.S. Department of Health and Human Services. https://www.cdc.gov/patientsafety/features/get-ahead-of-sepsis.html

DeMarco, S. (n.d.). *Wound and pressure ulcer management*. Johns Hopkins Medicine. https://www.hopkinsmedicine.org/gec/series/wound_care.html#wound_healing

Mayo Clinic Laboratories. (n.d.). *Test ID: SALCA*. https://www.mayocliniclabs.com/test-catalog/Clinical+and+Interpretive/37061

Mayo Foundation for Medical Education and Research. (2021, September 1). *Charcoal, activated (Oral route) side effects*. https://www.mayoclinic.org/drugs-supplements/charcoal-activated-oral-route/side-effects/drg-20070087

National Institute on Aging. (n.d.). *Providing care and comfort at the end of life*. U.S. Department of Health and Human Services. https://www.nia.nih.gov/health/providing-comfort-end-life

Prescribers' Digital Reference. (n.d.-a). *Flumazenil* [Drug information]. PDR Search. https://pdr.net/drug-summary/Flumazenil-flumazenil-1729

Prescribers' Digital Reference. (n.d.-b). *N-Acetylcysteine* [Drug information]. PDR Search. https://pdr.net/drug-summary/Acetylcysteine-acetylcysteine-668

Prescribers' Digital Reference. (n.d.-c). *Naloxone hydrochloride* [Drug information]. PDR Search. https://pdr.net/drug-summary/Naloxone-Hydrochloride-Injection--1-mg-mL--naloxone-hydrochloride-23987

Prescribers' Digital Reference. (n.d.-d). *Oseltamivir* [Drug information]. PDR Search. https://www.pdr.net/drug-summary/Tamiflu-oseltamivir-phosphate-2099.8269#14

Prescribers' Digital Reference. (n.d.-e). *Silver sufadiazine* [Drug information]. PDR Search. https://pdr.net/drug-summary/Silvadene-silver-sulfadiazine-2781

Schroeder, K., & Lorenz, K. (2018). Nursing and the future of palliative care. *Asia-Pacific Journal of Oncology Nursing*, 5(1), 4–8. https://www.ncbi.nlm.nih.gov/pmc/articles/PMC5763437

Singer, M., Deutschman, C. S., Seymour, C. W., Shankar-Hari, M., Annane, D., Bauer, M., Bellomo, R., Bernard, G. R., Chiche, J.-D., Coopersmith, C. M., Hotchkiss, R. S., Levy, M. M., Marshall, J. C., Martin, G. S., Opal, S. M., Rubenfeld, G. D., van der Poll, T., Vincent, J.-L., & Angus, D. C. (2016, February 23). The third international consensus definitions for sepsis and septic shock (sepsis-3). *Journal of the American Medical Association*, *315*(8), 801–810. https://www.ncbi.nlm.nih.gov/pmc/articles/PMC4968574

Torres, P. A., Helmstetter, J. A., Kaye, A. M., & Kaye, A. D. (2015). Rhabdomyolysis: Pathogenesis, diagnosis, and treatment. *The Ochsner Journal*, *15*(1), 58–69. https://www.ncbi.nlm.nih.gov/pmc/articles/PMC4365849

University of Rochester Medical Center. (n.d.). *Acetaminophen drug level*. https://www.urmc.rochester.edu/encyclopedia/content.aspx?contenttypeid=167&contentid=acetaminophen_drug_level#:~:text=The%20results%20of%20the%20acetaminophen,is%20risk%20for%20liver%20damage

11 BEHAVIORAL AND PSYCHOSOCIAL CONDITIONS

AGGRESSIVE/DISRUPTIVE/VIOLENT BEHAVIOR

Overview

- Acute agitation may be a symptom of many emergent health conditions. As such, a thorough investigation and assessment is needed to rule out physiological causes.
- Agitation that is caused by a variety of medical or psychiatric conditions can escalate into aggressive/violent behavior.
- The progressive care unit (PCU) team should assess all patients for risk for violence and attempt to facilitate therapeutic communication, provide diversionary activities, and utilize de-escalation techniques before a situation results in violence. The use of physical or chemical restraints should be a last resort.

COMPLICATIONS

Violent behavior places patients and caregivers at risk for injury. Agitation and threats of violence should be addressed proactively, and de-escalation of the agitated patient should be prioritized to reduce incidences of violence in the PCU.

Signs and Symptoms

- Compromised reality checking (such as with patients experiencing dementia and delirium, hallucinations and/or delusions, de-realization, and/or de-personalization)
- Restlessness, pacing, increased vocalization/volume and use of profanity or threatening language, aggressive gestures, and erratic or impulsive behavior
- Signs of intoxication or substance use
- Violent or threatening statements or actions toward self or others

Diagnosis

Labs

There are no labs specific to diagnose aggressive/disruptive/violent behavior. However, the following may be indicated based on the patient's clinical status:

- Complete blood count (CBC)
- Comprehensive metabolic panel (CMP)
- Ethanol (ETOH) level
- Urine drug screen
- Urinalysis

Diagnostic Testing

- Head CT scan to rule out underlying emergent medical condition
- X-rays as indicated for related injuries

Treatment

- De-escalation through practicing diversionary techniques, limiting external stimuli, and facilitating therapeutic communication
- Isolation of violent patients in an area where potential hazards can be removed to maintain patient/staff safety
- Medical or physical restraints if the patient does not respond to prior interventions and patient or staff harm is imminent
- Psychiatry consult as inpatient admission may be indicated once medically cleared
- Thorough evaluation to rule out possible emergent medical causes of behaviors
- Threats taken seriously
- Visualization of the patient utilizing 1:1 observation, if indicated

Nursing Interventions

- Administer medications as ordered (Table 11.1).
- Apply and monitor use of physical restraints as indicated by institutional protocols, as a last resort. Perform regular circulatory and neurovascular checks to restrained extremities. Provide assistance with oral intake and toileting as needed. Assess skin integrity per facility protocol to decrease the risk of complications related to restraint use or immobility. The patient may require a 1:1 sitter depending on facility protocol with the type of restraints required to maintain patient safety.
- Attempt to establish a therapeutic relationship.
- Continuously monitor for changes in vital signs.
- Facilitate de-escalation of the patient's behavior: Remain calm, use simple language, establish therapeutic communication if possible, and engage family members who may be present in de-escalation techniques if possible.
- Maintain an environment of safety: Remove items that could become weapons; reinforce/protect dressings, lines, and tubes as much as possible; obtain an order for restraint if needed.
- Maintain visual and situational awareness of the patient at all times.
- Remain calm and speak to the patient using simple language.
- Remove the patient to an appropriate location to maintain patient and staff safety.

[⚡] **ALERT!**

De-escalating a potentially violent patient can take time but is frequently successful if approached in the correct manner.

- First, ensure the environment is safe for the patient and staff involved.
- Speak calmly and objectively to the patient.
- Encourage conversation and attempt to form an alliance.
- Listen to what the patient has to say and respond in a respectful manner.
- Incorporate active listening into the conversation; use reflection to help the patient identify underlying feelings. Nonverbal communication can help establish a therapeutic relationship.
- If possible, stand next to the patient to appear less threatening.
- Remember, safety comes first. Do not attempt de-escalation alone, and always stand between the patient and the door.

Patient Education

- Identify ways to manage anger and stress, which may include physical exercise and relaxation techniques (deep breathing, meditation, yoga, etc.).
- If agitation or aggression is not the result of acute critical illness, consider following up with a counselor or therapist to address aggressive behavior.
- Limit alcohol and other substance use.
- Some medications have adverse reactions and may cause aggression or agitation. Alert all future providers to avoid administering this medication if it contributed to aggression.

[📝] **POP QUIZ 11.1**

What is the first step the nurse should take to respond to an agitated patient who is shouting and hitting the side of the bed?

TABLE 11.1 Psychiatric Medications

INDICATIONS	MECHANISM OF ACTION	CONTRAINDICATIONS, PRECAUTIONS, AND ADVERSE EFFECTS
Antidepressants, atypical (bupropion hydrochloride)		
• Major depression	• Dopamine norepinephrine reuptake inhibitor, inhibit presynaptic reuptake of dopamine, and norepinephrine (with a greater effect upon dopamine)	• Medication is contraindicated in seizure disorders or concurrent use with MAOIs. • Use caution in Tourette's (can cause worsening tics); major hepatic, renal, or cardiac disease; operating heavy machinery; or pregnancy. • Do not abruptly discontinue. • Adverse effects include anxiety, dry mouth, palpitations, restlessness, and difficulty sleeping.
Antidepressants: MAOIs (isocarboxazid)		
• Multiple psychiatric disorders, including treatment-resistant major depression	• Inhibit MAO through irreversible binding	• Medication is contraindicated in severe renal or liver impairments, concurrent use of medications known to interact with MAOIs, hypertension, or pheochromocytoma. • Use caution in concurrent use with contrast dye, procedures requiring general anesthesia, hyperthyroidism, diabetes, asthma, or seizure disorders. • Adverse effects include dry mouth, skin irritation/reactions, insomnia, increased risk for suicidal thoughts or actions following dosage change, and serotonin syndrome.
Antidepressants: SSRIs (citalopram, escitalopram, fluoxetine, paroxetine, and sertraline)		
• Moderate-to-severe depression • Anxiety disorders	• Increase levels of serotonin in the brain by blocking the reuptake of serotonin in neurons, making more available for transmitting signals	• Do not abruptly discontinue. • Adverse effects include nausea/vomiting, diarrhea, nervousness, agitation, restlessness, insomnia, weight loss or weight gain, sexual dysfunction, dry mouth, headache, serotonin syndrome, or suicidal thoughts or behaviors. • Use caution in pregnancy; heart, liver, and kidney disease; and bleeding disorders.
Antidepressants: SNRIs (duloxetine and venlafaxine)		
• Primarily as treatment for depression • Can be effective in treating anxiety disorders and chronic or nerve pain	• Block reuptake of serotonin and norepinephrine in the brain	• Taper gradually to discontinue. • Do not administer with MAOIs. • Adverse effects include headache, nausea, dizziness, increased perspiration, fatigue, constipation, insomnia, decreased appetite, sexual dysfunction, increased suicidal thoughts or behaviors, HTN, decreased liver functioning, and serotonin syndrome. • Use caution taking with blood thinners, if considering getting pregnant, or if pregnant.

(continued)

TABLE 11.1 Psychiatric Medications (*continued*)

INDICATIONS	MECHANISM OF ACTION	CONTRAINDICATIONS, PRECAUTIONS, AND ADVERSE EFFECTS
Antidepressants: Tricyclic (amitriptyline)		
• Fibromyalgia • Insomnia • Major depression • Painful diabetic neuropathy • Social phobia	• Mechanism of action not fully understood; thought to result from the decreased reuptake of norepinephrine and serotonin	• Medication is contraindicated in concurrent use with MAOIs or for patients in the acute recovery phase following acute MI. • Use caution in bipolar or mania, schizophrenia, alcoholism or CNS depression, seizure disorders, DM, geriatric populations, and pregnancy. • Do not abruptly discontinue. • Adverse effects include drowsiness, dry mouth, blurred vision, difficulty urinating or stooling, weight gain, or dizziness.
Antipsychotics: First generation (haloperidol)		
• Schizophrenia • Psychosis • Severe behavioral problems	• Mechanism of action not currently known; believed to block dopamine receptors	• Medication is contraindicated in coma or severe toxic CNS depression, Parkinson disease, and Lewy body dementia. • Use caution in cardiac, renal, liver, or pulmonary disorders; QT prolongation; seizure disorders; stroke; urinary retention; and pregnancy. • Do not abruptly discontinue. • Adverse effects include tremor, dyskinesias, anxiety, agitation, restlessness, diaphoresis, nausea, or vomiting. • IM formulary can be used for emergency treatment.
Antipsychotics: Second generation (e.g., risperidone)		
• Schizophrenia • Psychosis • Severe behavioral problems	• Exhibit effects through some dopamine blockade, but more from blockade of serotonin receptors	• Use caution in CNS depression; hematologic disease; tardive dyskinesia; cardiac, renal, or hepatic disease; seizure disorders; Parkinson disease; dementia; PKU; DM; and in older adult patients. • Do not abruptly discontinue. • Adverse effects include nausea, vomiting, diarrhea or constipation, weight gain, anxiety, dry or discolored skin, and decreased sexual function.
Anxiolytics: Benzodiazepines (e.g., alprazolam, chlordiazepoxide, clonazepam, diazepam, lorazepam, and midazolam)		
• Anxiety • Mood disorders	• Potentiate the effect of GABA, which increases the inhibition of the RAS system	• Do not abruptly discontinue. • Adverse effects include fatigue, nausea/vomiting, weight changes (loss or gain), sexual dysfunction, agitation, unsteady gait, slurred speech, or sedation. • Use caution in use with active suicidal ideation, psychosis or bipolar disorder, CNS depression, pulmonary disease, alcoholism or substance abuse, liver or renal disease, and geriatric populations.

(continued)

INDICATIONS	MECHANISM OF ACTION	CONTRAINDICATIONS, PRECAUTIONS, AND ADVERSE EFFECTS
TABLE 11.1 Psychiatric Medications (*continued*)		
Anxiolytics (buspirone)		
• Anxiety disorders	• Suppress serotonin while enhancing noradrenergic and dopaminergic cell firing to improve neurotransmission	• Medication is contraindicated in concurrent use with MAOIs. • Use caution in benzodiazepine dependence, renal or liver impairments, geriatric populations, or pregnancy. • Adverse effects include dizziness, headache, confusion, fatigue, nervousness, insomnia, mood changes, headache, palpitations, blurred vision, hives, or itching.
Opioid agonist (methadone)		
• Opioid withdrawal	• Bind to opiate receptor sites in CNS to alter perceptions of and response to painful stimuli, decreasing symptoms of withdrawal to opioids	• Medication is contraindicated in alcohol intolerance and concurrent use of MAOIs. • Use caution in heart disease; diuretic use; hypokalemia; hypomagnesemia; history of dysrhythmia; concurrent use with drugs that prolong QT interval; severe renal, hepatic, or pulmonary disease; and head trauma. • Adverse effects include confusion, sedation, hypotension, and constipation.
Opioid antagonist (naloxone)		
• Suspected opioid overdose • Opioid-induced respiratory depression	• Antagonize opioid effects by competing for the same receptor sites	• Use caution in patients with cardiovascular disease. • Adverse effects include ventricular dysrhythmias, hypertension, hypotension, nausea, and vomiting.
Vitamin B₁ supplements (thiamine)		
• Treatment of Wernicke–Korsakoff syndrome resulting from alcohol abuse • Vitamin B₁ deficiency	• Combine with ATP in the liver and kidneys to produce thiamine diphosphate, which acts as a coenzyme in carbohydrate metabolism allowing pyruvic acid to convert and enter the Krebs cycle	• Use caution in pregnancy. • Adverse effects include nausea, weakness, sweating, restlessness, or itching.

ATP, adenosine triphosphate; CNS, central nervous system; DM, diabetes mellitus; GABA, gamma-aminobutyric acid; HTN, hypertension; IM, imtramuscularly; MAO, monoamine oxidase; MAOI, monoamine oxidase inhibitors; MI, myocardial infarction; PKU, phenylketonuria; RAS, reticular activating system; SNRI, serotonin and norepinephrine reuptake inhibitor; SSRI, selective serotonin reuptake inhibitor.

ALTERED MENTAL STATUS
Overview

■ *Altered mental status (AMS)* can be described as an acute or chronic change in consciousness, arousal, self-awareness, expression, language, or emotions. ▶

COMPLICATIONS

Complications of AMS include impaired cognitive, behavioral, and physical functioning, which may lead to combative or agitated behavior and place the patient at risk for accidental self-harm (accidental removal of lines, drains, or tubes, falls, etc.). Alternately, it may lead to further central nervous system (CNS) depression, coma, or respiratory arrest.

Overview (*continued*)

■ AMS has a wide variety of causes ranging from metabolic derangements (e.g., alcohol withdrawal) to acute focal brain lesions (e.g., stroke) to chronic neurodegenerative diseases (e.g., Alzheimer dementia).

■ Often, AMS is the primary reason for admittance to the PCU.

Signs and Symptoms

■ Anxiety
■ Attention impairment
■ CNS depression and coma
■ Cognitive impairment
■ Confusion
■ Emotional withdrawal or emotional outbursts
■ Intermittent periods of lucidity
■ Irritability
■ Motor functioning changes
■ Slowed, slurred speech
■ Psychomotor agitation

Diagnosis

Labs

■ Possible indication based on patient's clinical status: An arterial blood gas (ABG) may indicate acidosis, hypercarbia, or hypoxia. A CMP may identify multiple issues. A CBC may indicate an elevated white blood cell (WBC) count if AMS is the result of an infection. Point of care glucose testing is used to assess for hypo- or hyperglycemia. Toxicology screening may be warranted if AMS is caused by drug or alcohol use. Urinalysis can be helpful (urinary tract infection [UTI] may cause confusion in an older adult).

Diagnostic Testing

■ Glasgow Coma Scale (GCS)
■ Head CT scan to rule out a neurologic abnormality
■ Mini-mental status examination
■ X-ray, if indicated

Treatment

Treatment of AMS is dependent on cause. This may include, but is not limited to:

■ Airway management with bilevel positive airway pressure (BiPAP) or intubation
■ Treatment of hypoglycemia (Chapter 4)
■ Treatment of intracranial hemorrhage or encephalopathy with appropriate neurologic intervention (Chapter 6)
■ Treatment of infection or septic shock with antibiotics (Table A.1), fluid resuscitation, and/or vasopressors (Table 2.3)
■ Management of AMS if no clear etiology: antipsychotics if indicated (Table 11.1), delirium precautions, and maintaining sleep–wake cycles

ALERT!

AMS could signal serious cerebral disease or illness including hemorrhage, tumors, abscesses, hematomas, or lesions. Any change in mental status should be thoroughly investigated.

ALERT!

Sundowning is a condition of late-day confusion in which a patient who is otherwise alert and oriented during the day becomes disoriented as the sun sets.

Nursing Interventions

- Administer medications as ordered to treat the underlying condition, pain/discomfort, and/or agitation.
- Assess vital signs for changes in hemodynamic stability, such as hypotension, tachycardia, or tachypnea.
- Build a trusting relationship.
- Consult psychiatry as needed.
- Create a safe environment: Consider using a bed or chair alarm to alert staff of unexpected ambulation or movement. If patient is at risk of self-harm or harm to someone else, consider utilizing a sitter to maintain patient safety and prevent unwitnessed ambulation. Place objects that can be used as projectiles or to harm self or someone else out of room. Lower the bed to decrease risk of falls. Position the call bell, telephone, and other personal items of importance near the patient. Protect or cover lines or tubes if the patient is attempting to pull at them.
- Engage in therapeutic communication.
- Maintain sleep hygiene and promote a regular sleep–wake cycle. Decrease environmental disruptions using sleep masks and do not disturb orders. Reschedule medications and lab draws to reduce sleep interruption, if possible.
- Perform neurologic assessment frequently. Regularly orient patient to current day and time with each interaction.
- Promote use of eyeglasses and hearing aids as needed.
- Provide urinal or assist to bedpan as needed.

Patient Education

- Depending on the level of mental status alteration, the patient may be unable to comprehend education provided by healthcare providers. However, make every effort to answer questions appropriately; communicate effectively; provide reassurance and therapeutically communicate; and reorient patient to person, place, time, and situation as needed/appropriate.
- If caregiver or family notices a sudden change in mental status, seek care through emergency services.
- If possible, avoid polypharmacy and taking unnecessary medications, especially if an older adult.
- Follow a regular sleep–wake cycle. Get at least 8 hr of undisturbed sleep.
- Limit alcohol consumption.

ANXIETY

Overview

- Anxiety involves fear and worry accompanied by a heightened physiologic response with symptoms ranging from mild to severe.
- Hospitalized patients often experience acute anxiety due to a threat to life or physical health, loss of control, and foreign environment.
- Pain, poor sleep quality, mobility changes, medical equipment/devices, and nightly interruptions have also been found to increase anxiety among hospitalized patients.
- Chronic anxiety may also be exacerbated by hospital admission.

 COMPLICATIONS

Anxiety in acute illness can result in irrational behavior and impaired cognition, leading to aggression, agitation, and inadvertent removal of important lines, drains, or tubes. Physiologic complications of anxiety also include vital sign changes including tachycardia and tachypnea. These changes can worsen health status while hospitalized.

Signs and Symptoms

- Behavioral: avoidance of triggers, impatient, fearful, frustrated, or quiet
- Cognitive: confusion, difficulty speaking, hyper-vigilance for threat, fear of loss of control, fear of physical injury or death, frightening mental thoughts or images, and poor concentration
- Physiologic: chest pain or pressure, diaphoresis, diarrhea, dizziness, dry mouth, dyspnea, nausea, numbness and tingling, palpitations, shaking, tachycardia, and weakness

Diagnosis

Labs

There are no labs specific to diagnose anxiety. However, the following may be indicated based on the patient's clinical status:

- ABG
- Blood cultures
- Basic metabolic panel (BMP)
- CBC
- Thyroid function test
- Toxicology screen
- Urinalysis

Diagnostic Testing

- Anxiety screening tools: GAD-7, or a hospital anxiety and depression screening tool
- Diagnostics to rule out physiologic causes: chest x-ray, EKG, and head CT scan

Treatment

- Medications (Table 11.1): antipsychotics, benzodiazepines, beta blockers (Table 2.3), buspirone, selective serotonin reuptake inhibitor (SSRIs), serotonin and norepinephrine reuptake inhibitor (SNRIs), and tricyclic antidepressants
- Nonpharmacologic interventions: distraction through use of conversation, television, or music; pet therapy; and therapeutic touch
- Psychotherapy if appropriate during the patient's PCU stay (may be deferred until transferred out of the unit)
- Ruling out underlying medical cause of anxiety symptoms
- Supplemental oxygen as needed for tachypnea or dyspnea

Nursing Interventions

- Administer scheduled antianxiety medications and assess the need for as needed (PRN) dosages as ordered. Notify the provider if the schedule and PRN dosage has not alleviated symptoms of anxiety.
- Assess for suicidal or homicidal ideation.
- Engage in therapeutic communication; listen to the patient and allow them to voice their fears and concerns. ▶

[🌐] NURSING PEARL

Family members or caregivers can bring in pictures or familiar and comforting items to the patient to decrease anxiety in the hospital setting.

[⚡] ALERT!

Use extreme caution when treating older adult patients with benzodiazepines. Use another pharmacologic agent if possible. Benzodiazepine use in older adult patients can impair mobility and cognition, increase the risk of falls, and enhance the risk of developing dementia and Alzheimer disease.

Nursing Interventions (*continued*)

- Establish rapport with the patient and build a trusting relationship.
- Monitor vital signs for anxiety-induced changes including tachycardia, tachypnea, and decreased oxygen saturation.
- Provide a safe, familiar environment.

Patient Education

- Consider following up with a therapist or psychologist following discharge.
- Practice good health habits: Get adequate sleep, eat a variety of foods, and exercise.
- Self-assess and identify what anxiety triggers may be. Remove or reduce triggers (if possible).
- Use nonpharmacologic anxiety-reducing techniques as needed, which include aromatherapy, guided imagery, meditation, music, slowed breathing, and yoga.

DELIRIUM

Overview

- *Delirium* is an alteration in mental status that is characterized by acute onset, fluctuating course, impaired attention, and either a disturbance in the level of consciousness or disorganized thinking.
- Delirium can manifest as hyperactive, hypoactive, or mixed.
- Patients experiencing critical illness and hospitalizations are at high risk for developing delirium, which manifests as an acute change in awareness or attention that appears over a short period of time.

COMPLICATIONS

Complications of delirium include aspiration pneumonia, decreased mobility and functioning, falls, combative behavior leading to accidental self-harm, malnutrition, fluid and electrolyte imbalance, pressure ulcers, and long-term cognitive impairment. Additionally, delirium increases the risk of medical complications, prolonged hospitalizations, functional decline, and dementia.

Signs and Symptoms

- Alterations in sleep–wake cycle
- Behavioral changes: emotional lability, hallucinations or delusions, irritability, psychomotor agitation, or unsafe behavior
- Cognitive impairment: anxiety, disorganized thinking, disorientation of consciousness, emotional liability, or fluctuating changes in awareness

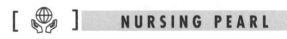
NURSING PEARL

Delirium coinciding with acute illness will often resolve with the treatment of underlying illness.

Diagnosis

Labs

There are no labs specific to diagnose delirium. Lab workup may be similar for patients with AMS as noted in the previous section.

Diagnostic Testing

- Head CT scan to rule out underlying etiology
- GCS
- Mini-mental status examination

Treatment

- Underlying etiology treatment if known cause of delirium, including glucose imbalances, hypoxia or hypercarbia respiratory issues, and infection
- See Altered Mental Status Treatment section for more information.

Nursing Interventions

See Altered Mental Status, Nursing Interventions.

Patient Education

See Altered Mental Status, Patient Education.

DEMENTIA

Overview

- Dementia is characterized by a slow and chronic deterioration in cognition and decline in functional activities.
- Patients with dementia will have memory difficulties in addition to personality changes and difficulty with abstract thinking, word recall, executive functioning, and social and special skills.

[ ]   **COMPLICATIONS**

Dementia complications include increased risk for infections (e.g., pneumonia or UTI), falls, fractures, inadequate nutrition and dehydration, depression, hallucinations, delusions, and death. Dementia is a progressive disease with high mortality rate.

- Patients with dementia are at high risk to develop a concomitant delirium, especially in the PCU setting.

Signs and Symptoms

- Behavioral changes: aggression, mood changes, self-neglect, and social withdrawal
- Cognitive impairments: communication difficulty, difficulty performing tasks, forgetfulness, hallucinations, and memory loss

Diagnosis

Labs

- CBC to rule out anemia
- Serum B_{12} level to rule out vitamin B_{12} deficiency
- Thyroid-stimulating hormone (TSH) to rule out hypothyroidism
- Additional routine labs to rule out other physiologic conditions if there is a specific suspicion for abnormality

Diagnostic Testing

- Autopsy examination of brain tissue to confirm Alzheimer/dementia diagnosis
- Head CT or MRI in the routine initial evaluation of patients with dementia

Treatment

- No cure is available. Treatments alleviate some symptoms; however, the disease inevitably progresses in all patients.
- Interventions to manage and maintain baseline functioning include avoidance of stimulants, daily exercise, medications (Table 11.1), pain control, and sleep hygiene.

[ ]   **ALERT!**

Behavior changes exhibited as a result of dementia can manifest as depression, anxiety, or psychosis. Treatment of these manifestations remains the same independent of a dementia diagnosis.

- In advanced dementia, a hospice and/or palliative care consult may be needed. Manage infection/fever as needed.

Nursing Interventions

- Alleviate physical discomfort: Administer medications as ordered, ambulate and mobilize as possible, and reposition frequently.
- Assist with frequent toileting and/or perineal care.
- Encourage safe oral by mouth (PO) intake.
- Engage in therapeutic communication.
- Provide nutritional support. Assist patient with meals and/or administer tube feedings as ordered/scheduled.
- Provide safe environment for patient.
- Provide support with decision-making and advance care planning.
- Provide symptom management relief.
- Reorient patient as needed.

Patient Education

- Consider respite care support or alternative care setting.
- Improve oral intake with finger foods, smaller portions, nutritional supplements, and alternating textures of food.
- Stay updated on current status, plan of care, advanced health directives, and healthcare proxy prior to end-stage dementia.
- Update family members on clinical course of delirium, treatments, and clinical course. Understand what to expect at the end stage of the disease.

DEPRESSION

Overview

- Depression is common among patients with chronic illness. Often, depression from a hospital admission or acute disease can lead to anxiety and posttraumatic stress disorder (PTSD).
- Depressive disorders are characterized by prolonged periods of a depressed mood most often related to a chemical imbalance.
- It can be difficult to diagnose as a patient may have mild symptoms resulting from a specific situation or trigger or severe symptoms consistent with a mood disorder.
- Major depression has a high morbidity and mortality rate. Identification and treatment of depression is essential to preventing complications.

Signs and Symptoms

- Appetite/weight changes
- Decreased or loss of interest in usual activities
- Decreased energy/fatigue
- Depressed mood
- Difficulty concentrating
- Fatigue
- Feelings of worthlessness
- Psychomotor disturbances
- Sleep disturbances
- Suicidal or recurrent thoughts of death

COMPLICATIONS

Depressed patients are at risk for impaired self-care, which can exacerbate preexisting physical conditions or lead to drug and alcohol abuse, self-harm, or suicide.

NURSING PEARL

Any verbalization of depression or suicidal thoughts in a critically ill patient should be taken seriously. A psychiatric consult and mood-stabilizing medications may be indicated.

Diagnosis

Labs

There are no labs specific to diagnose depression. However, the following may be helpful to rule out physiologic causes:

- CBC
- CMP
- ETOH level
- Rapid plasma reagin (RPR) to rule out syphilis
- TSH to rule out hypothyroidism
- Toxicology screen to rule out illicit drug use
- Vitamin B_{12} to rule out vitamin B_{12} deficiency

ALERT!

Use caution when starting depression treatments in the hospital setting. Often, these drugs take time to reach effectiveness, have multiple interactions with other medications, and should not be abruptly stopped. Request a psychiatric consult for a more in-depth evaluation.

Diagnostic Testing

There are no diagnostic tests specific to diagnose depression. However, the following may be indicated to rule out a neurologic mass or abnormality if physiologic pathology is a suspected cause:

- CT scan
- MRI

Treatment

- Assessment/treatment: suicidal ideations or attempts assessment and treatment
- Assessment/treatment: any electrolyte abnormalities and nutritional deficits
- Medications to manage symptoms (e.g., anxiety, depression, and insomnia; Table 11.1): atypical antidepressants, monoamine oxidase inhibitors (MAOIs), SSRIs, SNRIs, and tricyclic antidepressants
- Ruling out underlying medical condition
- Consult to social work and case management to ensure referrals and resources are in place for continued outpatient treatment
- Possibly indicated once patient is clinically stable: Consider electroconvulsive therapy (ECT) if antidepressant medications have not worked; consider psychotherapy to help treat depressive health problems by talking with a psychiatrist or other mental health provider, or transfer to a psychiatric unit.

Nursing Interventions

- Administer crystalloid fluids or nutritional supplements as indicated if underweight or malnourished.
- Administer medications as ordered.
- Arrange for a psychiatry consult.
- Assess for alcohol or drug use.
- Build a trusting relationship.
- Engage in therapeutic communication.
- Monitor vital signs continuously.
- Perform a focused psychological assessment.
- Provide a safe and familiar environment for the patient.

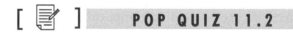

POP QUIZ 11.2

A patient is admitted to the PCU with hypertension due to medication noncompliance stemming from an untreated major depressive disorder. The provider starts the patient on an MAOI for his depression. The patient asks what other interventions are available to help treat his depression. What should the nurse's response be?

Patient Education

- If suicidal thoughts or feelings occur, reach out to close family or friends for support; refer the patient to support groups, therapists, or counselors; or call 911. ▶

Patient Education (*continued*)

■ Maintain a healthy lifestyle with exercise, a proper diet, and good sleep hygiene.

■ Pursue interventions to improve appetite if underweight, as well as weight loss programs if overweight.

■ Take medications as ordered, even if feeling better.

■ Understand the risk of abruptly stopping medication.

■ Understand the importance of follow-up care in an outpatient setting.

SUBSTANCE ABUSE

Overview

■ *Substance abuse* is the excessive use of alcohol or other drugs that activate the brain's reward system to reinforce behavior. This can include chronic drug or alcohol abuse or drug-seeking behavior, in addition to drug or alcohol withdrawal. It may lead to significant problems or distress, such as substance-related legal problems and impaired relationships with friends and family.

■ Patients in the PCU can be admitted as a direct result of their substance abuse (intoxication, withdrawal, etc.) or have a history of substance abuse. Acknowledgment of a substance abuse disorder is important to provide appropriate care.

[🧠]   COMPLICATIONS

Patients with substance or alcohol addiction are at risk for developing cardiovascular disease, cancer, stroke, lung disease, or mental disorders, land liver failure, or for contracting HIV/AIDS or hepatitis B and/or C. Additionally, patients are also at risk for seizure and death from withdrawal of certain substances.

Signs and Symptoms

■ Drug-seeking behavior includes aggressively complaining about the need for a specific drug, anger/irritability over detailed questioning about pain, asking for a specific drug by name/brand name at specific time, constant request for increased dose, claiming multiple allergies to alternate drugs, inappropriate self-medicating, inappropriate use of general practice, manipulative or illegal behavior, and/or resistant behavior.

■ Varied signs and symptoms may be observed, depending on the type of substance used. For depressants, these may include ataxia, CNS depression, coma, multiorgan failure, and slurred speech. For stimulants, symptoms may include anxiety, hypertension, psychosis, tachycardia, and tachypnea.

[⚡]   ALERT!

Alcohol withdrawal typically occurs 1 to 3 days following the patient's last drink. If possible, determine the date and time of last drink on admission. If date and time of last drink is unable to be determined and alcohol withdrawal is suspected, frequently monitor for condition changes consistent with alcohol withdrawal. Notify the provider and treat per institutional protocol.

■ Withdrawal signs may vary based on the substance. Alcohol withdrawal symptoms include agitation, anxiety, auditory disturbances, difficulty thinking, diaphoresis, headache, nausea and vomiting, tactile disturbances, tremor, and visual disturbances. Drug withdrawal symptoms vary by the drug. For barbiturates and benzodiazepines, they include psychotic symptoms, seizure, and rhabdomyolysis. For opiates, they include diarrhea, dilated pupils, nausea, sneezing, rhinorrhea, vomiting, and yawning. For cocaine and amphetamines, symptoms include depression, dysphoria, excessive sleep, hunger, psychomotor slowing, and sleep disturbances.

Diagnosis

Labs

There are no labs specific to diagnose substance abuse disorder. However, the following may be indicated based on the patient's clinical status:

- ABG to show acidosis, hypoxia, or hypercarbia
- CBC
- CMP to show abnormal electrolytes or altered renal or hepatic functioning, depending on the substance abused
- Toxicology screen

Diagnostic Testing

There are no diagnostic tests specific to diagnose substance abuse. However, the following may be helpful to determine medical conditions as a result of substance toxicity, route of administration, and high-risk behaviors (needle sharing, unprotected sexual encounters, poor hygiene, etc.):

- Screening tools specific to institution, such as the Alcohol Use Disorders Identification Test (AUDIT); the Addiction Severity Index (ASI); the Cut, Annoyed, Guilty, and Eye (CAGE) test; the Clinical Institute Withdrawal Assessment (CIWA); the Clinical Opiate Withdrawal Scale (COWS; and the tolerance, annoyance, cut down, eye opener (T-ACE) questions

Treatment

- Cognitive behavioral therapy
- Comprehensive mental health history
- Consult to psychiatry
- De-escalation techniques as first-line treatment for aggression: active listening, diversionary techniques, limiting external stimuli, and therapeutic communication
- Drug or addiction counseling, as indicated
- Medications as indicated (Table 11.1): antipsychotics provide supportive therapy for behavior changes related to drug or alcohol withdrawal; benzodiazepines assist with alcohol withdrawal; methadone aids in drug withdrawal; naloxone is used for opioid overdose; and thiamine is used for alcohol abuse
- Motivational interviewing/motivational enhancement
- Mutual health and support groups
- Ruling out organic causes for signs and symptoms
- Thorough substance abuse history, physical examination, family history, and review of social factors

Nursing Interventions

- Assess for suicidal or homicidal ideations.
- Administer medications as prescribed by provider to manage symptoms (e.g., anxiety, depression, and insomnia).
- Build a trusting relationship.
- Collaborate with social work to arrange resources at discharge.
- Engage in therapeutic communication. ▶

[🌐]   **NURSING PEARL**

Understanding the timing of the patient's last drink is essential to monitor and treat symptoms of alcohol withdrawal. Typically, patients can experience alcohol withdrawal 24 to 72 hr following their last drink.

[⚡]   **ALERT!**

Mental health issues often accompany addiction. Psychiatry involvement in care is often essential to provide the most comprehensive and holistic care possible.

[📝]   **POP QUIZ 11.3**

What is the time frame in which alcohol withdrawal symptoms typically manifest?

Nursing Interventions (*continued*)

- Frequently assess for symptoms of withdrawal (CIWA) and the potential for seizures; check for nausea or vomiting; check for signs of anxiety; monitor for visual, tactile, or auditory disturbances; look for tremors; and observe for signs of diaphoresis.
- If aggressive, maintain visual and situational awareness of the patient utilizing 1:1 observation, if indicated; facilitate de-escalation of the patient's behavior; and use medical and physical restraints if the patient does not respond to prior interventions and harm to the patient and/or staff is imminent.
- Instruct on measures to decrease/manage addiction and/or anxiety. Refer to online or in-person counseling or treatment options.
- Manage any underlying symptoms.
- Monitor vital signs to identify any hemodynamic changes requiring additional support.
- Notify the provider of new or worsening psychological conditions, including acts of self-harm, anxiety or depression, delusions or hallucinations, irrational or erratic behavior, self-destructive behavior including pulling at lines with intent to remove the lines despite education on importance to leave device intact (e.g., ripping at peripheral IVs, central lines, dialysis lines, and catheters), and verbalization or intent to harm themselves or others.
- Perform frequent physical assessments and a focused psychological assessment.
- Perform frequent screening assessments per institutional protocol.
- Provide a safe environment for the patient by removing any potentially harmful objects from the room.
- Offer nourishment as indicated for the patient's condition. For manic symptoms, feed high-calorie finger foods to meet the body's elevated caloric requirements. For depressive symptoms, encourage PO intake if patient's appetite is decreased. Supplement with nasogastric tube feeding if needed.

Patient Education

- Exercise regularly to help manage symptoms of depression.
- Follow up long term with outpatient providers and appointments to prevent relapse.
- Maintain good sleep hygiene practices.
- Obtain psychosocial support information, such as Alcoholics Anonymous/Narcotics Anonymous (AA/NA) support group resources or cognitive behavioral therapy resources.
- Report any disabling side effects so that medications can be adjusted. Do not stop taking the medications unless advised by provider.
- Take all medications as prescribed, even if symptoms improve.

[📝]   **POP QUIZ 11.4**

A patient with a substance abuse disorder asks the nurse what resources he has for long-term support to stay sober. What resources could the nurse discuss with the patient?

RESOURCES

James, J. (2016). Dealing with drug-seeking behaviour. *Australian Prescriber, 39*(3), 96–100. https://www.ncbi.nlm .nih.gov/pmc/articles/PMC4919169

Jesse, S., Bråthen, G., Ferrara, M., Keindl, M., Ben-Menachem, E., Tanasescu, R., Brodtkorb, E., Hillbom, M., Leone, M. A., & Ludolph, A. C. (2017). Alcohol withdrawal syndrome: Mechanisms, manifestations, and management. *Acta Neurologica Scandinavica, 135*(1), 4–16. https://www.ncbi.nlm.nih.gov/pmc/articles/PMC6084325

National Institute of Mental Health. (2018). *Anxiety disorders*. U.S. Department of Health and Human Services. https://www.nimh.nih.gov/health/topics/anxiety-disorders

Prescribers' Digital Reference. (n.d.-a). *Amitriptyline hydrochloride (amitriptyline hydrochloride)*. PDR Search. https:// www.pdr.net/drug-summary/Amitriptyline-Hydrochloride-amitriptyline-hydrochloride-1001

Prescribers' Digital Reference. (n.d.-b). *Buspirone hydrochloride tablets* [Drug information]. PDR Search. https://www.pdr.net/drug-summary/Buspirone-Hydrochloride-Tablets--USP--7-5-mg-buspirone-hydrochloride-1523#5

Prescribers' Digital Reference. (n.d.-c). *Duloxetine* [Drug information]. PDR Search. https://pdr.net/drug-summary/Cymbalta-duloxetine-288

Prescribers' Digital Reference. (n.d.-d). *Haldol (haloperidol)* [Drug information]. PDR Search. https://www.pdr.net/drug-summary/Haldol-haloperidol-942

Prescribers' Digital Reference. (n.d.-e). *Marplan (isocarboxazid)* [Drug information]. PDR Search. https://www.pdr.net/drug-summary/Marplan-isocarboxazid-1355

Prescribers' Digital Reference. (n.d.-f). *Methadone hydrochloride* [Drug information]. PDR Search. https://www.pdr.net/drug-summary/Dolophine-methadone-hydrochloride-727

Prescribers' Digital Reference. (n.d.-g). *Naloxone hydrochloride* [Drug information]. PDR Search. https://pdr.net/drug-summary/Naloxone-Hydrochloride-Injection--1-mg-mL--naloxone-hydrochloride-23987

Prescribers' Digital Reference. (n.d.-h). *Risperidone* [Drug information]. PDR Search. https://pdr.net/drug-summary/Risperidone-risperidone-3120

Prescribers' Digital Reference. (n.d.-i). *Thiamine (thiamine hydrochloride)* [Drug information]. PDR Search. https://www.pdr.net/drug-summary/Thiamine-thiamine-hydrochloride-2546#13

Prescribers' Digital Reference. (n.d.-j). *Wellbutrin (bupropion hydrochloride)* [Drug information]. PDR Search. https://www.pdr.net/drug-summary/Wellbutrin-bupropion-hydrochloride-237

Prescribers' Digital Reference. (n.d.-k). *Xanax (alprazolam)* [Drug information]. PDR Search. https://www.pdr.net/drug-summary/Xanax-alprazolam-1873#6

Wilber, S. T., & Ondrejka, J. E. (2016). Altered mental status and delirium. *Emergency Medicine Clinics of North America*, *34*(3), 649–665. https://doi.org/10.1016/j.emc.2016.04.012

12 PROFESSIONAL CARING AND ETHICAL PRACTICE

THE SYNERGY MODEL
Overview

- Nursing care should be implemented using the American Association of Critical-Care Nurses' (AACN's) *Synergy Model for Patient Care*. This patient-centered model focuses on the needs of the patient, the competencies of the nurse, and the synergy created when those needs and competencies match. This model ensures that nurses with appropriate ability and competency levels are paired with patients who require these skills and competencies in their care.
- Nursing competencies can evolve with increasing knowledge, skill, experience, and a nurse's desire for change. This includes advocacy and moral agency, caring practices, diversity and the nursing response, learning facilitation, collaboration, systems thinking, and clinical inquiry.
- Following the AACN's *Synergy Model for Patient Care* allows the nurse to provide high-quality professional and ethically appropriate care to any patient.

ADVOCACY AND MORAL AGENCY
Overview

- *Advocacy* is the support of another individual to promote their well-being, such as speaking on behalf of a patient whose voice is not represented. Advocacy is key in the progressive care unit (PCU), as these patients are vulnerable and often need help speaking up on their own behalf. The nurse's continuous presence at the bedside with the patient and family, as well as the ability to collaborate with the other members of the healthcare team, puts them in an ideal position to advocate for the patient.

[🌐] NURSING PEARL

Both advocacy and moral agency are essential aspects to the American Nurses Association's (ANA's) code of ethics. Provision 3 states, "The nurse promotes, advocates for, and protects the rights, health and safety of the patient."

- When the patient's family or nurse advocates on behalf of the patient, the nurse or family communicates the patient's ethical or clinical concerns related to their care, when they cannot. Hospitalization of a close family member may be a stressful and challenging time for families; in these situations, families may feel vulnerable or helpless if the patient cannot participate or if they are unsure of what decisions to make/what the patient would want at certain points in their care (e.g., code status). Families are always encouraged to act as the patient's advocate, similar to the nurse, speaking on their behalf. ▶

Overview (*continued*)

- *Moral agency* is the ability to continue to provide quality care despite obstacles. These obstacles may be physical, emotional, psychologic, or related to the healthcare system or unit status and/or access to resources (staffing, supplies, or technology). Moral agency occurs in the healthcare setting when the nurse helps to resolve potential ethical or clinical conflicts for the patient, regardless of the nurse's personal beliefs. To be an effective advocate and moral agent, the nurse needs to identify the patient's personal beliefs, values, and morals, as well as their own. Overall awareness influences how the nurse cares for their patients and ensures that the nurse is capable of incorporating ethical decision-making into their practice. Accepting differences allows the nurse to identify potential ethical conflicts that may affect their care so that they may advocate on behalf of the patient.

Ethical Principles

Nurses provide safe and compassionate care to the patient by incorporating four ethical principles of nursing into daily practice.

- *Nonmaleficence*: This means taking actions that do not cause harm. Nonmaleficence in nursing occurs when the nurse makes a choice or performs an action that prevents harm. One example of this can occur when holding a medication that may be causing adverse effects, discussing this with the provider, and finding an alternative treatment.
- *Beneficence*: This means taking actions that are in the best interest of the patient, or "doing good." Beneficence in nursing occurs when the nurse makes a choice that is moral and in the best interest of the patient. One example of this occurs when the nurse assists a patient with basic hygiene.
- *Autonomy*: This means respecting a patient and their right to choose. Autonomy in nursing occurs when the nurse supports a patient's choice, regardless of the nurse's personal beliefs. One example of this is accepting a patient's choice to decline blood transfusions for religious reasons with a low hemoglobin.
- *Justice*: This means caring for patients equally; in modern terms, acting in ways to reduce health disparity. Justice in nursing occurs when the nurse provides the same high level of care to all patients. One example of this is providing the same level of care to all patients admitted to the hospital.

Nursing Considerations

To promote advocacy and moral agency, the nurse must:
- Identify and discuss advance directives.
- Identify and support code status wishes.
- Identify and reconfirm goals of care.
- Promote informed decision-making.
- Promote patient and family-centered care.

Advance Directives

- *Advance directives* are legal documents that can be used as a framework to make choices or appoint another to make choices on behalf of the patient. These include the durable power of attorney and living wills. Not all patients need to have advance directives. If a patient wants to develop an advance directive, a social worker or case manager can help them create one during their hospital stay.
- *Durable power of attorney* is a legal document indicating an appointed person who is to make decisions on behalf of the patient and utilized in the event that the patient is unable to make their own decisions.
- A *living will* is a legal document that is written by the patient. This document states the patient's wishes should they find themselves unable to make their own decisions. ▶

Advance Directives (continued)

■ Both advance directives and living wills are typically completed before hospital admission (or critical illness) to verify the legality of the document; however, the patient can create one during a hospital admission. Patients should consult with legal counsel or may fill out a form independently. Notarization of forms ensures that they are legally completed.

Code Status

■ Code status should be identified and documented at the time of admission. If the code status is unknown, and no patient or next of kin is available to determine the code status, assume the patient is a full code.

■ Code status includes the following: *Full code* status indicates that in the event of cardiac or respiratory arrest, the patient has determined that they would like all interventions performed to resuscitate them. This includes CPR, intubation, defibrillation, emergency medication administration, central line insertion, nasogastric and/or orogastric tube (NGT/OGT) insertion, and possible emergency interventional procedure (cardiac catheterization lab, vascular interventional radiology, etc.). *Do not resuscitate (DNR)* orders indicate that in the event of a cardiac or respiratory arrest, the patient has determined that they do *NOT* want any resuscitation protocols or procedures to be performed on them. All other aggressive treatments aside from CPR/advanced cardiac life support (ACLS) protocols will be performed. *Do not intubate (DNI)* orders indicate that in the event of increasing oxygenation requirements or respiratory arrest, the patient does not want to be intubated. All other resuscitation protocols will be administered. *Comfort care* indicates that in the event of cardiac or respiratory arrest, the patient has determined that they want to pass without any aggressive treatment or intervention. This is typically ordered with a DNR but more accurately describes goals of care.

Goals of Care

■ Conversations regarding goals of care should occur at the time of admission to the facility or unit and throughout the hospital stay.

■ To advocate appropriately for the patient, understanding desired goals of care is essential.

■ Follow up and revisit goals of care with the patient as appropriate, especially if dealing with critical or chronic illness. These conversations can be difficult; however, it is important to remain impartial and nonjudgmental during these conversations. By doing this, the patient's autonomy and right to choose is supported.

■ The patient should be aware of their right to choose their treatment path (curative versus hospice/comfort). Curative treatment approaches will include all possible interventions to cure disease or achieve the highest level of functioning possible. Palliative treatment approaches shift the focus from curing to promoting quality of life. This may mean making choices that improve quality of life and comfort but accelerate illness or ultimate demise.

■ Per the patient/family request, consult the palliative and hospice care team to provide more information to the patient and families. *Palliative care* is a branch of specialized medicine that prioritizes optimizing quality of life and alleviating patient suffering. Hospice care and end-of-life care share common goals.

■ End-of-life or comfort care can occur for patients in the PCU setting and often coincides with removal of invasive respiratory or hemodynamic support. While end-of-life care occurs in the inpatient setting, the goals remain consistent with palliative and hospice care to alleviate suffering and allow for a peaceful death. In the inpatient setting, the nurse is responsible for administering continuous intravenous (IV) infusion of analgesic medication (commonly morphine), pushing IV anxiolytics and analgesics for breakthrough pain and anxiety, and preparing to administer an anticholinergic to help alleviate oral secretions and prepare to provide oral care and suctioning as needed. Be mindful of the signs and symptoms of death, which include decreased alertness and mental status, decreased appetite, vital sign changes, increase in respiratory and oral secretions, audible respiratory sounds (commonly referred to as the death rattle), and loss of bowel and urinary control. Communicate with the family to understand their support needs during this time and consult additional services as appropriate.

Informed and Ethical Decision-Making

- While it is the advanced practice provider's role to initiate a "goals of care" conversation with patients and family, the PCU nurse should be mindful and aware of the patient's or family's understanding surrounding the goals of care.
- Similar to the informed consent for procedures, it is the provider's responsibility to explain and review all pertinent information, such as treatment modalities, possible interventions/options, and the variations of goals of care and code status.
- The PCU nurse should be ready to reinforce education provided by the physician and provide additional opportunities for discussion as needed for the patient and family to feel comfortable in their decision. If possible, direct patients and family to community resources or appropriate online community resources to help supplement their understanding.

Patient and Family Rights

- The nurse should be aware of the Patient's Bill of Rights when providing care and advocating for them. Patients have the right to safe, considerate, and respectful care, consistent with their beliefs; confidential communications pertaining to records and plan of care; the opportunity to know and meet their coordinating physician; receive all information and education about their health status presented at their level of medical literacy; have a legally appointed representative when unable to receive information personally; receive informed consent that defines the procedure and identifies risks and alternatives prior to any procedure; obtain routine services during hospitalization, including treatment of any chronic conditions; know appointment times, as well as receive continuity of care; be involved in decisions about the assessment and treatment of pain; refuse to participate in research; transfer facilities pending insurance and clinical status; receive a medical summary at the end of care; and designate other physicians or organizations, at their request, to receive medical updates.
- Families and patients additionally have the right to determine code status; however, they are unable to demand the continuation of CPR if continuing has been determined to be medically futile per the overseeing provider (also known as "calling" the code).

Patient- and Family-Centered Care

- Allow family or friends to visit and stay with the patient if allowed per unit policy and when appropriate.
- Educate the family, as well as the patient, on the situation and any options to consider.
- Establish a family member or friend as a spokesperson who will update the rest of the family on the patient's status.
- Include family in meetings and "goals of care" discussions.

[🌐]   **NURSING PEARL**

The Nursing Alliance for Quality Care identifies these principles to ensure care is patient-centered:

- Patients should have an active partnership with their families as well as their healthcare providers.
- Patients have the right to make their own healthcare decisions.
- Patients, families, and providers need to share responsibility and accountability.
- Healthcare providers must always respect any privacy boundaries and ensure confidentiality.
- Information sharing and decision-making should be mutual.
- Patient engagement varies from patient to patient and may be influenced by culture or other individual elements.
- Patient advocacy is a critical feature of nursing.
- To fully engage with patients, the nurse needs to identify, appreciate, and acknowledge all cultural, racial, or ethnic backgrounds.
- It is essential to identify and individualize healthcare plans according to the patient's and family's educational, language, and literacy needs to ensure full comprehension.

CARING IN NURSING PRACTICE

Overview

- Theoretical knowledge alone is not enough to function effectively in the nursing profession.
- Caring is the central and most defining concept of nursing. Caring should be patient-centered to ensure the best outcomes for the patient.
- Though caring is not specifically addressed in the nursing code of ethics, it is integrated within each principle of the code.
- Caring in nursing practice promotes patient safety, comfort, and a compassionate, therapeutic, and supportive environment for patients, family, and other staff members. *Commitment* ensures that patients' rights and safety are at the forefront of decision-making and care delivery. *Communication* ensures that effective open communication is maintained to place the patients' needs and rights at the forefront of decision-making. *Compassion* ensures patients are treated well and provided with a positive supportive experience. *Competence* ensures that the nurse is held to a high standard of excellence and meets all legal, regulatory, and practice standards to provide quality care. *Conscience* ensures the best moral decision is made even when faced with challenges

ALERT!

The nurse's engagement with the patient is essential to ensure the safest and highest quality care is being delivered.

Nursing Considerations

- Nursing responsibilities to ensure patient safety include engagement, responsiveness, and vigilance.
- These characteristics promote a therapeutic and supportive environment, as well as promoting compassionate patient care: *Engagement* is the ability of the nurse to empower the patient to be involved in their own care and make informed decisions regarding their own health and healthcare. *Responsiveness* is the ability of the nurse to provide patient care that is respectful to the patient and addresses all their concerns. *Vigilance* is the ability of the nurse to identify any potential risks to the patient or signs of clinical deterioration and the ability to act in response to a change in condition.

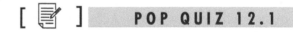

POP QUIZ 12.1

A nurse is caring for a 60-year-old male patient with a history of congestive heart failure (CHF), coronary artery disease (CAD), peripheral arterial disease (PAD), and type 2 diabetes mellitus (T2DM) who is requiring surgery for a coronary artery bypass grafting (CABG) the next day. The patient has been very anxious since hearing the news that he needs surgery. His wife has stayed with him to help alleviate his anxiety until visiting hr ended. The cardiovascular surgeon has come to obtain consent for the surgery; however, the patient is experiencing increased anxiety that his wife is not here for this conversation. How can the nurse effectively advocate for this patient?

Patient Safety

- Use precautions specific to the patient's needs to maintain safety (e.g., aspiration precautions, fall precautions, pressure ulcer precautions, seizure precautions, suicidal ideation precautions).
- Communicate these precautions to other members of the healthcare team to ensure they are maintaining the safety of the patient, especially if the patient is traveling to other areas of the hospital.
- Explain these precautions to the patient and family to include them in maintaining a safe environment.
- Update the patient's plan of care to reflect these precautions as their condition changes. Some patients may not need these precautions on admission but require them later in their care as their condition changes or vice versa.

Minimize Risk of Medical Errors

- Always use the five rights of medication administration: right patient, right drug, right dose, right route, and right time.
- Clarify orders with the physician or pharmacist if unsure or unfamiliar with order. For verbal orders, ask the physician to repeat or spell out the order to ensure it is correct. Limit distractions while taking orders.
- Practice good communication with all members of the healthcare team: active listening, documentation, and verbal communication.
- Utilize hospital policies and protocols to ensure accurate patient care.

Engagement

- It is important to build a therapeutic relationship with the patient and family in order to be able to engage with them at the fullest potential. Maintain an active and ongoing partnership with the patient and family by continually looking for social and nonsocial cues and careful assessment of the relationships throughout their care. Maintain an empathetic viewpoint of the patient and be careful to monitor the situation from their perspective. Support the patient as they learn to empower themselves. Offer emotional and mental presence as well as physical presence to build a therapeutic relationship with the patient. Be aware of cultural disparities and integrate cultural differences into practice. Maintain mutuality with the patient, which is essential for shared decision-making. Work with the patient, not just on behalf of the patient. Preserve patient dignity whenever possible. Actively listen to the patient. Be aware of the patient's educational needs and anticipate if resources are needed to assist the patient to fully understand their plan of care.
- Inspire the patient to become engaged in their own treatment once a therapeutic relationship has been established.
- Empower the patient to assume responsibility and accountability for actions that will improve their health and their care.
- Ensure that the patient and family are being heard and engaging in their care.

[⚡]　　　　**ALERT!**

Although it is important to build a therapeutic relationship with a patient, remember to maintain and respect privacy boundaries and confidentiality. It is also important for the nurse to take a step back when appropriate.

Responsiveness

Generally, the more responsive the nurse is to a patient, the more engaging the patient will be in their plan of care.

- Use a more flexible and responsive approach that is individualized to the needs of the specific patient population.
- Be available to respond to nonclinical needs or preferences.
- Ensure the patient can easily contact healthcare providers, utilizing new technology if desired.
- Adjust care as needed depending on specific groups of patients to fit their needs.
- Show integrity with patients and families.
- Maintain hourly rounding to ensure presence.

Vigilance

- Vigilance begins with a thorough patient physical, psychosocial, and environmental assessment.
- A vigilant assessment includes the following: Use clinical knowledge to anticipate the patient's physical examination depending on their condition. Compare knowledge of the condition to the patient's presenting symptoms. Anticipate what potential complications could arise with the patient depending on their condition. Identify what these complications would look like clinically, what changes to monitor for, and jump into action if these complications occur. Identify what interventions would be needed for ▶

Vigilance (continued)

treatment of the condition and any potential complications. Outweigh the risks and benefits of interventions for the patient. Recognize how the patient should respond to interventions. Ensure any potential patient changes are being accurately documented and reported to the healthcare team as necessary.

[SYNERGY EXAMPLE]

The nurse is providing care to a 24-year-old male patient in the PCU who was admitted for injuries resulting from a motor vehicle collision (MVC). The patient is now paralyzed from L2 down. The patient appears depressed, will not participate in therapy, and does not communicate with staff. The nurse who provides caring practice attempts to build a therapeutic relationship with the patient by addressing him as an individual and not by his injury. The nurse asks the patient about his likes, dislikes, friends, family, what interests him, and so forth, to help build a mutual relationship. Once a relationship has been built, the nurse also helps to identify short-term goals for the patient to help him participate in therapy and utilize his interests to motivate him. As the patient progresses through therapy, the nurse should ensure his safety precautions and goals are addressed as well.

DIVERSITY AND THE NURSING RESPONSE

Overview

- Respecting and valuing all patients is core to the nursing profession.
- Nurses are called on to respond with sensitivity and quality care to all patients, regardless of race, disability, socioeconomic status, religion, age, or sexual orientation.
- Knowledge of diversity and various cultural practices or values is essential to provide patient-centered care and to appropriately advocate and represent patients.
- Diversity in nursing ensures that all patients feel welcome and that they receive the care they deserve.

Nursing Considerations

- The PCU nurse should be familiar with the practices and cultures of the populations in their geographic area.
- Do not assume that the patient and/or family has the same values or beliefs: Get to know the patient on a personal level to identify any differences, explore these differences with the patient and their family, ask questions regarding any differences to improve understanding, and accept the information provided by the patient and family and modify the plan of care to fit their needs while still ensuring patient safety.
- Eliminate health disparities that may affect the patient, such as cultural, racial, and ethnic differences; mental status barriers; and socioeconomic disparities.
- Identify, respect, and address any differences in patients' values, preferences, or needs.

Age
- Use language that is appropriate for the patient's age group.
- Modify nursing care as needed to ensure it is appropriate for the patient.
- Utilize technology as a resource for the patient. Take into consideration that older adults may be less technologically inclined.

Culture

- Ensure the ordered diet meets what the patient needs nutritionally as well as maintains their cultural or religious beliefs.
- Remain open minded and respectful of cultural or religious practices. Allow cultural or religious practices that do not compromise patient or staff wellness or safety. For practices that may compromise patient or staff safety (lighting candles or opening windows), collaborate with the patient and family to identify alternative and acceptable solutions.
- Some cultures may use essential oils, lotions, teas, or medicinal herbs for healing purposes. Before allowing the patient or family to use these, ensure they do not have any potential interactions with any current medications.

Education

- Ensure communication to patients and families is at a level everyone can understand and fully comprehend.
- Utilize different techniques to educate patients, as everyone learns differently: handouts, verbal explanation, videos, and demonstration.

Ethnicity

- Ask the patient or family if there are any ethnic considerations that need to be considered while they are in the hospital.
- Be aware of certain risk factors and health conditions that may affect specific ethnicities more than others. For example, a disproportionate number of African American males are diagnosed with hypertension (HTN) when compared to the general population.
- Provide education or resources specific to the patient's and family's ethnic background if necessary.
- Identify any potential language barriers and make necessary accommodations to ensure accurate communication. Utilize medical interpreting services as needed.

Gender

- Respect privacy and boundaries as defined by the patient while still providing competent and safe care.
- Ask transitioning patients what name and pronouns they prefer and inform all essential members of the healthcare team.

Lifestyle

- Lifestyle choices can range from diet and exercise regimen to personal lifestyle choices such as sexual behaviors and use of illegal substances.
- Ask the patient about their lifestyle choices.
- If any poor choice is noted (alcohol, drug, tobacco, obesity, sedentary lifestyle, etc.) provide education and supportive resources to make lasting change.

Spirituality and Religious Beliefs

- Advocate from patient/family perspective, whether similar to or different from personal values.
- Ask the patient about their religion and if there are any special considerations that need to be taken while they are admitted.
- Allow the patient and family time to pray, openly practice their religion, or reflect depending on their religious needs as possible while following institutional guidelines and maintaining patient care.
- Allow religious objects in the room if requested.
- Support visitation with religious leader if requested while abiding by unit and institutional visitor policies.
- Consult chaplain services if requested by the patient or family to perform a prayer, last rites, and so forth.
- Support religious customs throughout patient's hospital stay.

Socioeconomics

- Ensure social work is consulted if necessary to follow up with discharge planning.
- Provide community resources to patients including outpatient exercise or diet programs, community food bank or donation centers, assistance with transportation, and/or securing medical devices or medication.

Values

- Identify what values are important to the patient and integrate them into their hospital care.
- If the patient's values pose a safety concern, collaborate with the patient, providers, and leadership to find an alternative solution that meets patient needs and maintains safety.

[ ]   **POP QUIZ 12.2**

The nurse is caring for a 72-year-old female of Chinese descent. She is day three post-op, recovering from an MVC where she required surgical repair of her right hip. The family arrives to visit, bringing her favorite foods, pictures from home, and a variety of medicinal healing herbs to assist with her recovery. What should the nurse's response be when the patient asks if she can take the herbal treatments brought from home?

[**SYNERGY EXAMPLE**]

The nurse is providing care to a 67-year-old male Muslim patient admitted for a cerebrovascular accident (CVA) post tissue plasminogen activator (TPA). The patient is improving and ready for transfer to the step-down unit. The staff is getting ready to transfer the patient at noon; however, the patient is requesting to wait as this is his time for prayer according to the Muslim religion. The nurse appropriately responds to diversity by accepting and accommodating the patient's beliefs, even though the nurse does not practice that same religion, and allows the transfer to wait until the patient has finished his prayers. The nurse communicates this to the other staff and provides the patient with privacy while he is praying.

FACILITATION OF LEARNING

Overview

- A key component of nursing care is the ability to facilitate learning between patients, families, nursing and other healthcare staff, and the community.
- Nurses can facilitate learning by engaging the patient in active learning, identifying any barriers to learning, and incorporating methods to overcome those barriers.
- Barriers to learning for patients may be cognitive, emotional, or psychosocial. These barriers must be identified and addressed before a patient is willing and able to receive new information.
- In addition to patient education, a large component of facilitation of learning applies to nurses educating other nurses in the field. This includes nurse preceptors and nursing educators providing education to new graduate nurses, new hires, or student nurses.

Nursing Considerations

- Both patients and new nurses use similar education concepts to facilitate learning: Adapt educational programs to fit the needs of the patient and family; work with the learner to set educational goals; coach and explain to patients and families at a level they will comprehend; support the ideas of the new learner and allow them to think of alternatives while offering feedback as needed; share information for the new learner to make an informed decision, rather than directing them to the answer; validate the experiences ►

Nursing Considerations (*continued*)

of the patient and/or student nurse; allow ample time for questions; identify what is most important to the patient and refocus their attention onto those things if they are overwhelmed; collaborate with other healthcare providers to incorporate the patient's goals; use creative ways to integrate education into patient care while providing evidence-based practice; use the teach-back method to verify learning has occurred; address barriers to learning and ways to overcome obstacles; and engage the learner in various ways.

■ Preceptors should also consider the following when teaching: Share stories—preceptors can share their experiences and passion for nursing to establish a relationship, as well as discuss how they faced and overcame the same challenges and fears. Assess clinical competency—new nurses may be fearful of making decisions independently; as a preceptor, give them tasks that allow them to develop clinical judgment skills while acting as a resource and standing by to prevent errors. Be an effective communicator. Allow time for reflection at the end of the shift. Be patient and understanding when learning new tasks or procedures. Have clear expectations and provide independent learning experiences—watching or shadowing cannot replace hands-on experience.

[SYNERGY EXAMPLE]

The nurse is caring for a patient with a new diagnosis of T2DM and needs to educate him and his wife on how to monitor blood glucose at home. As a competent facilitator of learning, the nurse knows that people learn in different ways. The nurse decides to provide educational pamphlets, videos, and online resources for the patient and his wife. The nurse also demonstrates to the patient and his wife how to use the glucometer to check blood glucose and how to draw up and inject insulin.

To further facilitate his learning, the nurse watches the patient check his blood glucose using his new glucometer while providing feedback. The nurse informs the patient care technician that the patient should be checking his own blood glucose from now on. Collaborate with the assistant to ensure the patient is performing this correctly and asking staff any questions he may have.

COLLABORATION

Overview

■ In healthcare, *collaboration* is defined as the ability to work with others toward the same common goal. It is essential in critical care. Collaboration requires all members of the healthcare team to work together, sharing responsibility for problem-solving and decision-making. It also requires active listening, effective communication, trust, and a sharing of ideas between all stakeholders (patients, families, and the medical care team).

■ Collaboration occurs among all professionals and leaders in the healthcare team, patients, and family. Taking care of critically ill patients utilizes staff from all fields, such as physicians, psychologists, pharmacists, respiratory therapists, occupational therapists, physical therapists, registered dieticians, physician assistants, nurse practitioners, and certified technicians. Many critically ill patients have diseases and medical problems that affect multiple body systems. This may require physicians from all levels and specialties, working together to ensure the health and well-being of the patient. ▶

Overview (*continued*)

■ The nurse is instrumental in promoting collaboration between different members of the healthcare team to eliminate potential knowledge gaps, facilitating information sharing and decision-making, and identifying any barriers to the health and safety of the patient.

Nursing Considerations

■ Collaboration cannot effectively take place without open communication between the patient, family, and interdisciplinary staff. Effective communication occurs when the healthcare team, who may have different backgrounds, experience, education levels, skill levels, or specialties, can discuss information, ideas, and opinions openly with one another. Participation in daily rounds with the healthcare team promotes collaboration across all skill levels. It also provides focused communication about the patient's treatment plan.

■ At the core of collaboration is also trust. Trust needs to be evident in the relationships between team members (how work is done, how words are spoken, and how the results are accounted for). Without trust, collaboration can fall apart quickly. In order to work together to effectively care for the patient, the nurse needs to trust the skills, knowledge, and training of the interdisciplinary team. This is especially important in high-stress patient situations, as well as for basic nursing tasks, such as helping with patient bathing or turns, covering for each other during lunch, and answering each other's questions. Team learning involves everyone working together toward one common goal and improving patient care using best practice evidence.

■ Collaborative leadership allows members of a leadership team to work together to make decisions to keep the unit thriving. This style of leadership among charge nurses, preceptors, assistant nurse managers, and unit managers offers an environment of openness, trust, and comfort, which in turn allows nurses to freely share different perspectives, voices, opinions, and ideas. This is a necessary step for innovation.

[📝]   **POP QUIZ 12.3**

A patient has vocalized feelings of sadness and depression that have worsened throughout their critical illness. Though the patient's clinical status has improved, they still require 35% oxygen via trach collar during the day and ventilator support overnight. Therefore, they are unable to be transferred to the PCU per this hospital's policy. Family and staff have tried engaging to improve the patient's mood, but nothing has made real change. The nurse asks the patient if they would like to go on a "field trip" to see something other than her hospital room and unit. The patient is excited by this and asks when they can go.

Before taking this patient off the unit, what collaborative actions must the nurse take?

[SYNERGY EXAMPLE]

Interdisciplinary rounding is a good example of collaboration between health disciplines. During interdisciplinary rounding, while each institution may have their own protocol for the flow and order, generally the medical doctor (MD), nurse practitioner (NP), and/or physician assistant (PA) gives a brief overview of the patient's history and physical and then reviews the events of hospital admission. Nursing presents the overnight or daily events and brings up new issues or concerns to the team. Pharmacy reviews medications, dosages, and labs to ensure medications are still appropriate for the clinical condition, while the dietician reviews diet orders, weight gain or loss, and tube feeding composition, if applicable. When new issues arise, they are discussed together, considering all angles and points of view before moving forward with new interventions. This process allows the patient to receive high-quality collaborative care.

SYSTEMS THINKING

Overview

- Systems thinking takes into consideration the entire healthcare system's process while providing care for patients.

- It is a holistic approach to advancing healthcare or identifying problems on a global or large system scale. This includes understanding the patient or whole person within a system, public domain, regional health trends (e.g., increased incidence of diabetes in southern states, regional vaccination rates), national health data (e.g., increased incidence of childhood obesity), and world or global health (e.g., increase access to OB/GYN or midwifery care in all nations).

- Systems thinking can be applied to providing care for patients, discharge planning, policy creation, and root cause analysis of adverse or sentinel events.

Nursing Considerations

- To be a systems thinker, nurses must consider unintended consequences, fully consider issues while taking the systems functioning into consideration, identify cause and effect relationships within the system, make meaningful connections between aspects of the system, observe how aspects of a system change over time, note patterns and trends within these changes, recognize and understand that a systems structure generates behavior, and seek to understand the big picture.

- When using systems thinking to identify root cause, the nurse must first identify the problem, identify involved parties, collect data from charting and/or interviewing, determine factors which could lead to problems, identify solutions and/or corrective actions to causative factors, implement solutions, and identify other areas where this solution could be implemented.

[SYNERGY EXAMPLE]

A CT scan was completed on a patient over 12 hr after the order was placed, leading to a delay in treatment. A member of the quality control committee performed a root cause analysis to identify the cause of the delay in care. The involved parties include the patient, the family, the assigned nurse, and the providers. After a chart review, additional information was identified. The order was placed at the change of shift, and the oncoming nurse admitted a new patient. Once the order was recognized by the nurse a few hr later, transport was called. However, transportation logs showed over an hr delay. Additionally, CT had to delay this patient's scan because they were overloaded with emergent scans from the emergency department. The investigating nurse identified that a challenging patient assignment, paired with transport delays, and an increased acuity in the emergency department resulted in a delayed scan. A possible solution includes the physician changing the order of the scan from "routine" to "STAT," to prioritize this patient's scan. Also, the CT technician can call the nurse to plan a scheduled time for both the CT scan and transportation.

CLINICAL INQUIRY

Overview

- Clinical inquiry is the process of questioning and evaluating practice to advance evidence-based and informed practice. ▶

Overview (*continued*)

- It involves the continual progression of nursing care through questioning and evaluating healthcare practice.
- The nurse can create effective change by practicing evidence-based practice, conducting research, and implementing experiential knowledge.
- The goal is to stay up to date with the most recent professional literature and share this information with others.

Nursing Considerations

The PCU nurse should be familiar with the best practice by engaging in clinical inquiry. This can be performed by doing the following:

- Review and compare research/literature findings to current practice and engage in evidence-based practice or quality improvement projects. This can be done independently or in collaboration with an individual mentor, a like-minded group, or a unit committee. If a research or best practice committee exists within the unit or hospital, consider joining to routinely engage in research or literature findings to identify current best practice. If the unit or hospital does not currently have a research or evidence-based practice committee, speak with unit leadership about possibly starting one.
- Gather knowledge. This can be done by basic internet searches or through rigorous searching of nursing journals or databases.
- Conduct unit-specific research. Consider collaborating with unit leadership or a best practice committee to conduct unit-specific research to identify possible improvements to policy, procedure, or the care process. Quality improvement projects involve live monitoring and evaluation of the quality of services provided to patients. Shortcomings and solutions are identified and then tested through additional data collection. Evidence-based practice (EBP) studies are more scholarly experiences focused on literature and research review. Once EBP procedures are identified, they are then implemented into unit practice and procedures and monitored for outcomes.
- Advocate for practice changes to align with research-based practice recommendations. Be observant of the policies, procedures, or care processes that could be improved or made more efficient. Identify and discuss findings to unit leadership and/or providers to create meaningful change.
- Share findings with the unit leadership, nurse educator, clinical nurse specialist, and staff as appropriate. Present findings as appropriate through presentations at unit meetings, emails, or hand-outs posted throughout the breakroom or nursing station. Continue disseminating this information until meaningful and positive change is achieved.

[SYNERGY EXAMPLE]

During a monthly article review, the nurse learns that chlorhexidine-impregnated dressings can reduce central line-associated bloodstream infections (CLABSIs) and increase cost effectiveness in the healthcare setting. During the last unit meeting, the nurse educator described the increased rates of patients with CLABSIs in the hospital. The nurse advocates for an increase in the supply of chlorhexidine central line dressings and disinfecting caps for the needleless connectors on the IV tubing. The nurse educates other nurses on the unit to keep the sterile dressing clean, dry, and occlusive, and to change the dressing every 7 days or when soiled.

RESOURCES

Albert, T. (2019). *Why you need to be a systems thinker in health care*. American Medical Association. https://www
.ama-assn.org/education/accelerating-change-medical-education/why-you-need-be-systems-thinker-health-care

American Nurses Association. (2015). *Code of ethics for nurses with interpretive statements*. https://www
.nursingworld.org/coe-view-only

Chan, T. W., Poon, E., & Hegney, D. (2011). What nurses need to know about Buddhist perspectives of end-of-life
care. *Progress in Palliative Care*, *19*, 61–65. https://doi.org/10.1179/1743291X10Y.0000000010

Epstein, B., & Turner, M. (2015). The nursing code of ethics: Its value, its history. *Online Journal of Issues in Nursing*,
20(2), Manuscript 4. https://doi.org/10.3912/OJIN.Vol20No02Man04

Ervin, J. N., Kahn, J. M., Cohen, T. R., & Weingart, L. R. (2018). Teamwork in the intensive care unit. *The American
Psychologist*, *73*(4), 468–477. https://www.ncbi.nlm.nih.gov/pmc/articles/PMC6662208

Gaines, K. (2021). What is the nursing code of ethics? *Nurse.org*. https://nurse.org/education/nursing-code-of
-ethics

Gaylord, N., & Grace, P. (1995). Nursing advocacy: An ethic of practice. *Nursing Ethics*, *2*(1), 11–18. https://doi
.org/10.1177/096973309500200103

Grace, P. (2018). Enhancing nurse moral agency: The leadership promise of doctor of nursing practice preparation.
The Online Journal of Issues in Nursing, *23*(1), Manuscript 4. https://doi.org/10.3912/OJIN.Vol23No01Man04

Hardin, S. R., & Kaplow, R. (2016). *Synergy for clinical excellence: The AACN synergy model for patient care*. American
Association of Critical-Care Nurses.

Institute for Patient- and Family-Centered Care. (n.d.). *Patient- and family-centered care. What is PFCC?* https://www
.ipfcc.org/about/pfcc.html

Meyer, G., & Lavin, M. A. (2005). Vigilance: The essence of nursing. *Online Journal of Issues in Nursing*, *10*(3), 8.
https://doi.org/10.3912/OJIN.Vol10No03PPT01

Mick, J. (2017). Funneling evidence into practice. *Nursingcenter.com*. https://www.nursingcenter.com/wkhlrp/
Handlers/articleContent.pdf?key=pdf_00006247-201707000-00009

NIH Clinical Center. (n.d.). *Patient bill of rights*. U.S. Department of Health and Human Services. https://
clinicalcenter.nih.gov/participate/patientinfo/legal/bill_of_rights.html

O'Daniel, M. (2008). Professional communication and team collaboration. In R. G. Hughes (Ed.), *Patient safety and
quality: An evidence-based handbook for nurses*. Agency for Healthcare Research and Quality. https://www.ncbi
.nlm.nih.gov/books/NBK2637/#:~:text=Collaboration%20in%20health%20care%20is,out%20plans%20for
%20patient%20care

Six Sigma. (2017, March 10). *Root cause analysis (RCAa) – Important steps*. https://www.6sigma.us/etc/root-cause
-analysis-important-steps

Tarrant, C., Angell, E., Baker, R., Boulton, M., Freeman, G., Wilkie, P., Jackson, P., Wobi, F., & Ketley, D. (2014).
Responsiveness of primary care services: Development of a patient-report measure – qualitative study and
initial quantitative pilot testing. *Health Services and Delivery Research*, *2*(46). https://www.ncbi.nlm.nih
.gov/books/NBK263682

Welch, J., & Fournier, A. (2018). Patient engagement through informed nurse caring. *International Journal for Human
Caring*, *22*(1), 1–10. https://doi.org/10.20467/1091-5710.22.1.pg5

13 PRACTICE TEST QUESTIONS

1. The nurse is caring for a patient who has overdosed. The patient has a heart rate of 44 BPM and a blood pressure of 90/50 mmHg. The patient is dizzy and having difficulty breathing. Which of the following drugs caused the overdose?
   A. Acetaminophen
   B. Fentanyl
   C. Metoprolol
   D. Carbon monoxide

2. Which electrolyte abnormality is commonly seen in patients with a kidney injury?
   A. Hypokalemia
   B. Hypophosphatemia
   C. Hypocalcemia
   D. Hypernatremia

3. While reviewing a patient's hemodynamic profile when monitoring digitalis levels, which value would the nurse note as abnormal?
   A. Central venous pressure of 6
   B. Stroke index of 50 mL/m2/beat
   C. Pulmonary artery pressure of 25/10
   D. Mean arterial pressure of 105 mmHg

4. Which diagnostic test is most useful to evaluate heart failure?
   A. MRI
   B. Chest x-ray
   C. 2D echocardiogram
   D. 12-lead echocardiogram

5. Which of the following mandates the scope of practice and behaviors of professional nurses?
   A. The National Council of State Boards of Nursing
   B. The Nurses Bill of Rights
   C. The Nurse Practice Act of the state in which the nurse practices
   D. The American Nurses Association

6. Which hemodynamic change will occur with mitral stenosis?
   A. Tachycardia
   B. Exaggerated A waves
   C. Decreased cardiac output
   D. Large V wave pulmonary artery occlusive pressure tracing

7. The nurse has a patient in first-degree atrioventricular block. Which treatment is used for this arrhythmia?
   A. Intravenous adenosine
   B. Transcutaneous pacing
   C. No treatment is required
   D. Synchronized electrical cardioversion

8. A patient is having an anaphylactic reaction. The provider orders epinephrine to be administered. Which dose would the nurse prepare?
   A. 1:1,000 dilution 0.2 to 0.5 mg
   B. 1:10,000 dilution 0.2 to 0.5 mg
   C. 1:1,000 dilution 0.5 to 0.9 mg
   D. 1:10,000 dilution 0.5 to 0.9 mg

9. Which of the following situations would require the enactment of a patient's durable power of attorney for healthcare?
   A. The patient is having a surgical procedure that requires anesthesia.
   B. The patient cannot afford to pay healthcare bills.
   C. The patient has a stroke and is on life support.
   D. The patient is being cared for by an adult child.

10. Which intervention will the nurse implement first for a patient with suspected endocarditis?
    A. Assess need for antiplatelet therapy.
    B. Initiate anticoagulant therapy.
    C. Remove infected implanted devices.
    D. Start effective antimicrobial therapy.

11. Which of the following measures is most effective in preventing aspiration of tube feeding in an unconscious, mechanically ventilated patient?
    A. Frequent, scrupulous mouth care
    B. Blue food coloring in the feeding solution
    C. Patient positioned on the left side
    D. Head of the bed elevated 30 to 45 degrees, unless contraindicated

12. A 57-year-old male patient has a low hemoglobin due to slow gastrointestinal bleeding. The patient's medical history includes diabetes and congestive heart failure. The patient's last set of vital signs were temperature of 98.3°F (36.8°C), heart rate of 75 BPM, respiratory rate of 36 BPM, and SpO$_2$ of 94% on 2 L/NC. The patient has slight crackles in the bases and chest x-ray is consistent with mild pulmonary edema. Hemoglobin has been steady at 9 for the past 24 hours. Which intervention should the nurse prepare?
    A. Metoprolol IV
    B. 100% O$_2$ via face mask
    C. Dobutamine infusion
    D. Diltiazem IV infusion

13. The nurse has a patient who is a fall risk. The patient has tried to get out of bed unassisted three times during the nurse's shift. The nurse should:
    A. Restrain the patient
    B. Continue to monitor the patient every 4 hours
    C. Administer a sedative
    D. Remind the patient of their risk of falls and ask them to not get out of bed again

14. A patient is admitted with a new myocardial injury. How often would the nurse draw cardiac enzymes?
    A. Every 2 hours
    B. Every 4 hours
    C. Every 6 hours
    D. Every 8 hours

15. The physician orders blood cultures on a patient with suspected endocarditis. Which method would the nurse use to obtain the cultures?
    A. Administer antibiotics and obtain one culture from one venipuncture site.
    B. Administer antibiotics and obtain two cultures from two venipuncture sites.
    C. Wait to start antibiotics and obtain one culture from one venipuncture sites.
    D. Wait to start antibiotics and obtain two cultures from two venipuncture sites.

16. Which nursing action constitutes the conditions of malpractice?
    A. The nurse fails to assess and monitor a patient receiving a blood transfusion and a reaction occurs.
    B. The nurse attempts an intravenous line start and misses the vein.
    C. The nurse lowers the bed and places the side rails up per policy, but the patient climbs over the rails and falls to the floor.
    D. The nurse places a "nothing by mouth" sign on a patient's door, but the patient obtains food from a visitor.

17. When assessing if a procedural risk to a patient is justified, the ethical principle underlying the dilemma is known as what?
    A. Justice
    B. Beneficence
    C. Self-determination
    D. Nonmaleficence

18. Which patient situation would prompt the nurse to activate the rapid response team?
    A. Blood pressure of 202/110 mmHg
    B. Patient complains of sudden, severe headache
    C. Sudden change in alertness of a patient
    D. Patient vomiting coffee ground emesis

19. Which factors are considered when assessing stroke volume?
    A. Contractility, preload, and afterload
    B. Compliance, impedance, and heart rate
    C. Blood volume, viscosity, and impedance
    D. Cardiac output, heart rate, and compliance

20. Which process describes the mode of action of famotidine in patients at risk for upper gastrointestinal bleed?
    A. Famotidine is an H2 blocker and reduces acidic secretions.
    B. Famotidine stimulates the release of gastrin.
    C. Famotidine protects the mucosal barrier by coating the barrier.
    D. Famotidine lowers esophageal sphincter pressure.

21. An insulin-dependent diabetic complains of nervousness and appears confused. One hour earlier, the patient had a blood glucose level of 240 and received 4 units of insulin lispro. Which priority intervention should the nurse perform?
    A. Administer a rapid-acting carbohydrate.
    B. Ask the patient about recent food intake.
    C. Give the patient a sandwich with meat.
    D. Draw a stat blood glucose test.

22. A patient with a history of diabetes has serum ketones and a serum glucose level above 300 mg/dL. Which condition is characterized by these findings?
    A. Diabetes insipidus
    B. Diabetic ketoacidosis
    C. Hypoglycemia
    D. Somogyi phenomenon

23. The nurse is caring for a patient following an exacerbation of his chronic obstructive pulmonary disease (COPD). The nurse is educating the patient on how to use pursed lip breathing. Which correctly describes how pursed lip breathing assists a patient with COPD?
    A. Pursed lip breathing increases carbon dioxide, which stimulates breathing.
    B. Pursed lip breathing decreases the amount of air trapping and resistance.
    C. Pursed lip breathing helps to liquefy secretions.
    D. Pursed lip breathing prolongs inspiration and shortens expiration.

24. A bounding pulse is indicative of which condition?
   A. Septic shock
   B. Hypovolemia
   C. Pericardial tamponade
   D. Hypertrophic cardiomyopathy

25. A nurse calls out from a room in which a patient has a cardiac monitor, yelling that the patient has no pulse and to bring a defibrillator immediately. Which arrhythmia is the patient MOST LIKELY experiencing?
   A. Atrial fibrillation
   B. Ventricular fibrillation
   C. Asystole
   D. Pulseless electrical activity

26. A 44-year-old patient is admitted to the step-down unit following a left lateral thoracotomy. The patient has a history of substance abuse but has been sober for 14 years. The patient is in a great deal of pain. Which postoperative pain management orders would the nurse anticipate?
   A. Pain medication prescribed for different levels of pain
   B. Acetaminophen only
   C. Patient-controlled analgesia
   D. Anti-inflammatory medications for severe pain

27. The nurse is caring for a patient who is experiencing an anaphylactic reaction. Which drug will the nurse administer for initial intervention?
   A. Diphenhydramine
   B. Prednisone
   C. Epinephrine
   D. Normal saline

28. The nurse is asking an experienced colleague about the unit's dressing change guidelines and what has been done in the past. This nurse is practicing which nursing dimension of the American Association of Critical-Care Nurses Synergy Model?
   A. Collaboration
   B. Clinical inquiry
   C. Systems thinking
   D. Clinical judgment

29. A patient with a severe traumatic brain injury patient has very limited use of his left side, cannot speak, and is currently relying on a ventilator for minimal respiratory support. What is this patient's level of resiliency?
   A. The patient's resiliency cannot be determined at this time and will need to be reassessed.
   B. The patient has very low resiliency.
   C. The patient has moderate resiliency.
   D. The patient has high resiliency.

30. Which of the following is an important cultural consideration when caring for a patient who is Chinese?
   A. Body language is important.
   B. Patient may not disagree with others in public.
   C. Excessive eye contact indicates rudeness.
   D. An upturned palm is considered offensive in communication.

31. The nurse is caring for a patient who has acute respiratory distress syndrome. Which intervention would be included in the plan of care?
   A. Administer low-flow oxygen continuously via nasal cannula.
   B. Encourage oral intake of at least 3,000 mL of fluids per day.
   C. Offer high-protein and high-carbohydrate foods frequently.
   D. Place in a prone position.

32. Which of the following blood pressure measurements would be considered a hypertensive crisis?
   A. 140/90 mmHg
   B. 185/115 mmHg
   C. 160/100 mmHg
   D. 200/100 mmHg

33. The nurse is treating a patient with Stage 4 breast cancer. The patient has two adolescent daughters and fears that they are predisposed to the same diagnosis. Which action by the nurse is appropriate when providing care to this patient and family?
   A. The nurse provides information about genetic counseling.
   B. The nurse assures the patient that her daughters are not at increased risk of cancer.
   C. The nurse informs the patient that stress will hinder treatment progress.
   D. The nurse asks a chaplain to visit with the family.

34. Following abdominal surgery, a patient develops stridor and hypoxia despite vigorous respiratory effort. The nurse requests a chest x-ray to confirm which complication?
   A. Pneumothorax
   B. Pulmonary edema
   C. Diffuse atelectasis
   D. Pulmonary embolism

35. The nurse has a patient admitted for hypertensive emergency. Which of the following is an important goal when caring for this patient?
   A. Provide weight loss and nutritional counseling.
   B. Reduce blood pressure in increments of 10% to 20% over the course of several hours.
   C. Start oral antihypertensive medication after administering bolus IV fluids.
   D. Return patient's blood pressure to within normal range within the first hour.

36. The nurse is monitoring a patient who was recently admitted to a step-down unit following a cardiac catheterization. Which of the following orders is the nurse's priority?
   A. Assess heart rate.
   B. Assess urinary output.
   C. Assess pulses distal to insertion site.
   D. Assess pulses proximal to insertion site.

37. The nurse has given dobutamine and fluids to a patient in cardiogenic shock with hypotension. The hypotension has not improved, and the patient is still unstable. Which medication would the nurse administer next?
   A. Dopamine
   B. Nitroglycerin
   C. Norepinephrine
   D. Sodium nitroprusside

38. A nurse unintentionally commits a dietary error which necessitates the cancellation of a scheduled test for the patient. The nurse follows policy and procedures in the reporting and management of the error. The nurse is demonstrating:
   A. Social justice
   B. Accountability
   C. Reliability
   D. Confidentiality

39. The nurse is performing an assessment on a patient who is sitting up in bed and appears comfortable. The pulse oximetry monitor begins to alarm and shows a reading of 78%. Which assessment finding would suggest that this is not a mechanical malfunction?
   A. The pulse oximetry monitor has not been plugged in.
   B. The patient's apical pulse is 76, and the pulse oximetry reading shows a pulse of 144.
   C. The patient states he is cold.
   D. The pulse oximetry reading shows no pulse.

40. The nurse is to receive a patient for observation to a stepdown unit who has a diagnosis of class IV heart failure. For which symptoms would the nurse monitor?
   A. Minimal discomfort with exertion
   B. Chest pain and shortness of breath only with exertion
   C. Increased blood pressure and pulse rate
   D. Chest pain and shortness of breath not relieved by rest

41. Which of the following drugs is a reversal agent for a benzodiazepine overdose?
   A. Naloxone
   B. Flumazenil
   C. Sodium bicarbonate
   D. *N*-Acetylcysteine

42. During which stage of hemorrhagic pancreatitis does extra-pancreatic inflammation occur?
    A. Stage I
    B. Stage II
    C. Stage III
    D. Stage IV

43. The nurse is assisting with an emergency intubation and auscultates lung sounds only on the right side. Which is the most appropriate initial action by the nurse?
    A. Prepare for chest tube insertion.
    B. Advance the endotracheal tube 1 cm.
    C. Pull the endotracheal tube back 1 cm.
    D. Increase oxygen concentration.

44. When examining a patient for suspected upper gastrointestinal bleed, which assessment would the nurse consider a priority?
    A. Medication administration
    B. Hemodynamic compromise
    C. Nutritional intake
    D. Mallory-Weiss syndrome

45. To provide effective nursing care, the nurse should engage in what type of communication with the patient and family?
    A. Purposive communication
    B. Intrapersonal communication
    C. Metacommunication
    D. Therapeutic communication

46. A patient is admitted to the unit with a traumatic head injury. The nurse evaluates the following lab values: Serum sodium of 150 mEq/L, serum potassium of 3.2 mmol/L, and normal glucose levels. The patient complains of intense thirst and the urine specific gravity is less than 1.005. Urine output is greater than 300 mL per hour. The nurse should further evaluate in the patient for which diagnosis?
    A. Hyperthyroidism
    B. Hypothyroidism
    C. Diabetes mellitus
    D. Diabetes insipidus

47. If a patient's PaO_2 is 90 on 30% FiO_2, what is the PaO_2/PiO_2 ratio?
    A. 0.3
    B. 3
    C. 30
    D. 300

48. Which of the following assessment findings indicate a systemic reaction to inflammation?
    A. Erythema and edema
    B. Functional impairment
    C. Pain and warmth
    D. Tachypnea and tachycardia

49. When assessing a patient for diffuse parenchymal lung disease, which components of the lungs would be included in the assessment?
    A. Pleura, airway, and bronchioles
    B. Trachea, bronchus, and pleura
    C. Bronchus, bronchioles, and alveoli
    D. Alveoli, alveolar ducts, and bronchioles

50. The nurse on a step-down unit has been assigned a patient with dyspnea and tachypnea. Arterial blood gas results are pH 7.32, $PaCO_2$ 55, and HCO_3 24. The patient is experiencing:
    A. Metabolic acidosis
    B. Metabolic alkalosis
    C. Respiratory acidosis
    D. Respiratory alkalosis

51. In a stable, septic patient, the nurse would perform which of the following actions first?
    A. Obtain blood cultures.
    B. Administer antibiotics.
    C. Insert a urinary catheter.
    D. Administer a fluid bolus.

52. The nurse is caring for an older adult patient with congestive heart failure following a hypertensive crisis. The patient is receiving an angiotensin-converting enzyme inhibitor in addition to spironolactone. Initial lab results indicate severe hypokalemia and mild hypomagnesemia. For which event would the nurse monitor closely when reviewing the patient's electrocardiogram?
    A. Cardiac arrhythmias
    B. Previous myocardial infarction
    C. Complete heart block
    D. Unstable angina

53. A patient is considered tachycardic if they have which heart rate?
    A. 40 beats per minute
    B. 60 beats per minute
    C. 100 beats per minute
    D. 120 beats per minute

54. Which of the following best describes the pathophysiology of anaphylaxis?
    A. Blood clots form causing organ damage or a blockage in an artery.
    B. The body loses heat faster than it can produce heat, producing a dangerously low body temperature.
    C. Type I immunoglobulin E (IgE)-mediated hypersensitivity reaction involves mast cells and basophils that are suddenly released into the body.
    D. A disturbance of calcium homeostasis occurs in skeletal muscle.

55. A patient's central venous pressure is 10 and pulmonary arterial occlusion pressure is 14. The nurse assesses for:
    A. Left atrial failure
    B. Right atrial failure
    C. Left ventricle failure
    D. Right ventricle failure

56. The nurse is preparing to administer reteplase (rPA) to a patient with a ST-elevation myocardial infarct. Which dose would the nurse give the patient?
    A. 1.5 million U over 30 to 60 minutes
    B. Two 10-U bolus doses given 30 minutes apart
    C. A dose based on the patient's weight
    D. 15-mg bolus followed by a 0.75-mg/kg dose given over 30 minutes

57. Which of the following is a sign or symptom of both hypocalcemia and hypomagnesemia?
    A. Seizures
    B. Excessive thirst
    C. Abdominal pain
    D. Hypertension

58. A patient who is 1-week post–myocardial infarction suddenly becomes agitated, restless, and diaphoretic. Pulse pressure drops to 20 mmHg. Assessment also reveals faint radial and apical pulses that weaken significantly on inspiration. Which complication is the patient most likely experiencing?
    A. Mitral valve rupture
    B. Pulmonary embolism
    C. Pulmonary edema
    D. Cardiac tamponade

59. A 65-year-old male is being evaluated for recurrent syncopal episodes present for the past 4 months. A cardiac workup is unrevealing until he becomes symptomatic in the middle of the night. EKG reveals atrial fibrillation with a heart rate of 144 beats/minute. What is the appropriate next step?
    A. Amiodarone drip
    B. Intravenous line heparin with immediate transthoracic cardioversion
    C. Intravenous line metoprolol
    D. Adenosine push

60. The nurse evaluates a patient with random seizure activity followed by nausea and vomiting. Which lab result indicates the possible cause for these symptoms?
    A. Triglyceride level of 200 mg/dL
    B. Serum potassium of 3.8 mEq/L
    C. Serum sodium level of 110 mEq/L
    D. Blood glucose level of 156 mg/dL

61. An older adult is scheduled for an invasive procedure. The patient has a designated personal representative who is requesting information regarding the procedure. According to the Health Insurance Portability and Accountability Act, what is the nurse's responsibility to the patient in this situation?
    A. The nurse should request that the personal representative contact the administrator.
    B. The nurse should forward the request to the facility's ethics committee.
    C. The nurse should provide the personal representative with information about the procedure.
    D. The nurse should ask the personal representative to contact the patient's healthcare provider.

62. Noninvasive ventilation provides which of the following advantages?
    A. Less antibiotic use
    B. Airway protection
    C. Decreased risk of aspiration
    D. Increased ability to clear secretions

63. The nurse is evaluating the results of arterial blood gases on a patient: pH of 7.36, $PaCO_2$ of 68 mm/Hg, HCO_3 of 36 mEq/L. What do the lab values represent?
    A. Uncompensated respiratory acidosis
    B. Uncompensated metabolic acidosis
    C. Compensated respiratory acidosis
    D. Compensated metabolic alkalosis

64. The nurse has a patient whose cardiac monitor shows atrial flutter. Which incidence would cause this arrhythmia?
    A. Inflammation
    B. Left ventricle failure
    C. Sympathetic overstimulation of the left atria
    D. Inferior or posterior wall myocardial infarction

65. Which laboratory result is the most accurate indicator of improved kidney function in a patient with an acute kidney injury?
    A. Decreased serum creatinine
    B. Decreased white blood cell count
    C. Decreased blood urea nitrogen level
    D. Increased serum creatinine and blood urea nitrogen

66. Which intervention is indicated for an unstable patient in ventricular tachycardia?

  A. Administer adenosine.

  B. Administer amiodarone.

  C. Administer atropine.

  D. Administer unsynchronized cardioversion.

67. Which ethical principle requires that a nurse's actions inflict no harm?

  A. Veracity

  B. Autonomy

  C. Beneficence

  D. Nonmaleficence

68. The nurse works with a respiratory and physical therapist to help a patient achieve their goal of completing a lap around the nurse's station. Which characteristic is the nurse exhibiting?

  A. Advocacy

  B. Caring practice

  C. Collaboration

  D. Communication

69. Which condition is consistent with increased residual lung volume in a patient with obstructive lung disease?

  A. Lung cancer

  B. Emphysema

  C. Bronchitis

  D. Allergic rhinitis

70. A patient is scheduled for an invasive procedure that requires additional informed consent. What elements must be included for the nurse to determine that informed consent was achieved?

  A. Type of anesthesia, risks of procedure, length of recovery

  B. Length of recovery, expected outcomes, name of healthcare provider

  C. Voluntary consent, insurance coverage, benefits of the treatment

  D. Voluntary consent and risks, benefits, alternatives of treatment

71. The nurse is caring for a patient on a ventilator who has a cervical fracture that has rendered the diagnosis of brain death. The healthcare provider has recommended that the ventilation tube be removed, and the family has agreed with this decision. The nurse experiences distress when asked to discontinue the ventilation tube. The nurse:

  A. Fears legal repercussions

  B. Is experiencing a conflict with personal values

  C. Does not believe in euthanasia

  D. Is experiencing a cultural crisis

72. What is a common finding in acute pulmonary embolism?
    A. Bradycardia
    B. Tachypnea
    C. Subconjunctival hemorrhage
    D. Bradypnea

73. The nurse has been assigned to care for a 66-year-old patient who has developed rapid atrial fibrillation. The patient has been weaned from intravenous (IV) diltiazem to oral administration and now has developed new onset of hallucinations, agitation, and disorientation. Which is the appropriate initial nursing action?
    A. Obtain an order for lorazepam every 6 hours.
    B. Assess the patient's SpO_2 and neurologic status.
    C. Obtain an order for IV haloperidol.
    D. Consult pharmacy for a possible drug interaction.

74. The nurse is caring for a postoperative orthopedic patient. Which primary laboratory tests should the nurse review prior to initiation of nonsteroidal anti-inflammatory drug therapy?
    A. Serum amylase, electrolytes, blood urea nitrogen
    B. Electrolytes and fasting blood sugar
    C. Creatinine clearance, complete blood count, liver function tests
    D. Complete blood count, metabolic profile

75. An older adult patient is admitted with a blood glucose of 688 mg/dL, which is reduced from initial testing of 765 mg/dL. Skin turgor is poor, and the patient is confused and weak. What is the priority response in treating this patient?
    A. Initiate intravenous regular insulin.
    B. Initiate intravenous solution of D5W.
    C. Initiate a sliding-scale insulin every 4 hours.
    D. Assess the patient for a distended bladder/urinary retention.

76. Which of the following is one of the four essential components of a clinical pathway?
    A. Order set
    B. Timeline
    C. Short-term outcome criteria
    D. Patient response

77. The nurse has a patient complaining of fatigue. Upon closer assessment, the nurse also finds peripheral edema, a cough, hepatomegaly, and a respiratory rate of 28 breaths per minute. Which diagnosis does the nurse suspect?
    A. Cardiogenic shock
    B. Left-sided heart failure
    C. Right-sided heart failure
    D. Hypertrophic cardiomyopathy

78. The nurse is managing a patient postoperatively after an aortic repair with graft placement. Which action is the nurse's priority of care for this patient?
    A. Administration of antibiotics
    B. Correct coagulopathy
    C. Prevention of fluid overload
    D. Blood pressure management

79. The nurse is caring for a patient on the ventilator who has soft wrist restraints. The patient's need for restraints is no longer present, so the nurse removes them. What ethical principle is being employed?
    A. Beneficence
    B. Utilitarianism
    C. Autonomy
    D. Justice

80. Which mean pulmonary artery pressure (mPAP) and pulmonary artery occlusion pressure (PAOP) findings are consistent with primary pulmonary arterial hypertension?
    A. mPAP of 30 mmHg and PAOP of 10 mmHg
    B. mPAP of 25 mmHg and PAOP of 15 mmHg
    C. mPAP of 30 mmHg and PAOP of 20 mmHg
    D. mPAP of 20 mmHg and PAOP of 10 mmHg

81. The severity of a pulmonary obstruction is determined by forced expiratory volume in 1 second (FEV1). Which value indicates a moderate obstruction?
    A. Greater than 80% predicted
    B. 60% to 79% predicted
    C. 40% to 59% predicted
    D. Less than 40% predicted

82. Which assessment findings are most consistent with peritonitis?
    A. Hypoactive bowel sounds and slow and irregular pulse
    B. Hyperactive bowel sounds, vomiting, and diarrhea
    C. Abdominal pain, fever, and rigid board-like abdomen
    D. Lethargy, hypothermia, and slow respirations

83. A 20-year-old female patient is admitted after ingesting approximately 25 acetaminophen tablets. After assessing airway, breathing, and circulation, the nurse should:
    A. Administer acetylcysteine
    B. Establish two large-bore intravenous lines
    C. Obtain an EKG
    D. Administer dopamine

84. A patient being treated with radiation therapy for stomach cancer suddenly develops severe right flank pain that radiates to the groin. The patient is nauseous and afebrile and bent over with pain. Urinalysis shows marked hematuria and no casts. What is the nurse's most appropriate first step in treating this patient?
    A. Narcotic analgesia
    B. CT scan of the abdomen
    C. Lithotripsy procedure
    D. Providing the patient with a strainer

85. What is the most common cause of a transudative pleural effusion?
    A. Pneumonia
    B. Congestive heart failure
    C. Pulmonary embolus
    D. Nephrotic syndrome

86. Which arrhythmia is caused by sympathetic overstimulation of the left atrium?
    A. Atrial flutter
    B. Bradycardia
    C. Third-degree atrioventricular block
    D. Ventricular tachycardia

87. Which medication is recommended for prophylactic management of bleeding in a patient with esophageal varices?
    A. Simvastatin
    B. Propranolol
    C. Vasopressin
    D. Octreotide

88. When caring for older adult patients, what structural changes to the respiratory system would the nurse observe?
    A. Weakened respiratory muscles
    B. Increased gag reflexes
    C. Decreased snoring at night
    D. Increased elasticity in lungs

89. A patient is 6 hours post thyroid surgery for cancer. The nurse examines the patient and notes blood soaking the gown. What is the priority response in treating this patient?
    A. Assess the patient for breath sounds and respiratory effort.
    B. Reassure the patient and change the gown.
    C. Reinforce the dressing and notify the surgeon.
    D. Raise the head of the bed to high Fowler's position.

90. The nurse asks a patient to make a tight fist with their hand. What is the nurse trying to elicit within the patient's cardiovascular system?
    A. Increased venous return and increased ventricular volume
    B. Decreased venous return and decreased ventricular volumes
    C. Increased systemic vascular resistance and increased venous return
    D. Increased cardiac output and increased left ventricular filling pressures

91. Which sign would be monitored for in a patient at risk for upper gastrointestinal bleed?
    A. Hematemesis
    B. Left upper quadrant pain
    C. Hematochezia
    D. Bradycardia

92. The nurse inspects a wound that a patient sustained during a motor vehicle crash and determines that a portion of the dermis is intact, so the nurse cleans and bandages the wound. Which wound classification will the nurse document on the patient's health record?
    A. Unintentional, partial-thickness wound
    B. Intentional, full-thickness wound
    C. Intentional, partial-thickness wound
    D. Unintentional, full-thickness wound

93. Which mineral deficiency would the nurse anticipate in lab findings for the patient presenting with lethargy, weight gain, bradycardia, and a goiter?
    A. Fluoride
    B. Calcium
    C. Sodium
    D. Iodine

94. A patient's electrocardiogram shows findings consistent with an ST-segment elevation myocardial infarction. Which treatment would be recommended?
    A. Cardiopulmonary bypass
    B. Revascularization procedure
    C. Intravenous thrombolytic agent
    D. Coronary balloon angioplasty with stenting

95. The nurse is evaluating a patient with subclinical hypothyroidism. Which set of lab values is most consistent with this disorder?
    A. Normal thyroid-stimulating hormone (TSH), decreased free T3, decreased free T4
    B. Increased TSH, normal free T3, normal free T4
    C. Decreased TSH, decreased free T3, decreased free T4
    D. Normal TSH, decreased free T3, normal free T4

96. During defecation, a patient experiences decreased cardiac output related to the Valsalva maneuver. What does the nurse know to expect when taking the patient's vital signs immediately after defecation?
    A. The patient will have a decrease in respirations.
    B. The patient will experience tachypnea.
    C. The patient's blood pressure will decrease.
    D. The patient's blood pressure will increase.

97. The nurse is caring for a patient diagnosed with syndrome of inappropriate antidiuretic hormone secretion. What precautions should the nurse initiate?
    A. Hypertensive crisis precautions
    B. Carbohydrate precautions
    C. Seizure precautions
    D. Fall precautions

98. A young adult male is admitted due to an acute onset of fatigue, vomiting, diarrhea, and anorexia after being found unconscious in his home. His blood pressure is low, and he has a fever. History reveals a recent acute non-bloody gastroenteritis that cleared after 2 days of treatment with high-dose antibiotics. Blood chemistry reveals decreased sodium, increased potassium, and glucose level of 52 mg/dL. For what does the nurse further assess?
    A. Onset of type 1 diabetes
    B. Myxedema
    C. Adrenal insufficiency
    D. Diabetic ketoacidosis

99. The nurse is caring for a patient with a blood pressure of 190/90 mmHg, heart rate of 88 beats/minute, central venous pressure of 10, body surface area of 1.8 m2, and a cardiac output of 4 L. The patient's stroke volume is:
    A. 123 mmHg
    B. 45 mL/beat
    C. 2,260
    D. 2.2 L/min/m2

100. The nurse has a patient in diabetic ketoacidosis and just started a low-dose continuous insulin infusion. What procedure would the nurse anticipate performing next?
    A. Urinary catheter placement
    B. Nasogastric tube placement
    C. Intravenous line (IV) placement
    D. Central line placement

101. Which of the following is the most definitive tool for diagnosis of thoracic aortic aneurysm?
    A. Chest x-ray
    B. Ultrasound
    C. Arteriogram
    D. CT scan

102. Which lab results correspond with a patient in postrenal failure?
     A. Urine output of less than 0.5 mL/kg/hr for more than 3 consecutive hours
     B. Urine output of less than 0.5 mL/kg/hr for more than 6 consecutive hours
     C. Serum creatinine that decreases by 0.3 mg/dL or more within 48 hours
     D. Serum creatinine that rises by 0.3 mg/dL or more within 72 hours

103. The nurse is monitoring a patient with signs of early intestinal obstruction. The nurse would assess for which of the following during auscultation?
     A. Absent bowel sounds
     B. Hyperactive bowel sounds
     C. Low-pitched, rumbling bowel sounds
     D. Diminished bowel sounds

104. The nurse has a patient who is septic. Which fluid would the nurse anticipate the provider ordering for initial resuscitation?
     A. Albumin
     B. Hetastarch
     C. Crystalloids
     D. Packed red blood cells

105. The nurse asks a medical assistant to monitor a patient's urine output every 4 hours and record the volume in the patient's chart. The nurse is demonstrating which Right of Delegation?
     A. Right task
     B. Right direction
     C. Right supervision
     D. Right circumstance

106. The nurse is caring for a patient in acute pain. The nurse administers 2 mg of morphine at 6:00 a.m. The medication will be eliminated from the patient's system at what time?
     A. 9:00 a.m.
     B. 12:00 p.m.
     C. 3:00 p.m.
     D. 10:00 p.m.

107. Which level of resiliency is present if a patient can initiate some degree of compensation?
     A. Level 1
     B. Level 3
     C. Level 4
     D. Level 5

108. A patient refuses treatment and states that he wants to be left alone to die. Which ethical principle supports his right to die?
    A. Self-determination
    B. Justice
    C. Autonomy
    D. Veracity

109. Which patient is a candidate for noninvasive ventilation?
    A. A patient in status asthmaticus
    B. A patient with altered mental status
    C. A patient with swallowing abnormalities
    D. A patient who is not able to control secretions

110. A patient presents with a pulse that alternates between strong and weak. Which diagnosis would be considered?
    A. Septic shock
    B. Hypovolemia
    C. Pericardial tamponade
    D. Hypertrophic cardiomyopathy

111. Upon auscultation of a patient's lungs, the nurse hears loud, high-pitched sounds over the larynx. What term will the nurse use in documentation to describe these breath sounds?
    A. Rhonchi
    B. Normal
    C. Vesicular
    D. Bronchial

112. The nurse applies 2 liters of oxygen to a patient complaining of shortness of breath. What respiratory diagnosis prevents the nurse from providing a higher level of oxygen to this patient?
    A. Pulmonary edema
    B. Asthma
    C. Rhinitis
    D. Chronic obstructive pulmonary disease

113. A 69-year-old, 80-kg patient exhibits the following signs and symptoms: temperature: 102.6°F (39.2°C), heart rate: 136 BPM, blood pressure: 90/50 mmHg, urine output for last hour: 40 mL/hour, white blood cell count: 10,000, lactate: 2 mmol/L, pan cultures: negative. The nurse suspects the patient is developing:
    A. Systemic inflammatory response syndrome
    B. Cardiogenic shock
    C. Septic shock
    D. Multiple organ dysfunction syndrome

114. The nurse is assessing a patient with acute respiratory distress syndrome. Which data indicates the patient is experiencing a complication related to the ventilator?
    A. Urine output of 110 mL over a 4-hour period
    B. Pulse oximetry reading of 96%
    C. Telemetry that shows sinus bradycardia
    D. Asymmetrical chest expansion

115. Which patient would be most likely to have the following arterial blood gas result: pH of 7.6, $PaCO_2$ of 23 mmHg, PaO_2 of 70 mmHg, and HCO_3 of 21 mEq/L?
    A. A patient experiencing a panic attack
    B. A patient experiencing a morphine overdose
    C. A patient experiencing prolonged vomiting
    D. A patient with uncontrolled type 1 diabetes

116. The nurse notes an area of tissue injury on a patient's sacral area. The wound presents as a shallow open injury with a red–pink wound bed and partial-thickness loss of dermis. The wound is a:
    A. Stage I pressure injury
    B. Stage II pressure injury
    C. Stage III pressure injury
    D. Stage IV pressure injury

117. Which abnormal lab value is a predictor of poor outcomes in a patient with dilated cardiomyopathy?
    A. Hypokalemia
    B. Hyponatremia
    C. Hypocalcemia
    D. Hypomagnesemia

118. The nurse has a patient with a urinary catheter. Which action would the nurse take to prevent a urinary tract infection?
    A. Maintain an open drainage system.
    B. Place the collection bag on the floor.
    C. Empty the collection bag only when it is full.
    D. Keep the collection bag lower than the bladder.

119. Following percutaneous coronary intervention (PCI) for an ST-elevated myocardial infarction (STEMI), a patient complains of shortness of breath. The nurse auscultates crackles in all lung fields. Vital signs are documented as follows: blood pressure 72/50 mmHg, heart rate 124 beats/minute, respiratory rate 32 breaths/minute, and SpO_2 88% on 2L O_2 nasal cannula. Which goal for treatment would the nurse initiate for this patient?
    A. Volume to enhance venous return
    B. Diuresis to reduce myocardial workload
    C. Antiarrhythmics to restore electrical stability
    D. Thrombolytics to eliminate pulmonary embolus

120. The nurse is using a hospital translator to explain diagnostic procedures to a patient whose preferred language is not English. The nurse determined the patient's language through a:
    A. Learning needs assessment
    B. Culture competency assessment
    C. Vulnerability assessment
    D. Competency assessment

121. The nurse is caring for a patient who practices Hinduism. Based on their religious beliefs, the patient may:
    A. Request same-sex caregivers
    B. Refuse all medical care
    C. Refuse blood transfusions
    D. Request that their face be turned toward the right after they die

122. A stable patient in ventricular tachycardia asks the nurse what is causing the arrhythmia. Which response would the nurse give the patient?
    A. "Your left ventricle has failed."
    B. "You are in cardiogenic shock."
    C. "You have inflammation in your heart."
    D. "You have electrolyte abnormalities."

123. A patient who is a Jehovah's Witness refuses a blood transfusion based on religious beliefs and practices. Which ethical principle is the nurse following when honoring this patient's wishes?
    A. The right to die
    B. Advance directive
    C. The right to refuse treatment
    D. Substituted judgment

124. The nurse is evaluating a patient admitted with right upper-quadrant abdominal pain, a temperature of 102.4°F (39.1°C), and jaundice. Upon further assessment, it is revealed the patient has been treated for chronic pancreatitis and is a self-reported alcoholic. Based on these symptoms, for which diagnosis would the nurse further assess?
    A. Ascending cholangitis
    B. Acute pyelonephritis
    C. Acute appendicitis
    D. Choledocholithiasis

125. Which of the following is a sign or symptom of hypophosphatemia?
    A. Nausea
    B. Vomiting
    C. Gait disturbances
    D. Excessive thirst

1. **C) Metoprolol**

   Beta-adrenergic blockers produce bradycardia and hypotension with overdose. Metoprolol is a beta blocker. Carbon monoxide poisoning symptoms are headache, dizziness, weakness, upset stomach, vomiting, chest pain, and confusion. Acetaminophen overdoses are manifested by abdominal pain, upset stomach, appetite loss, coma, seizures, diarrhea, irritability, jaundice, nausea, vomiting, and sweating. Fentanyl (opioid) overdose symptoms include constricted pupils, changes in level of consciousness, scratching, or slurred speech.

2. **C) Hypocalcemia**

   Electrolyte abnormalities commonly seen in patients with a kidney injury are hyperkalemia, hyperphosphatemia, hypocalcemia, and hyponatremia.

3. **B) Stroke index of 50 mL/m2/beat**

   The abnormal lab value is a stroke index of 50 mL/m2/beat, which is an elevated measure found in patients taking digitalis or dopamine. A normal range would be 25 to 45 mL/m2/beat. Central venous pressure within the range 2 to 6 is considered normal. A normal pulmonary artery pressure is 25/10. A mean arterial pressure within normal limits is 70 to 105 mmHg.

4. **C) 2D echocardiogram**

   The most useful diagnostic test to evaluate heart failure is a 2D echocardiogram. The 2D echocardiogram can determine whether the abnormality is with the myocardium, heart valves, or pericardium. An MRI can evaluate the size, ventricular mass, right ventricular dysplasia, and pericardial disease. A chest x-ray is unable to determine left ventricle function or valvular abnormalities. A 12-lead echocardiogram is unable to determine the mechanical function of the ventricles.

5. **C) The Nurse Practice Act of the state in which the nurse practices**

   Nursing scope of practice refers to professional nursing activities as defined by state law. Each state's Nurse Practice Act (NPA) is determined through the boards of nursing. Nurses use the scope of practice to guide them in varying work environments to ensure they are practicing and providing care within the confines of the law. The National Council of State Boards of Nursing (NCSBN) is an independent, not-for-profit organization through which nursing regulatory bodies counsel together on matters of common interest and concern affecting public health, safety, and welfare, including the development of nursing licensure examinations. The American Nurses Association Bill of Rights asserts the rights that registered nurses must have to provide high-quality patient care in a safe work environment. The American Nurses Association is a professional organization to advance and protect the profession of nursing.

6. **B) Exaggerated A waves**

Mitral regurgitation will show exaggerated A waves. Aortic stenosis will show a decreased cardiac output. Aortic regurgitation will show tachycardia, decreased cardiac output, widened pulse pressure, and exaggerated A waves in pulmonary artery occlusion pressure (PAOP) tracing. Mitral stenosis will have a large V wave in PAOP tracing.

7. **C) No treatment is required.**

A patient in first-degree atrioventricular (AV) block does not require any treatment. Adenosine would be given if the patient were in paroxysmal supraventricular tachycardia. Transcutaneous pacing is required with second-degree Mobitz Type II AV block. Synchronized electrical cardioversion would be performed on an unstable patient with atrial fibrillation or atrial flutter.

8. **A) 1:1,000 dilution 0.2 to 0.5 mg**

Epinephrine is the initial drug used to treat an anaphylactic reaction. Epinephrine 1:1,000 dilution at 0.2 mg to 0.5 mg dose can be administered subcutaneously or intramuscularly. Administering at a higher dose would have adverse effects on the patient (e.g., arrythmias). A concentration of 1:10,000 is more diluted and will not effectively treat an anaphylactic reaction.

9. **C) The patient has a stroke and is on life support.**

A durable power of attorney for healthcare is a legal document that allows a person to designate someone else to make healthcare decisions in the event they are unable to do so themselves. It provides instructions about preferred medical treatment. Many states have laws that specify qualifying conditions/situations, or they can be specified in the legal document itself. A durable power of attorney for healthcare would be invoked when a patient is on life support. A patient who requires anesthesia or is in the care of an adult child is not necessarily unable to make healthcare decisions. More information would be required to make that determination. A patient's ability to afford the cost of healthcare has no bearing on the patient's ability to make healthcare decisions.

10. **D) Start effective antimicrobial therapy.**

Prompt diagnosis and institution of effective antimicrobial therapy to reduce the risk of complications and development of indications for surgery is the priority. Management of antithrombotic therapy is important as well, but it is not a primary intervention. Neither anticoagulant therapy nor antiplatelet therapy is indicated to reduce the risk of thromboembolic complications. Assessment of the need for removal of any infected implanted devices would be an intervention that would be implemented later after risk for infection has been reduced.

11. **D) Head of the bed elevated 30 to 45 degrees, unless contraindicated.**

The Centers for Disease Control and Prevention recommends that the head of bed (HOB) be elevated to at least 30 degrees to prevent ventilator-associated pneumonia (VAP). Research has shown that keeping the HOB at 30 degrees is effective in reducing VAP by preventing oral secretions from collecting on the cuff of the tube and entering the lungs. Oral care is recommended to keep the mouth moisturized, but brushing the plaque is necessary to help prevent VAP. Turning the patient on their left side will not prevent VAP; the patient should be turned every 2 hours to prevent skin breakdown. Blue food coloring should not be added to tube feedings.

12. **C) Dobutamine infusion**

    Dobutamine is an inotrope that improves oxygen delivery by increasing cardiac output with beta-receptor stimulation. Metoprolol and diltiazem are negative inotropes that decrease cardiac output and oxygen delivery to end organs. 100% O_2 via face mask will not provide a significant amount of oxygenation over the current method of delivery since perfusion is the problem.

13. **D) Remind the patient of their risk of falls and ask them to not get out of bed again.**

    It is recommended that alternative patient management strategies be explored before deciding to restrain. The nurse should start with the least restrictive method. Many times, patients need reminders not to get out of bed unassisted. If the nurse just continues to reassess, this is not providing an intervention for the situation. Administering a sedative or restraining the patient should be considered if the least restrictive method is not successful.

14. **D) Every 8 hours**

    To rule out a myocardial infarction, cardiac enzymes are commonly drawn every 8 hours for 24 hours. Intervals of 2, 4, or 6 hours are too brief to show changes.

15. **D) Wait to start antibiotics and obtain two cultures from two venipuncture sites.**

    Two to three sets of blood cultures should be obtained from separate venipuncture sites. These should be obtained before initiation of empiric antibiotic therapy sites.

16. **A) The nurse fails to assess and monitor a patient receiving a blood transfusion and a reaction occurs.**

    Malpractice is defined as improper or unethical conduct or unreasonable lack of skill by a holder of a professional or official position. To establish a nursing malpractice claim, the following conditions must be demonstrated: (a) The nurse had an obligation to the patient, (b) the nurse did not meet the appropriate standard of care, (c) the nurse breached that standard of care, (d) the breach in the standard of care led to an injury, and (e) the injuries and damages suffered are documented. An example of malpractice is failing to assess and monitor a patient receiving a blood transfusion and a reaction occurs. Missing a vein is common and not considered malpractice. If a patient climbs over the rails that were properly in place per policy, it is not malpractice. There was no breach of standard on the nurse's part. Placing a "nothing by mouth" sign on the patient's door is a correct nursing action. The visitor providing food to this patient is not related to the actions of the nurse, and no injury occurred.

17. **D) Nonmaleficence**

    Nonmaleficence refers to preventing or minimizing harm to an individual, as patients have a right to no harm. Nonmaleficence requires that nurses avoid causing harm to patients. Assisting patients with tasks that they are unable to perform on their own, keeping side rails up for fall precautions, or providing medications in a quick and timely manner are all examples of beneficence. Self-determination is important for respecting patients' wants and abilities to make their medical decisions on treatments and outcomes. All patients have a right to be treated fairly and equally by others. Justice involves how people are treated when their interest competes with others.

18. **C) Sudden change in alertness of a patient**

The rapid response should be called if a patient has a sudden change in alertness. This can indicate a neurologic or metabolic emergency that requires immediate intervention and possible resuscitation. An elevated blood pressure should prompt a call to the provider, as should a severe headache or vomiting of coffee ground emesis, but these situations do not require a STAT team activation.

19. **A) Contractility, preload, and afterload**

Stroke volume is dependent on three factors: preload, contractility, and afterload. Cardiac output consists of two elements, stroke volume and heart rate, and is the product of these two elements (cardiac output = stroke volume × heart rate). Preload is the initial stretching of the cardiac myocytes (muscle cells) prior to contraction. It is related to ventricular filling. Afterload is the force or load against which the heart must contract to eject blood. Contractility is the intrinsic strength of the cardiac muscle independent of preload, but a change in preload will affect the force of contraction. Compliance describes how easily a chamber of the heart or the lumen of a blood vessel expands when it is filled with a volume of blood. Cardiac impedance is a measurement of the mechanical activation of the heart. Blood volume refers to the total amount of fluid circulating within the arteries, capillaries, veins, venules, and chambers of the heart at any time. The components that add volume to blood include red blood cells (erythrocytes), white blood cells (leukocytes), platelets, and plasma. Blood viscosity is a measurement of the thickness and stickiness of an individual's blood. It is a direct measure of the ability of blood to flow through the blood vessels.

20. **A) Famotidine is an H2 blocker and reduces acidic secretions.**

Famotidine is a histamine-2 (H2) receptor antagonist that reduces acid secretion by inhibiting gastrin secretion but does not lower esophageal sphincter pressure. Antacids neutralize acid, and mucosal barrier fortifiers protect the mucosal barrier.

21. **A) Administer a rapid-acting carbohydrate.**

Insulin lispro peaks in 30 to 90 minutes; therefore, a hypoglycemic reaction should be suspected. A rapid-acting carbohydrate is required immediately. A bedside blood glucose test is a fast way to verify the suspicion. Since the patient is confused, asking about food consumption is important after responding to the immediate need. Giving the patient a sandwich with meat is not the priority, as the glucose must be elevated quickly, and the patient is confused. A stat blood glucose test is a verification of the blood glucose, but the nurse should not wait on the results to treat the patient. A long-acting carbohydrate and protein source should be provided to prevent a reoccurrence of the hypoglycemic reaction.

22. **B) Diabetic ketoacidosis**

Patients with serum ketones and serum glucose levels above 300 mg/dL could be diagnosed with diabetic ketoacidosis. Diabetes insipidus is an overproduction of antidiuretic hormone and doesn't create ketones in the blood. Hypoglycemia causes low blood glucose levels. The Somogyi phenomenon is rebound hyperglycemia following an episode of hypoglycemia.

23. **B) Pursed lip breathing decreases the amount of air trapping and resistance.**

    Pursed lip breathing is a technique that helps people living with asthma or chronic obstructive pulmonary disease (COPD) when they experience shortness of breath. Pursed lip breathing helps control shortness of breath and provides a quick and easy way to slow the pace of breathing, making each breath more effective. Exhaling through pursed lips creates a smaller opening for air movement, effectively slowing and prolonging expiration, which prevents air from being trapped in the alveoli and decreases resistance to exhalation. Increasing carbon dioxide levels to stimulate breathing is the natural stimulus for a person without COPD to breathe. Prolonging inspiration and shortening expiration does not assist the patient because exhalation is difficult for the COPD patient. Humidification and fluid intake help to liquefy secretions.

24. **A) Septic shock**

    A bounding pulse is indicative of septic shock. A weak and thready pulse is indicative of hypovolemia. A patient with a pericardial tamponade will have a pulse that alternates between strong and weak. A patient with hypertrophic cardiomyopathy will have pulsus bisferiens.

25. **B) Ventricular fibrillation**

    Defibrillation is required for ventricular fibrillation. Defibrillation is not utilized for atrial fibrillation, asystole, or pulseless electrical activity.

26. **A) Pain medication prescribed for different levels of pain**

    The patient has a history of substance abuse and has been sober for 14 years. The level of pain the patient is experiencing indicates a need for differentiated pain medication management and that an opioid pain medication is likely needed. With a 14-year history of sobriety, the patient has a low risk for addiction. The opioid should be used only when pain is severe. Administration of acetaminophen or anti-inflammatories is not adequate pain control for a thoracotomy. Patient-controlled analgesia has a great deal of risk of overuse of opioid medications in a patient with a history of substance abuse.

27. **C) Epinephrine**

    Epinephrine is the initial drug used to treat an anaphylactic reaction. Epinephrine 1:1,000 dilution at an 0.2- to 0.5-mg dose can be administered subcutaneously or intramuscularly. If hypotension is present, it is treated with fluid resuscitation (e.g., normal saline), vasopressors, and supplemental oxygen. Steroids (e.g., prednisone) and an antihistamine (e.g., diphenhydramine) can sometimes provide greater symptom relief, but this is not an initial intervention.

28. **B) Clinical inquiry**

    Clinical inquiry occurs when a nurse questions and evaluates practices. The nurse can then provide informed innovation through research and experimental learning. Clinical judgment would be the nurse using critical thinking, nursing skills, and a global grasp of the situation to make an informed decision. Collaboration is interprofessional teamwork that promotes a person's contributions to a patient goal. Systems thinking allows the nurse to see the care environment from a perspective of a holistic interrelationship.

29. C) The patient has moderate resiliency.

The American Association of Critical-Care Nurses (AACN) Synergy Model evaluates a patient on eight characteristics: resiliency, vulnerability, stability, complexity, resource availability, participation in care, participation in decision-making, and predictability. Patients are assigned a numeric value based on their capacity in each category—1 (very low), 3 (moderate), or 5 (high). A resiliency evaluation assesses a patient's ability to return to a baseline level of functioning after an illness or injury. The patient is rated a level 1 if the patient has a very low level of resiliency, 3 for moderate resiliency, and 5 for a high level of resiliency. This patient currently has a moderate resiliency level.

30. C) Excessive eye contact indicates rudeness.

In the Chinese culture, individuals may nod their head to indicate yes or shake their head for no. Excessive eye contact indicates rudeness, and excessive touch is considered offensive. Body language is important to Native Americans, and they will seldom disagree with others in public. Vietnamese Americans consider an upturned palm offensive.

31. D) Place in a prone position.

Acute respiratory distress syndrome (ARDS) is an acute respiratory failure in which the patient remains hypoxic despite the administration of 100% oxygen. Oxygenation in patients who have ARDS is improved when they are placed in the prone position. Frequent and consistent turning of the patient is also beneficial and can be accomplished by the use of specialty beds. Patients with ARDS require high concentrations of oxygen, usually by mask or ventilator. Diuretics and fluid restrictions help minimize pulmonary edema. ARDS patients are at high risk for malnutrition. Nutritional needs will be met through enteral or parenteral means.

32. B) 185/115 mmHg

A blood pressure measurement with systolic pressure greater than 180 mmHg and diastolic pressure greater than 110 mmHg is considered a hypertensive crisis.

33. A) The nurse provides information about genetic counseling.

A nurse's role as an advocate is crucial and providing the patient with information on genetic counseling may put the patient's mind at ease. Inaccurate reassurance or avoidance does not respect patient rights. Providing appropriate alternatives and options for the patient and the daughters are correct responses to the patient's concerns.

34. B) Pulmonary edema

Stridor and hypoxia are common in pulmonary edema, which is a complication post-intubation. Pneumothorax would present as profound dyspnea with absence of lung sounds on the affected side. Diffuse atelectasis is a chest x-ray finding indicating pneumonia or fluid. Pulmonary embolism is manifested by chest pain and extreme shortness of breath.

35. B) Reduce blood pressure in increments of 10% to 20% over the course of several hours.

Secondary causes of hypertension are more common in patients who have a hypertensive emergency. The most important aspect of care for the patient with a hypertensive emergency is assuring that high-quality outpatient follow-up is available. Many of the presenting problems may improve greatly if the blood pressure is well controlled. Weight loss is not a priority of care at this point. Starting an oral antihypertensive medication may not be indicated at this time, and the patient may still be on intravenous medications. The nurse should not lower the blood pressure too quickly or too much because ischemic damage can occur in vascular beds.

36. C) Assess pulses distal to insertion site.

Although all vital signs should be monitored on an ongoing basis, assessment of the pulses distal to the insertion site is the priority intervention to ensure adequate tissue perfusion to the limb. Heart rate and urinary output are monitored, but not at a higher priority than the pulses distal to the insertion site. Pulses proximal to the insertion site are not a priority.

37. C) Norepinephrine

The first line of intervention in managing hypotension in a patient with cardiogenic shock is administering an inotrope. Dobutamine is an inotrope. Vasoconstrictors should not be used initially to treat hypotension in cardiogenic shock because of increased systemic vascular resistance. If vasoconstrictors are needed, it is recommended that norepinephrine be used with caution instead of dopamine. Nitroglycerin and sodium nitroprusside are vasodilators and will worsen the patient's condition.

38. B) Accountability

Accountability involves accepting responsibility for the consequences of one's actions, as the nurse did by following policy for reporting and managing the error. Reliability implies that a nurse is dependable. Social justice involves upholding moral, legal, and humanistic principles. Confidentiality is a required and lawful principle that limits healthcare information to designated providers and parties.

39. B) The patient's apical pulse is 76, and the pulse oximetry reading shows a pulse of 144.

The pulse oximetry may be reading artifact or external movements as pulse beats. The patient may also be experiencing arrhythmias, which can alter the accuracy of the pulse oximetry monitor. Comparing the apical heart rate with the rate reported on the pulse oximetry can help determine if the reading is accurate. If the pulse oximetry monitor is unplugged, this could be a low battery indication. The patient reporting that he is cold can lead to false readings, but would more likely result in inability to obtain a reading. A pulse oximeter that shows no pulse on an awake, alert patient should be checked for accuracy.

40. D) Chest pain and shortness of breath not relieved by rest

Class IV heart failure is characterized by chest discomfort at rest and inability to complete activities of daily living. Class I heart failure involves no symptoms or limitations. Class II heart failure involves slight symptoms and limited activity. Class III involves discomfort during any activity that is relieved by rest.

41. B) Flumazenil

Flumazenil is used to reverse sedation and respiratory depression caused by accidental or intentional benzodiazepine overdose. Naloxone is used to rapidly reverse an opioid overdose, sodium bicarbonate is used to treat cardiovascular complications associated with tricyclic antidepressant toxicity, and *N*-Acetylcysteine is used to treat acetaminophen overdoses.

42. **C) Stage III**

Extra-pancreatic inflammation occurs during stage III of hemorrhagic pancreatitis. In stage I, premature activation of trypsin occurs, digestive enzymes are activated, and autodigestion of the pancreas begins. In stage II, intrapancreatic inflammation occurs due to activated neutrophils and macrophages. There is no stage IV.

43. **C) Pull the endotracheal tube back 1 cm.**

Absence of lung sounds on the left side of a newly intubated patient indicates that the endotracheal tube is likely advanced into the right main bronchus, thus only ventilating the right lung. Pulling the tube back 1 cm and re-auscultating is the appropriate initial action. Chest tube insertion might be indicated if pneumothorax is suspected, but this is not an appropriate initial action. Advancing the endotracheal tube will result in a farther right main bronchus intubation. Increasing oxygen concentration will not deliver oxygen to both lungs.

44. **B) Hemodynamic compromise**

When examining a patient with suspected upper gastrointestinal (UGI) bleed, assessing for hemodynamic compromise is critical as the first priority is to address blood loss. While medication and food could cause a patient to experience melena and hematemesis, this is typically not the cause and would not be considered a priority. Mallory-Weiss syndrome is caused by a tear in the gastroesophageal junction and can cause bleeding, so this would be the second priority once blood loss has been stabilized.

45. **D) Therapeutic communication**

Therapeutic communication facilitates interactions focused on the patient and the patient's and family's concerns. Therapeutic communication is defined as the face-to-face process of interaction that focuses on advancing the physical and emotional well-being of a patient. Nurses use therapeutic communication techniques to provide support and information to patients and families. Purposive communication intends to fulfill a conscious purpose or design or to effect a useful function, but not as a result of planning or design. Intrapersonal communication can be defined as communication with one's self that may include self-talk, acts of imagination and visualization, and even recall and memory. Metacommunication involves nonverbal cues (e.g., tone of voice, body language, gestures, facial expression) that carry meaning that either enhance or negate what is said in words.

46. **D) Diabetes insipidus**

The patient likely has diabetes insipidus (DI) caused by the traumatic head injury. The acute head trauma can lead to dysfunction of the hypothalamic neurons secreting antidiuretic hormone (ADH) or of the posterior pituitary gland causing posttraumatic DI. With DI, the kidneys can pass 3 to 20 quarts of urine a day. As a result, a person with DI may feel the need to drink large amounts of liquids. DI and diabetes mellitus (DM) are unrelated. DM causes high blood glucose (blood sugar), resulting from the body's inability to use blood glucose for energy. Hyperthyroidism is the production of too much thyroxine hormone. Symptoms include unexpected weight loss, rapid or irregular heartbeat, sweating, irritability, and an increased metabolism. Hypothyroidism's deficiency of thyroid hormones can disrupt heart rate, body temperature, and all aspects of metabolism.

47. **D) 300**

When calculating the PaO_2/PiO_2 ratio, use a decimal point for the FiO_2: 90 divided by 0.3 is 300. The value 0.3 is the decimal form of 30%. The ratio would be 3 if the nurse forgot to change 30% to a decimal and just divided the two numbers.

48. **D) Tachypnea and tachycardia**

Systemic manifestations of infection include elevated or abnormally low temperature, tachycardia, tachypnea, and leukocytosis. Erythema, warmth, pain, edema, and functional impairment all indicate a local reaction.

49. **D) Alveoli, alveolar ducts, and bronchioles**

The parenchyma is responsible for gas exchange and includes the alveoli, alveolar ducts, and bronchioles. The respiratory system divides into airways and lung parenchyma. The airways consist of the bronchus, which bifurcates off the trachea and divides into bronchioles and then further into alveoli. Therefore, in diffuse parenchymal lung disease, also referred to as interstitial lung disease, the parenchyma would be assessed including the alveoli, alveolar ducts, and bronchioles.

50. **C) Respiratory acidosis**

Normal range for $PaCO_2$ is 35 and 45. Normal range for pH is 7.35 to 7.45. An increase in $PaCO_2$ with an accompanying decrease in pH signifies respiratory acidosis caused by a retention of CO_2. Normal range for HCO_3 is 22 to 26. This may be elevated or below normal, but will not contribute to a respiratory acidosis.

51. **A) Obtain blood cultures.**

Antibiotics are the main treatment for sepsis and should be started early; however, they should be started only if cultures have been obtained first (as long as it does not cause a significant delay in antibiotic administration). The patient is stable, so cultures should be collected first. If antibiotics are administered before a culture is obtained, they may affect the culture results. Inserting a urinary catheter can cause infection and should be avoided if possible. Administering a fluid bolus depends on the patient's hemodynamic status.

52. **A) Cardiac arrhythmias**

Older adult patients with congestive heart failure and angiotensin-converting enzyme (ACE) inhibitor medication therapy have a higher incidence of symptomatic cardiac arrhythmias. This is largely due to electrolyte disturbances induced by diuretic therapy for hypertension and heart failure. The major electrolyte disturbance implicated in arrhythmogenesis is diuretic-induced hypokalemia. A previous myocardial infarction finding would indicate ischemic disease or changes in heart muscle and was present prior to the admission. In complete heart block, there is complete absence of atrioventricular conduction where none of the supraventricular impulses are conducted to the ventricles. This condition does not follow hypokalemia and mild hypomagnesemia. Angina (angina pectoris) describes the pain, discomfort, ache, or other associated symptoms that occur when blood flow to heart muscle cells does not meet its energy needs.

53. **D) 120 beats per minute**

    A normal heart rate (HR) is 60 to 100 beats per minute. An HR of more than 100 beats per minute (e.g., 120 beats per minute) is considered tachycardia. An HR of 40 beats per minute would be considered bradycardia.

54. **C) Type I immunoglobulin E (IgE)-mediated hypersensitivity reaction involves mast cells and basophils that are suddenly released into the body.**

    Anaphylaxis is an acute, potentially life-threatening Type I immunoglobulin E (IgE)-mediated hypersensitivity reaction, involving the release of mediators from mast cells, basophils, and recruited inflammatory cells. When blood clots form in the body, it may be disseminated intravascular coagulation (DIC), a condition that causes too many blood clots to form. It could also be deep vein thrombosis, which is a blood clot that forms in a vein deep in the body. Most deep vein clots occur in the lower leg or thigh. If the vein swells, the condition is called thrombophlebitis. A deep vein thrombosis can break loose and cause a pulmonary embolism. Hypothermia is a medical emergency that occurs when the body loses heat faster than it can produce heat, causing a dangerously low body temperature. Malignant hyperthermia is a potentially lethal inherited disorder characterized by disturbance of calcium homeostasis in skeletal muscle.

55. **C) Left ventricle failure**

    If a patient's central venous pressure (CVP) and the pulmonary arterial occlusion pressure (PAOP) are elevated, it may be due to left ventricular failure or volume overload. Normal CVP is 2 to 6. Normal PAOP is 4 to 12. Right ventricle failure will result in an elevation of CVP and lower PAOP. These values do not reflect an atrial diagnosis.

56. **B) Two 10-U bolus doses given 30 minutes apart**

    Reteplase (rPA) is a thrombolytic agent and would be given in two 10-U boluses given 30 minutes apart. A streptokinase dose is 1.5 million U over 30 to 60 minutes. Tenecteplase doses are weight based. Alteplase is given as a 15-mg bolus followed by 0.75 mg/kg given over 30 minutes and then 0.5 mg/kg over 1 hour.

57. **A) Seizures**

    Seizures are a sign of hypocalcemia and hypomagnesemia. Excessive thirst, abdominal pain, and hypertension are signs of hypercalcemia and hypermagnesemia.

58. **D) Cardiac tamponade**

    One-week post–myocardial infarction patients may face increased risk for a number of complications, including cardiac tamponade. The weakened pulse pressure on inspiration is pulsus paradoxus, which is most commonly caused by cardiac tamponade. Mitral valve rupture would present as an S3 murmur, pulmonary embolus as chest pain and shortness of breath, and pulmonary edema as heart failure symptoms.

59. **C) Intravenous line metoprolol**

    Immediate treatment of atrial fibrillation with rapid ventricular response is a beta blocker such as metoprolol. Amiodarone drip is indicated for continued rate control. Intravenous line (IV) heparin and immediate transthoracic cardioversion is indicated for an unstable, critical situation with ongoing rapid rate. Adenosine push is used for supraventricular tachycardia (SVT), not atrial fibrillation.

60. **C) Serum sodium level of 110 mEq/L**

A normal blood sodium level is between 135 and 145 mEq/L. Hyponatremia occurs when the sodium in the blood falls below 135 mEq/L. Sodium is an essential electrolyte that helps maintain the balance of water in and around the body's cells. Sodium is important for proper muscle and nerve function. Losing sodium quickly is a medical emergency. It can cause loss of consciousness, seizures, and coma. Other common symptoms of low blood sodium include weakness, fatigue, headache, nausea and vomiting, muscle spasms, confusion, and irritability. The normal serum potassium level falls between 3.5 and 5.5 mEq/L. Normal triglycerides levels are 40 to 200 mg/dL. A normal blood glucose level is 70 to 110 mg/dL.

61. **C) The nurse should provide the personal representative with information about the procedure.**

The nurse should provide the personal representative with information about the procedure. The Health Insurance Portability and Accountability Act (HIPAA) Privacy Rule establishes a foundation of federally protected rights that permit individuals to control certain uses and disclosures of their protected health information. Under the Rule, a person authorized to act on behalf of the individual in making healthcare-related decisions is the individual's "personal representative." The nurse should address the patient's representative directly and not ask the representative to contact the administrator or the healthcare provider. It is not necessary to involve the facility's ethics committee.

62. **A) Less antibiotic use**

The use of noninvasive ventilation (NIV) helps lessen the use of antibiotics; however, it increases the patient's risk for aspiration, does not provide airway protection, and decreases the patient's ability to clear secretions.

63. **C) Compensated respiratory acidosis**

The pH of 7.36 is on the acidic side of normal (normal pH is 7.35 to 7.45) rather than the basic side. The $PaCO_2$ is elevated, which indicates a primary respiratory acidosis. The HCO_3 (sodium bicarbonate) is elevated, but the pH is almost normal; therefore, it is compensated. If the HCO_3 were normal, it would represent uncompensated respiratory acidosis. Uncompensated metabolic acidosis is associated with a low pH and a low HCO_3 level. Compensated metabolic alkalosis would be associated with a pH near 7.45.

64. **C) Sympathetic overstimulation of the left atria**

Sympathetic overstimulation of the left atria causes atrial flutter. Atrial fibrillation is caused by left ventral failure. Inflammation causes paroxysmal supraventricular tachycardia. Inferior or posterior wall myocardial infarction causes bradycardia.

65. **A) Decreased serum creatinine**

Creatinine is found in serum, plasma, and urine. It is excreted by glomerular filtration at a constant rate and in the same concentration as in plasma. Creatinine is a more reliable indicator of renal function than blood urea nitrogen because it is less influenced by other factors such as diet and hydration. White blood cell counts do not measure kidney function. An increase in serum creatinine and blood urea nitrogen is abnormal and could indicate renal failure.

66. D) Administer unsynchronized cardioversion

For an unstable patient in ventricular tachycardia, unsynchronized cardioversion is indicated. Administer adenosine for a patient with paroxysmal supraventricular tachycardia, and administer amiodarone for a patient in atrial fibrillation. Atropine is administered for severe bradycardia and cardiac arrest.

67. D) Nonmaleficence

The ethical principle that requires that the nurse's actions inflict no harm is nonmaleficence. The nurse also has a duty to tell the truth, which is called veracity. Autonomy stipulates that patients have the right to determine their own care and the right to refuse treatment. Beneficence refers to the nurse's responsibility to maximize benefit to patient.

68. C) Collaboration

Working with respiratory and physical therapists to help a patient achieve their goal of completing a lap around the nurse's station is an example of collaboration. Nurses exhibit caring practice when they create a compassionate, supportive, and therapeutic environment that emphasizes comfort and healing. Nurses exhibit advocacy when they implement measures to preserve human dignity, promote patient equality, and provide freedom from suffering. While effective communication is an integral component to successful collaboration, it is not demonstrated in this particular scenario.

69. B) Emphysema

Chronic obstructive lung disease is a disorder in which subsets of patients may have dominant features of chronic bronchitis, emphysema, or asthma. The result is airflow obstruction that is not fully reversible. Residual volume is the amount of air left in the lungs at the end of a maximal expiration and is typically increased due to the inability to forcibly expire and remove air from the lungs. Increased lung volumes, particularly residual volume (RV), are commonly observed in airway obstruction. Residual volume is also increased in younger people affected by any condition that causes increased airway resistance, such as bronchitis, asthma, or emphysema. Airway obstruction is the most common cause of reduction in FEV1. Chronic lung diseases associated with a decreased forced vital capacity (FVC) include chronic obstructive pulmonary disease (COPD), emphysema, chronic bronchitis, pulmonary fibrosis, inflammatory lung diseases, and restrictive and obstructive airway diseases.

70. D) Voluntary consent and risks, benefits, alternatives of treatment

Informed consent is the process in which a healthcare provider educates a patient about the risks, benefits, and alternatives of a given procedure or intervention. The patient must be competent to make a voluntary decision about whether to undergo the procedure or intervention. Informed consent is both an ethical and legal obligation of the healthcare provider. For informed consent to be achieved, the patient should receive the diagnosis or condition that requires treatment, purposes of the treatment, what the patient can expect to feel and experience, intended benefits of the treatment, risks, and what could occur if the surgery is not performed or if alternatives to the treatment are chosen. The patient must not be coerced in any manner. Type of anesthesia, length of recovery, and insurance coverage are not elements required of informed consent because these are done prior to the procedure and patients are informed and educated prior. In addition, in most cases, insurance has already been preapproved for the procedure prior to scheduling.

71. **B) Is experiencing a conflict with personal values**

    The nurse is distressed because the situation is creating a conflict with her personal values. Values are described as an individual's set of personal beliefs and attitudes that guide one's behavior. The decision is within ethical principles and institutional policy, so it will not produce legal repercussions. This is not a case of euthanasia because the patient is not able to participate in this decision. In addition, cultural values are not a component of this scenario.

72. **B) Tachypnea**

    Tachypnea is a respiratory condition that results in fast and shallow breathing. It is commonly seen in patients experiencing a pulmonary embolism (PE). A pulmonary embolus can cause permanent damage to the lungs and low oxygen levels in the blood. Common signs and symptoms of PE include dyspnea, pleuritic chest pain, tachycardia, and tachypnea. Recurrent short episodes of bradycardia and hypotension are rarely reported as clinical manifestations of an acute PE. The main symptom of bradycardia is a heart rate less than 60 BPM. This abnormally low heart rate can cause the brain and other organs to become oxygen deprived. Subconjunctival hemorrhage is the term for a broken blood vessel on the surface of the eye that is usually caused by trauma, straining, contact lenses, or routine anticoagulant therapy. Bradypnea is an abnormally slow breathing rate. This is the opposite of tachypnea, which is common in an acute pulmonary embolus.

73. **B) Assess the patient's SpO$_2$ and neurologic status.**

    Diltiazem is a calcium channel blocker. When the route of administration is changed from intravenous (IV) to oral administration, the uptake is slowed. Cardiac output may be compromised and not adequate to sustain oxygen delivery to the brain. If the SpO$_2$ is low, the dose may need to be increased or resumption of IV therapy initiated. Lorazepam or haloperidol will only mask the neurologic symptoms of hypoxia and would be contraindicated. A drug interaction could be considered, but this is not the appropriate initial nursing action.

74. **C) Creatinine clearance, complete blood count, liver function tests**

    Nonsteroidal anti-inflammatory drugs (NSAIDs) are medications widely used to relieve pain, reduce inflammation, and bring down a high temperature. NSAIDs are generally not recommended for people with kidney disease, heart failure, or cirrhosis, or those who take diuretics. It is important to assess the patient's creatinine clearance to determine kidney function, as well as liver function tests and complete blood count, prior to initiation of NSAID therapy. There is no need to assess the patient's electrolytes or serum amylase because neither of these levels are affected by NSAIDs.

75. **A) Initiate intravenous regular insulin.**

    The patient should be treated for hyperosmolar hyperglycemic nonketotic syndrome (HHNS). A hyperosmolar hyperglycemic state is a metabolic complication of diabetes mellitus characterized by severe hyperglycemia, extreme dehydration, hyperosmolar plasma, and altered consciousness. It most often occurs in older type 2 diabetic patients, often in the setting of physiologic stress. A hyperosmolar hyperglycemic state is diagnosed by severe hyperglycemia and plasma hyperosmolality and absence of significant ketosis. Treatment is intravenous (IV) saline solution and regular insulin.

76. B) Timeline

Clinical pathways are detailed, evidence-based protocols for delivering care to patients with specific conditions. They are used to guide the provision of quality and efficient patient care, improve patient safety, and minimize healthcare costs. A clinical pathway includes four essential components: timeline, categories of care and associated interventions, intermediate and long-term outcome criteria (not short-term), and variance record. An order set is a clinical decision support tool that helps healthcare providers prescribe appropriate treatments using predefined sets of applicable drugs and recommended dosages. Order sets may be incorporated into a clinical pathway; however, they are not an essential component. Patient response is not a component of a clinical pathway.

77. C) Right-sided heart failure

The patient is having symptoms consistent with right-sided heart failure: jugular vein distention, hepatomegaly, splenomegaly, elevated central venous pressure, peripheral edema, decreased cardiac output, and tachycardia. Left-sided heart failure will manifest with tachypnea, crackles, cough, pink frothy sputum, and tachycardia. Symptoms of cardiogenic shock include tachycardia, cool clammy skin, decreased urine output, tachypnea, and altered mental status. Hypertrophic cardiomyopathy will manifest with electrocardiogram changes, dyspnea, and an S4 gallop.

78. D) Blood pressure management

Blood pressure management during post-op care of a patient with an aortic repair with graft placement is the priority to prevent disruption of the graft, dissection, and hemorrhage. Hemodynamic monitoring, prevention of fluid overload, correct coagulopathies, and administering of antibiotics to prevent infections are also components of management.

79. A) Beneficence

The ethical concept of beneficence is the obligation to help the patient by removing or preventing harm and promoting good. The nurse has a duty to remove wrist restraints when they are no longer needed. Utilitarianism is the obligation to act in such a way to be useful or beneficial to the majority. Justice is the quality of being fair and acting without bias. Autonomy refers to the obligation to ensure that mentally competent patients have the right to make their own health decisions.

80. A) mPAP of 30 mmHg and PAOP of 10 mmHg

Hemodynamic findings of pulmonary arterial hypertension (PAH) are mean pulmonary artery pressure (mPAP) of more than 25 mmHg and pulmonary artery occlusive pressure (PAOP) of less than 15 mmHg.

81. C) 40% to 59% predicted

A moderate obstruction is identified by a forced expiratory volume in 1 second (FEV1) that equals 40% to 59% predicted. A FEV1 greater than 80% predicted is considered normal. A FEV1 of 60% to 79% predicted would indicate a mild obstruction, and less than 40% would indicate a severe obstruction.

82. C) Abdominal pain, fever, and rigid board-like abdomen

Peritonitis is inflammation of the peritoneum, which is the lining of the inner wall of the abdomen that covers organs in the abdomen. Positive assessment findings in peritonitis can include acute abdominal pain, elevated temperature, and involuntary guarding due to severe pain. The abdominal muscles are tense and board-like upon palpation. Early in peritonitis, bowel sounds can be heard on auscultation, but these sounds tend to disappear as the inflammation progresses. Hypoactive bowel sounds and slow and irregular pulse are not correct because peritonitis causes tachycardia. Hyperactive bowel sounds, vomiting, and diarrhea are incorrect, as bowel sounds tend to subside. Lethargy, hypothermia, and slow respirations would not be correct due to the inflammatory process which increases the temperature.

83. A) Administer acetylcysteine

Acetylcysteine is the appropriate initial treatment for acetaminophen overdose. Multiple large-bore intravenous lines (IVs) are appropriate for trauma or hypovolemia. EKG is not an initial action for acetaminophen overdose. Dopamine is not used in the treatment of acetaminophen overdose.

84. A) Narcotic analgesia

Narcotic analgesia is the most appropriate first response. The symptoms suggest that an obstruction of the urinary tract is present, which can be due to scar tissues from radiation therapy. The pain of an obstruction is excruciating. A CT scan of the abdomen can be helpful in diagnosing the problem. High-speed or dual energy CT may reveal scar tissues and even tiny stones. Simple abdominal x-rays are used less frequently because this kind of imaging test can miss scar tissue or small stones. Lithotripsy may be ordered if there is a conclusive diagnosis of stones, but this would not be indicated in patients with scar tissue. Providing the patient with a strainer to catch passed stones will not treat the pain being experienced by the patient, nor will it identify any other cause of pain.

85. B) Congestive heart failure

Congestive heart failure accounts for 90% of transudative pleural effusions. A transudative pleural effusion is caused by a fluid shift out of the capillaries due to increased hydrostatic pressure or decreased oncotic pressure. Pneumonia would cause an exudative effusion due to leaky capillary walls caused by inflammation or infection. Although possible, nephrotic syndrome and pulmonary embolus are not common causes of transudative pleural effusions.

86. A) Atrial flutter

Atrial flutter is caused by sympathetic overstimulation of the left atrium. Acid–base disturbances cause ventricular tachycardia. Bradycardia is caused by an inferior or posterior wall myocardial infarction or vagal stimulation. Third-degree atrioventricular (AV) block is caused by an anterior or inferior wall infarct.

87. B) Propranolol

Propranolol is a beta blocker used to treat high blood pressure, irregular heart rate, tremors, and other conditions. It is the treatment of choice to prevent recurrent episodes of esophageal varices. Simvastatin is used to treat patients with elevated low-density lipoprotein (LDL) cholesterol levels and is considered the best choice in lowering LDL levels. Vasopressin is used to treat diabetes insipidus and to treat or prevent certain conditions of the stomach after surgery or during abdominal x-rays. Vasopressin is used in emergency settings to raise blood pressure in adults who are in shock. Octreotide is an octapeptide that mimics natural somatostatin pharmacologically, though it is a more potent inhibitor of growth hormone, glucagon, and insulin than the natural hormone. Octreotide is often given as an infusion for management of acute hemorrhage from esophageal varices in liver cirrhosis on the basis that it reduces portal venous pressure.

88. **A) Weakened respiratory muscles**

Structural changes to the respiratory system as individuals age include weakened respiratory muscles, the chest wall becomes stiffer as a result of calcification of the cartilage, kyphosis may occur, and arthritic changes to the costovertebral joints can be seen. Likewise, the lungs become smaller and less elastic. Diminished coughing and gag reflexes and increased mouth breathing and snoring are functional changes to the respiratory system in older adults.

89. **A) Assess the patient for breath sounds and respiratory effort.**

A soaked gown indicates that the incision is bleeding excessively. This could indicate edema and pressure in the surgical site, thus affecting the patient's breathing. Blood could be compromising the airway. Assessing the patient for breath sounds and respiratory effort is the priority. Reassuring the patient and changing the gown can be done after the airway is secured. Reinforcing the dressing and calling the surgeon should be completed after the airway is secured. Raising the head of the bed is dependent on the airway assessment.

90. **D) Increased cardiac output and increased left ventricular filling pressures**

A handgrip will increase systemic vascular resistance, cardiac output, and left ventricle filling pressures. The Valsalva maneuver decreases venous return and ventricular volumes. Taking a breath (inspiration) will increase venous return and ventricular volumes. Leg elevation will increase systemic vascular resistance and venous return.

91. **A) Hematemesis**

In an upper gastrointestinal (UGI) bleed, patients will experience vomiting of blood (hematemesis) that often resembles coffee ground-like blood. Tachycardia, not bradycardia will also be noted. Left upper quadrant pain most often is due to diseases of the pancreas, spleen, and heart, not UGI bleed.

92. **A) Unintentional, partial-thickness wound**

The patient sustained an unintentional, partial-thickness wound. An unintentional wound is an accidental wound. A partial-thickness wound is characterized by all or a portion of the dermis remaining intact. A full-thickness wound is characterized by severing of the entire dermis, sweat glands, and hair follicles.

93. **D) Iodine**

Iodine is a central component of thyroid hormones that regulate growth, development, and metabolic rate. A patient will present with weight gain, lethargy, and a goiter. Low iodine levels result in hypothyroidism. If deficient in calcium, the patient presents with impaired growth and osteoporosis.

When deficient in fluoride, the patient presents with dental decay and is subject to osteoporosis. A sodium deficiency presents as restlessness, irritability, muscle weakness, cramps, and possibly nausea and vomiting.

94. **D) Coronary balloon angioplasty with stenting**

The patient is having electrocardiogram changes associated with ST-segment elevation myocardial infarction (STEMI). An emergency coronary balloon angioplasty with stenting is recommended for STEMI. Thrombolytic therapy remains an important option for hospitals without the capability of balloon angioplasty. Cardiopulmonary bypass is indicated when repair of the aorta is needed. Revascularization is performed to manage cardiogenic shock.

95. **B) Increased TSH, normal free T3, normal free T4**

Subclinical hypothyroidism is an early, mild form of hypothyroidism, a condition in which the body does not produce enough thyroid hormones. It is called subclinical because only the serum level of thyroid-stimulating hormone from the front of the pituitary gland is a little bit above normal. Thyroid-stimulating hormone (TSH) levels change before free T3 and free T4, making TSH levels the best screening test for thyroid dysfunction. Increased TSH indicates a hypothyroid state. The normal free T3 and T4 indicate a subclinical picture. These patients may develop overt hypothyroidism. Normal TSH, decreased free T3, decreased free T4 is considered hypothyroidism (not subclinical). Decreased TSH, decreased free T3, and decreased free T4 is hypothyroidism. Normal TSH, decreased free T3, and normal free T4 constitutes central hypothyroidism. A low TSH and low T4 indicate hypothyroidism due to a problem involving the pituitary gland. A low TSH with an elevated T4 is found in individuals who have hyperthyroidism. T3 tests are often useful to diagnosis hyperthyroidism or to determine the severity of the hyperthyroidism.

96. **D) The patient's blood pressure will increase.**

The Valsalva maneuver is the performance of forced expiration against a closed glottis. Activities such as straining during defecation entail performance of the Valsalva maneuver. The key event occurring during the maneuver is increasing intrathoracic pressure leading to the reduction of preload to the heart. The onset of strain is associated with a transient rise in blood pressure (BP) because of emptying of some blood from the large veins and pulmonary circulation. When a patient bears down to defecate, the increased pressures in the abdominal and thoracic cavities result in a decreased blood flow and a temporary decrease in cardiac output. Once the bearing down ceases, the pressure is lessened, and a larger than normal amount of blood returns to the heart, which elevates the patient's BP.

97. **C) Seizure precautions**

Seizure precautions should be in place. Syndrome of inappropriate antidiuretic hormone secretion (SIADH) is a condition in which the body makes too much antidiuretic hormone (ADH). This hormone helps the kidneys control the amount of water the body loses through urination. SIADH causes the body to retain too much water. This process upsets the body's balance of electrolytes, causing hyponatremia. With a severe and acute fall in sodium concentration, headache, lethargy, obtundation, and seizures can occur. A hypertensive crisis is not associated with SIADH. Carbohydrate precautions would be associated with blood sugar values. All patients in the unit would be under fall precautions, but this is not based on late symptoms of SIADH.

98. **C) Adrenal insufficiency**

Adrenal insufficiency, including Addison's disease, is a disorder that occurs when the adrenal glands do not make enough of certain hormones. These include cortisol, sometimes called the "stress hormone," which is essential for life. Patients with adrenal insufficiency experience fatigue, muscle weakness, loss of appetite, weight loss, and abdominal pain. Hyponatremia, hyperkalemia, and hypoglycemia are often present. Adrenal insufficiency is considered a medical emergency. Onset of type 1 diabetes would not present with hypoglycemia. Patients with myxedema present with weight gain, although they may have hyponatremia and hypoglycemia. Diabetic ketoacidosis signs and symptoms often develop quickly, sometimes within 24 hours. Symptoms may be the first indication of having diabetes and include excessive thirst, frequent urination, nausea and vomiting, abdominal pain, weakness or fatigue, shortness of breath, fruity-scented breath, and confusion. Blood sugar levels will be high, and ketones appear in the urine.

99. **B) 45 mL/beat**

Stroke volume = cardiac output/heart rate (× 1,000). This patient's stroke volume = 45. Mean arterial pressure = (systolic blood pressure – diastolic blood pressure/3) + diastolic blood pressure. This patient's mean arterial pressure = 123 mmHg. Cardiac index = cardiac output/body surface area. For this patient, it is 2.2 L/min/m2. Systemic vascular resistance = (mean arterial blood pressure – central venous pressure) x 80/cardiac output. For this patient, that is 2,260.

100. **A) Urinary catheter placement**

A patient in diabetic ketoacidosis (DKA) will have increased urine output. Output needs to be monitored closely as the glucose levels are decreased, so a urinary catheter will likely be placed. A nasogastric tube may be placed later if necessary but will not be the next procedure. The patient should already have an intravenous line (IV) because the insulin infusion has been started. A central line is not indicated at this point since the patient has the IV access required for current treatment.

101. **C) Arteriogram**

An arteriogram is the gold standard tool for diagnosing a thoracic aortic aneurysm. CT scans and chest x-rays are used for screening, not diagnosis. Ultrasound is not used in the diagnosis of thoracic aortic aneurysm.

102. **B) Urine output of less than 0.5 mL/kg/hr for more than 6 consecutive hours**

Postrenal failure results in kidney injury. Acute kidney injury (AKI) is an abrupt or rapid decline in renal function. Criteria for AKI is urine output less than 0.5 mL/kg/hr for more than 6 consecutive hours, serum creatinine that rises by 0.3 mg/dL or more within 48 hours, or serum creatinine that rises by 1.5 times or more from normal.

103. **B) Hyperactive bowel sounds**

Hyperactive bowel sounds are often found before a blockage. It is quite common to find one quadrant with hyperactive bowel sounds and one with none or hypoactive ones. This is because the intestine is attempting to clear the blockage with increased peristalsis. The nurse may also hear high-pitched sounds and rushing noises. Obstipation or absent bowel sounds are seen in late bowel obstruction. High-pitched sounds may be heard in the early stages of a bowel obstruction, but not low-pitched, rumbling bowel sounds, or diminished sounds.

104. C) Crystalloids

The initial fluid resuscitation recommendation for sepsis is crystalloids. If the patient requires substantial amounts of fluids to meet the goal of volume resuscitation, then albumin can be added. Blood is a colloid, not a crystalloid. Hetastarch is not recommended for sepsis due to the worsening effect it has on the kidneys.

105. B) Right direction

In the progressive care environment, nurses will often delegate tasks to unlicensed assistive personnel. When delegating, the nurse should always follow the five Rights of Delegation: right task, right circumstance, right person, right direction, and right supervision. First, the nurse must determine if it is the right task—one that is appropriate to delegate and is delegable according to all necessary rules and regulations. The nurse must also ensure that the right circumstances are in place (e.g., setting is appropriate, resources are available) for successful completion of the delegated task. The nurse must then consider whether they are delegating to the right person (i.e., one that has the skills required to successfully complete the task), as well as ensure that the delegatee understands which patient requires assistance. Providing the medical assistant with clear explanations of the task and expectations, as demonstrated in the scenario, is providing the right direction. The final step in the process is the right supervision. This occurs when the nurse carefully monitors, provides feedback, evaluates, and intervenes as required until the task is complete.

106. D) 10:00 p.m.

The half-life of morphine is 3 hours. There would be 5 half-lives to a 3-hour half-life, which calculates to 15 hours. The morphine would be expected to be eliminated from the patient's body by 10:00 p.m.

107. B) Level 3

In Level 3 resiliency, a patient can mount a moderate response with some degree of compensation. If the patient were unable to mount a response, didn't have any compensatory mechanism, and had minimal reserves, they would be classified at a Level 1 (minimally resilient). A patient who can mount and maintain a response with intact compensatory mechanisms and strong reserves would be considered a Level 5, or highly resilient. There is not a Level 4 when referring to resiliency.

108. C) Autonomy

Autonomy means that patients are able to make independent decisions and that they have been made aware of all information in order to make informed independent decisions. Nurses do not influence the patient's choice. Self-determination is a concept that refers to each person's ability to make choices and manage one's own life and allows people to feel that they have control over their choices and lives. Justice is being fair and acting without bias. Veracity is the basis of the trust relationship established between a patient and a healthcare provider. It ensures that honesty and all information was provided and allows for patients to make good decisions.

109. A) A patient in status asthmaticus

A patient in status asthmaticus is a candidate for noninvasive ventilation (NIV). NIV is not recommended for patients with altered mental status, swallowing abnormalities, or an inability to control secretions due to the risk of aspiration. These patients should be intubated and placed on a ventilator.

110. **C) Pericardial tamponade**

A patient with pericardial tamponade will have a pulse that alternates between strong and weak. The nurse should consider septic shock on a patient with a bounding pulse. Hypovolemia should be considered on a patient with a weak and thready pulse. A patient with hypertrophic cardiomyopathy will have pulsus bisferiens.

111. **D) Bronchial**

Bronchial breath sounds are loud, high-pitched sounds heard primarily over the trachea and larynx. A normal breath sound is similar to the sound of air. Rhonchi is a low-pitched breath sound. Vesicular breath sounds are low-pitched, soft sounds heard over the peripheral lung fields. Vesicular, bronchial, and bronchovesicular breath sounds are normal breath sounds.

112. **D) Chronic obstructive pulmonary disease**

In patients diagnosed with chronic obstructive pulmonary disease, oxygen toxicity related to high carbon dioxide content in the blood (hypercapnia) leads to drowsiness (narcosis), deranged acid–base balance due to respiratory acidosis, and death. The brain does not recognize high levels of carbon dioxide as a stimulus to breathe, so giving high levels of oxygen further removes this stimulus as the brain must experience oxygen hunger. Administering oxygen at 2 L/min is considered a safe rate of supplemental oxygen. Pulmonary edema is a condition caused by excess fluid in the lungs. Asthma is a condition in which a person's airways become inflamed, narrow and swell, and produce extra mucus, which makes it difficult to breathe. Rhinitis is inflammation and swelling of the mucous membrane of the nose, characterized by a runny nose and stuffiness and usually caused by the common cold or a seasonal allergy.

113. **A) Systemic inflammatory response syndrome**

By process of elimination, systemic inflammatory response syndrome (SIRS) is the correct answer. Data doesn't support septic, cardiogenic shock, or multiple organ dysfunction syndrome (MODS). This data does meet the definition of SIRS because there are at least two SIRS signs and symptoms being reported: fever and tachycardia. It cannot be determined whether the patient is septic. White blood cells are high normal and cultures are negative, but sepsis can be suspected. Shock is not yet present as evidenced by the normal lactate level in the presence of a low normal blood pressure with adequate urine output = 0.5 mL/kg/hr. MODS is not correct because that would be the sequelae to shock, and there is only one possible organ involvement reported.

114. **D) Asymmetrical chest expansion**

Asymmetrical chest expansion can indicate the presence of a pneumothorax, a complication of mechanical ventilation. The normal urine output is 30 mL/hr. The urine output of 110 mL over 4 hours is within normal limits. The pulse oximetry reading of 96% is within normal limits. Sinus bradycardia would not be a ventilator complication.

115. **A) A patient experiencing a panic attack**

This is an example of hyperventilation as seen in patients experiencing a panic attack. The pH of 7.6 means the patient is alkalotic; the $PaCO_2$ of 23 mmHg is low and consistent with respiratory alkalosis; the bicarbonate is low in the attempt to compensate. The patient is blowing off CO_2. A patient experiencing a morphine overdose would have respirator depression, leading to respiratory acidosis. A patient experiencing prolonged vomiting would have metabolic alkalosis due to extracellular fluid depletion from the gastrointestinal tract. A patient with uncontrolled type 1 diabetes would experience metabolic acidosis.

116. **B) Stage II pressure injury**

A stage II pressure injury is defined as a partial-thickness loss of dermis presenting as a shallow open ulcer with a red–pink wound bed. Stage I is defined as intact skin with a localized area of nonblanchable redness, usually over a bony prominence. Stage III is defined as full-thickness loss without exposed bone, tendon, or muscle. Stage IV is defined as full-thickness tissue loss with exposed bone, tendon, and muscle.

117. **B) Hyponatremia**

Hyponatremia matches the severity of heart failure within dilated cardiomyopathy. This is because of the release of antidiuretic hormone and volume overload. Hypomagnesemia is a feature of heart failure associated with complex ventricular arrhythmias. Hypokalemia increases the risk of cardiac arrythmias and reduces survival in patients suffering from a myocardial infarction. Hypocalcemia is a relatively uncommon but reversible cause of congestive heart failure.

118. **D) Keep the collection bag lower than the bladder.**

To reduce the risk of urinary tract infection, the collection bag should be kept lower than the bladder. The risk of infection is higher with an open drainage system and/or when the bag is emptied only when it is full. The bag should not be placed on the floor.

119. **B) Diuresis to reduce myocardial workload**

The decreased SpO_2, along with crackles in all lung fields and increased pulse, indicates the patient has a fluid volume overload. The patient needs diuretics to reduce the myocardial workload and optimize cardiac output. Enhancing venous return will not restore stability as the problem is an inadequate cardiac output. Antiarrhythmics are not indicated because the problem is fluid volume. The increased heart rate, crackles, and reduced SpO_2 indicate increased myocardial workload rather than a pulmonary embolism, which usually manifests as chest pain and shortness of breath.

120. **A) Learning needs assessment**

All patients require a learning needs assessment admission; preferred language is a question within the assessment. Vulnerability and competency are part of patient characteristics in the American Association of Critical-Care Nurses (AACN) Synergy Model and do not provide the patient's language preference. The nurse shows cultural competency by trying to assess and determine the patient's needs related to their culture, but not language.

121. **A) Request same-sex caregivers**

A Hindu patient may request same-sex caregivers. A patient who is a Christian Scientist may refuse all medical care. A patient who is a Jehovah's Witness may refuse blood transfusions. A Muslim patient may request that their face be turned toward the right after they die.

122. **D) "You have electrolyte abnormalities."**

Causes of ventricular tachycardia include electrolyte abnormalities, hypoxia, and acid–base disturbances. Cardiogenic shock causes ventricular fibrillation. Atrial fibrillation can be caused by pericarditis and left ventricle failure.

123. **C) The right to refuse treatment**

The right to refuse treatment is grounded in the ethical principle of respect for autonomy of the individual. The patient has the right to refuse treatment if the patient is competent and is made aware of the risks and complications associated with refusal of treatment. The right to die involves whether to initiate or withhold life-sustaining treatment for a patient who is irreversibly comatose, vegetative, or suffering with end-stage terminal illness. Substituted judgment is an ethical principle used when the decision is made for an incapacitated patient based on what is best for the patient. An advance directive is a document used as a guideline for starting or continuing life-sustaining medical care of patients with a terminal disease or disability who can no longer communicate their own wishes.

124. **A) Ascending cholangitis**

These symptoms are consistent with ascending cholangitis. Cholangitis is an infection of the biliary tree that requires prompt diagnosis and treatment. Most patients have fever, jaundice, and right upper-quadrant pain (Charcot triad). Cholangitis can quickly become an acute, septic, life-threatening infection that requires rapid evaluation and treatment. Acute pyelonephritis is a sudden and severe kidney infection. Common symptoms include a fever greater than 102°F (38.9°C); pain in the abdomen, back, side, or groin; painful or burning urination; and fishy-smelling, cloudy, or bloody urine. Acute appendicitis presents with pain near the belly button and then the right lower quadrant, accompanied by nausea, vomiting, poor appetite, fever, and chills. Choledocholithiasis refers to the presence of gallstones within the common bile duct without infection or acute symptoms.

125. **C) Gait disturbances**

Gait disturbances are a sign or symptom of hypophosphatemia due to bone pain that is caused by alterations in bone metabolism and bone material structure. Nausea and vomiting are symptoms of hyponatremia. Excessive thirst can be caused by hypercalcemia and hypermagnesemia.

CHAPTER 2

POP QUIZ 2.1

The nurse's next action would be to increase the patient's oxygen to obtain a saturation >90%. The nurse should then notify the provider of the new ST elevation noted on the EKG and worsening symptoms and vital sign changes.

POP QUIZ 2.2

The nurse's next action should be to auscultate the heart and lungs. Pericarditis after acute chest trauma can quickly progress into a pericardial effusion and/or cardiac tamponade. When auscultating the heart, muffled heart sounds or a pericardial friction rub may be present. These assessment findings, in addition to the patient's presentation, are hallmark signs of acute pericarditis.

POP QUIZ 2.3

The nurse should request activity orders and pain relief medication. Activity and movement may elevate blood pressure (BP) greater than the 110-mmHg goal. Confirm with the provider what activity orders are appropriate for your patient. Patients with suspected aortic aneurysms should be treated with pain medication and antihypertensives. While this patient's aortic aneurysm was asymptomatic, he did sustain a rib fracture. The pain associated with his acute trauma may contribute to a BP increase and jeopardize the integrity of the aneurysm. Bedside monitoring is also indicated for BP management and sudden vital sign changes in the patient.

POP QUIZ 2.4

This patient has three-vessel disease, which is a contraindication to stent placement or balloon angioplasty. She requires a coronary artery bypass grafting to treat her coronary artery disease and lesions. You should expect cardiothoracic surgery to place orders to urgently prep this patient for surgery.

POP QUIZ 2.5

Notify the provider. This is a surgical emergency, which requires prompt evacuation of the extra fluid from the pericardial sac.

POP QUIZ 2.6

Notify the provider that the patient requires a higher level of care. Vasopressors are not typically administered in the progressive care unit. This patient requires central-line placement, vasopressors, and continuous arterial blood pressure monitoring. Call a rapid response if necessary to gather additional support staff to facilitate a quick transfer.

POP QUIZ 2.7

Patients with HIV are at risk to develop left ventricular dysfunction, which often progresses to dilated cardiomyopathy and presents with little to no symptoms. If this patient's HIV antibody test comes back positive, then the etiology of his cardiomyopathy has likely been identified. This patient can begin highly active antiretroviral therapy. Prophylaxis for opportunistic infection, which could worsen the clinical condition, can now be administered.

POP QUIZ 2.8

The nurse should notify the provider immediately, call for a rapid response, and prepare for transfer to the ICU.

POP QUIZ 2.9

Patients taking loop diuretics are at risk for developing hypokalemia. If hypokalemia develops in the context of digoxin therapy, patients are at risk for developing digoxin toxicity. Digoxin toxicity manifests with gastrointestinal symptoms (nausea, vomiting, and anorexia), visual disturbances (blurred vision, photophobia, yellow-tinged vision, and halos), central nervous system symptoms (fatigue and headache), and dysrhythmia, which can result in cardiac arrest.

POP QUIZ 2.10

Patients with hypertension (HTN) and their family must be educated on the importance of following a low-sodium diet to help achieve blood pressure control. Patients and family may hear that sodium should be avoided; however, many do not understand which foods have high sodium and may need education on what should be avoided. Chinese takeout and fast food have elevated levels of sodium, which can be dangerous for patients with HTN. Advise the wife to bring a breakfast item that adheres to the Dietary Approaches to Stop Hypertension (DASH) diet.

POP QUIZ 2.11

Notify the provider immediately and call for necessary support team members depending on the situation (rapid response, code stroke, code team, etc.). Prepare to transfer to a higher level of care.

POP QUIZ 2.12

Patients with mitral valve stenosis and atrial fibrillation are at high risk for embolism development, pulmonary embolism, deep vein thrombosis, or stroke. Anticoagulation or antiplatelet therapy is indicated to prevent these additional complications.

POP QUIZ 2.13

Administer vitamin K as ordered and monitor for excessive bleeding.

CHAPTER 3

POP QUIZ 3.1

Barotrauma occurs from overdistention of the alveoli during mechanical ventilation through increased tidal volumes or high positive end-expiratory pressure settings. Barotrauma can lead to pneumothorax, tension pneumothorax, and subcutaneous emphysema.

POP QUIZ 3.2

Intubation and mechanical ventilation are the next steps if the patient becomes unresponsive to standard treatment.

POP QUIZ 3.3

Patients with no history of smoking or secondhand smoke inhalation should be worked up for alpha 1 antitrypsin deficiency. This is a genetic disorder that can cause chronic obstructive pulmonary disease.

POP QUIZ 3.4

Respiratory depressants (including opioids, sedatives, alcohol, or other drugs) should be avoided, as they can worsen sleep apnea.

POP QUIZ 3.5

The nurse should clarify the procedure being performed related to the diagnosis with the student. Needle decompression is an appropriate treatment for a tension pneumothorax, but not hemothorax.

POP QUIZ 3.6

Daily oral care with oral cleaning solution is an essential daily intervention.

POP QUIZ 3.7

Lung transplant is considered the last option for treatment of pulmonary hypertension (HTN). Despite this option, there is the potential for recurrence of pulmonary HTN post lung transplant.

POP QUIZ 3.8

Although the patient wakes up complaining of pain, the respiratory rate is concerning. Providing additional pain medication is contraindicated based on mental status and alertness, oxygen saturation, and respiratory rate (RR). Hold any additional narcotics until the patient's RR and mental status improve. Consider a reversal agent if the patient continues to be difficult to arouse.

POP QUIZ 3.9

Proning patients who are mechanically ventilated can improve ventilatory status. If no improvement is observed with proning, the patient can be considered a candidate for extracorporeal membrane oxygenation.

POP QUIZ 3.10

This is correct. Atelectasis following a thoracic procedure can be an emergency. If chest tube and intubation are indicated and not possible in your current setting, call for immediate transfer to the ICU.

CHAPTER 4

POP QUIZ 4.1

Call 911, make sure the patient is in a safe place while waiting for emergency medical services (EMS) with a patent airway, check the patient's blood sugar, and utilize the emergency glucagon kit.

POP QUIZ 4.2

A fasting blood glucose >125 is concerning for diabetes. While there are other reasons for an elevated fasting blood glucose in the inpatient setting (such as stress or acute illness), the provider should be notified of this finding. Treat as ordered and continue to monitor throughout the course of their progressive care unit (PCU) admission.

POP QUIZ 4.3

The patient is hypernatremic. Notify the provider and request fluids be exchanged to 0.45% normal saline.

POP QUIZ 4.4

Untreated hyperglycemia can result in microvascular damage. This most commonly includes neuropathy, retinopathy, and nephropathy. Large vessel damage includes coronary artery disease, peripheral vascular disease, and cerebrovascular disease.

POP QUIZ 4.5

Notify the provider, then follow institutional protocol for hypoglycemia. Provide the patient with another 4 oz of juice or bolus of intravenous dextrose and recheck blood glucose in 15 minutes. Repeat this process until the patient's blood glucose is >70 mg/dL.

CHAPTER 5

POP QUIZ 5.1

The nurse should notify the provider immediately of a suspected gastrointestinal (GI) bleed. Although this patient is receiving intravenous iron replacement for his iron deficiency anemia, his vital sign changes, abdominal pain, and stool volume, consistency, and distinct odor are consistent with an acute GI bleed. Urgent intervention is needed.

POP QUIZ 5.2

Check the patient's chart to make sure the provider has obtained consent for blood product administration. Verify the patient has an active type and screen prior to administering any blood products. Protocols may vary among institutions, but the patient will most likely need a larger-bore intravenous line (IV) to receive his blood products. Insert a large-bore IV or consult the IV therapy team to assist with IV placement. If unsuccessful, the provider may have to place a central line. During an emergency, the blood may be initiated via the 22 gauge IV and switched to larger-bore IV when more access is obtained.

POP QUIZ 5.3

The provider will order the immediate discontinuation of heparin.

CHAPTER 6
POP QUIZ 6.1

Patients with hepatic encephalopathy and elevated ammonia levels should routinely and regularly take lactulose to decrease ammonia level through excretion. It is important to engage in therapeutic communication and reeducate patients on the importance of adhering to these medication orders. If unsuccessful, notify the provider.

POP QUIZ 6.2

The next step is to call for assistance, lay the head of the bed down, and position the patient on their side. The nurse should not insert anything into the patient's mouth during the seizure (tongue blade, suction catheter, etc.). Make sure the patient is free from injury.

POP QUIZ 6.3

Prior to administering their first oral by mouth intake/meal, the nurse should confirm that a swallow study has taken place and that the provider diet order allows for the type of food brought in by the family. If a swallow study has not been conducted or the current diet order does not allow for a milkshake, explain this process to the daughter and offer to store the milkshake in the freezer until the swallow study has been completed or the diet order has been appropriately modified based on clinical condition. Consult speech–language pathology to assist with completing the swallow study per hospital protocol.

CHAPTER 7
POP QUIZ 7.1

Large bowel obstruction is suspected. Intermittent feculent vomiting with diffuse abdominal pain and constipation are symptoms of large bowel obstruction.

POP QUIZ 7.2

Gastric residuals should be checked by aspirating and measuring gastric contents. If gastric residuals are >250 mL prior to initiating tube feed, the tube feed should be held, and the provider should be notified.

POP QUIZ 7.3

The rigid abdomen with worsening abdominal and back pain, tachycardia, and hypotension indicate that the patient may be bleeding postoperatively. The nurse should call the provider, who will evaluate the need to return to surgery to repair the bleed.

POP QUIZ 7.4

Each hospital and program are different; however, many liver transplant programs do not list patients with history of alcohol abuse unless they have at least 6 months of sobriety. Refer to the transplant coordinator for further questions and explanation.

POP QUIZ 7.5

Minimal fasting before surgery, ambulation soon after surgery, returning to normal eating and drinking within a day of surgery, and multimodal analgesia with appropriate opioid all help decrease the risk of post-operative ileus.

POP QUIZ 7.6

Eggs are a good choice because they do not fall under the FODMAP category. Foods that fall under the FODMAP category include dairy, fruit, highly fermentable carbohydrates, onions, sorbitol, certain vegetables, and wheat.

POP QUIZ 7.7

CT angiography is the gold standard for diagnosing bowel ischemia.

CHAPTER 8

POP QUIZ 8.1

This patient needs urgent dialysis to lower the potassium level. Transfer to a higher level of care is indicated to monitor for EKG changes and for initiation of hemodialysis or continuous renal replacement therapy (if hemodynamically unstable).

POP QUIZ 8.2

While healthy, these meals are high in potassium. Patients with chronic kidney disease should limit the amount of potassium in their daily diet. The patient should be educated on the importance of minimizing dietary potassium in addition to adhering to medication therapy.

POP QUIZ 8.3

Patients with hypokalemia may also experience concurrent hypomagnesemia. Hypomagnesemia can exacerbate hypokalemia or make routine supplementation ineffective. Be sure to treat both electrolyte abnormalities to achieve normal values.

CHAPTER 9

POP QUIZ 9.1

Based on this information, the patient displays physical, environmental, and sensory risk factors for falling. Physical risk factors for falls include a history of diabetes and atrial fibrillation. Environmental risk factors include loose rugs and stairs in his house. Sensory risk factors include a history of impaired vision and wearing glasses.

POP QUIZ 9.2

Medication therapy (carbidopa/levodopa), deep brain stimulation, and a combination of exercise programs and cognitive training will help patients improve mobility and stability.

POP QUIZ 9.3

Physical activity helps decrease the risk for developing pneumonia, pressure ulcers, and blood clots.

CHAPTER 10

POP QUIZ 10.1

Although the patient is complaining of pain, she is still experiencing the effects of medications given in the operating room/post-anesthesia care unit. To provide additional narcotics for a patient with a respiratory rate of 8, on 4 LNC setting at 92%, responsive only to touch, who is unable to keep eyes open for prolonged periods, may be unsafe and place the patient at risk for further respiratory depression. Consider alternative nonnarcotic medications and nonpharmacologic interventions, such as heating pads, ice, or repositioning to manage this patient's pain until she becomes more awake following surgery.

POP QUIZ 10.2

Notify the provider and gather materials to draw stat blood cultures. It is important that two sets of blood cultures be obtained using sterile technique. Each set should include both an anaerobic and aerobic bottle.

POP QUIZ 10.3

If the patient was unresponsive to medical management for hyperkalemia and has decreased urine output, the patient may require dialysis.

CHAPTER 11

POP QUIZ 11.1

The nurse should attempt to de-escalate the situation before the patient becomes more violent by remaining calm and speaking to the patient reassuringly. The nurse should first attempt to engage the patient in conversation and establish a therapeutic relationship. The nurse should incorporate nonverbal communication strategies to appear less threatening. If these techniques are unsuccessful, administer medications or utilize restraints to protect the patient and staff.

POP QUIZ 11.2

Additional medications can be added in combination to address the patient's depression. Once stable, the patient can also undergo psychotherapy or electroconvulsive therapy as recommended by the provider.

POP QUIZ 11.3

Be alert for alcohol withdrawal symptoms to develop anywhere between 24 to 72 hr after the patient's last drink.

POP QUIZ 11.4

The nurse could discuss Alcoholics Anonymous or Narcotics Anonymous, depending on substance abuse disorder. The nurse could also discuss the possibility of inpatient or outpatient rehabilitation programs and the potential for using behavioral health resources like therapists or psychologists to support their recovery.

CHAPTER 12

POP QUIZ 12.1

The nurse should explain to the surgeon that the patient has been anxious all day and to allow the wife to meet with and talk to the surgeon to provide the best patient- and family-centered care. Suggest that the surgeon be on speakerphone with the wife while explaining the surgery to the patient. This would allow the wife to hear about the procedure, as well as ask any questions she may have. This will promote collaboration between the patient, family, and surgeon, as well as ease any anxiety the patient or his wife may have.

POP QUIZ 12.2

Before allowing the patient or family to use any medicinal herbal treatments to assist in her recovery, explain to the family the unit policy for using medicinal herbs. Gather the names and quantities of herbal remedies and consult the pharmacy and the provider to determine if there may be any interaction with medications the patient is currently taking. If medicinal herbs are not allowed, collaborate with the family to identify an acceptable alternative solution that allows the patient to practice her cultural beliefs while allowing hospital staff to provide safe care.

POP QUIZ 12.3

The nurse must first discuss and collaborate with the overseeing provider to determine whether her clinical status will allow for this travel. If the provider believes the patient is clinically stable enough for travel, the necessary orders to travel off unit should be obtained. Second, because this patient is trached requiring supplemental 35% oxygen via trach collar, a respiratory therapist should travel with the patient and nurse. If available, a patient care tech may also accompany the patient, nurse, and respiratory therapist as an additional set of hands. An emergency travel bag/equipment should be taken with the nurse in the event of an emergency. Once all orders are obtained and staff members are identified, a time and destination for travel should be chosen.

APPENDIX A: COMMON MEDICATIONS IN THE PROGRESSIVE CARE UNIT

TABLE A.1 Common Antibiotic and Antifungal Medications

GENERAL INDICATIONS	GENERAL MECHANISM OF ACTION	GENERAL CONTRAINDICATIONS, PRECAUTIONS, AND ADVERSE EFFECTS
Aminoglycosides (e.g., gentamicin, streptomycin, neomycin, etc.)		

Common indications among aminoglycosides:
 	
• Bacteremia and sepsis
• Bone and joint infections
• CAP
• Empiric treatment for febrile neutropenia
• Infective endocarditis
• Intra-abdominal infections
• Lower respiratory tract infections
• Nosocomial pneumonia
• Ophthalmic infections
• Surgical infection prophylaxis
 	
Specific indications for gentamicin:
 	
• Complicated UTIs
• Meningitis and ventriculitis
• PID
• Pyelonephritis
• Skin and skin structure infections
 	
Specific indications for streptomycin:
 	
• Gram-negative bacillary bacteremia, meningitis, or lower respiratory tract infections in combination with other antimicrobials
• UTI
• Drug susceptible tuberculosis
• Specific indications for neomycin:
  ◦ Adjunctive therapy for hepatic encephalopathy
  ◦ Infectious diarrhea
	• Inhibit bacterial protein synthesis, causing bactericidal effect	• Medication is contraindicated in administration for organisms resistant to aminoglycosides.
		• Use caution in administering to patients with inflammatory bowel disease, as there is a high likelihood for developing pseudomembranous colitis or *Clostridium difficile*.
		• Monitor closely for nephrotoxicity or neurotoxicity, including ototoxicity in all aminoglycoside medications. Nephrotoxicity or ototoxicity development requires dose adjustment or discontinuation.
		• Additional adverse effects include nausea, vomiting, auditory disturbances, headache, skin irritation, rash, anemia, and elevated liver enzymes.

(continued)

TABLE A.1 Common Antibiotic and Antifungal Medications (*continued*)

GENERAL INDICATIONS	GENERAL MECHANISM OF ACTION	GENERAL CONTRAINDICATIONS, PRECAUTIONS, AND ADVERSE EFFECTS
Antibiotic, sulfonamide derivative (TMP-SMX, also known as co-trimoxazol)		
• UTI • Pyelonephritis • Pneumocystic pneumonia • Otitis media • Acute bacterial exacerbations of chronic bronchitis	• Inhibits enzymes in folic acid synthesis pathway, causing bactericidal effects	• Medication is contraindicated in folate deficiency, megaloblastic anemia, G6PD deficiency, severe renal impairment, and hepatic disease. • Use caution in patients with hypothyroidism, colitis or GI disturbances, HIV/AIDS, cardiac disease, and dysrhythmia. • Adverse effects include megaloblastic anemia, aplastic anemia, hemolytic anemia, TTP, angioedema, Stevens-Johnson syndrome, exfoliative dermatitis, anaphylactic reaction, anuria, hyperkalemia, rhabdomyolysis, seizures, hemolysis, leukopenia, QT prolongation, chest pain, dyspnea, nausea, vomiting, itching, fever, and chills.
Antiprotozoals, respiratory (pentamidine)		
• Pneumocystis pneumonia • Leishmaniasis • Oral inhalation antifungal agent used for various fungal infections	• Mechanism of action not clearly known; thought to interfere with fungal DNA and RNA replication	• Use caution if administering rapidly, as it can lead to hypotension. • Use caution in patients with renal, hepatic, or cardiac disease, asthma, or pregnancy. • Adverse effects include dysrhythmia, bronchospasm, elevated AST/ALT, hypoglycemia, tremor, cough, fever, itching, diarrhea, headache, or night sweats.
Azoles (e.g., fluconazole, etc.)		
• Cutaneous leishmaniasis • Cutaneous or lymphocutaneous sporotrichosis • Skin or skin structure infection caused by *Candida* • Talaromycosis, coccidioidomycosis, or histoplasmosis prophylaxis in HIV-infected patients • Primary pulmonary histoplasmosis • Bacterial vaginosis	• Alter fungal cell membrane to inhibit fungal reproduction and growth through fungistatic action	• Use caution in cardiac, hepatic, or renal conditions. • Avoid use during pregnancy except in severe, life-threatening emergencies. • Adverse effects include dizziness, rash, diarrhea, nausea, and headache.

(continued)

TABLE A.1 Common Antibiotic and Antifungal Medications (*continued*)

GENERAL INDICATIONS	GENERAL MECHANISM OF ACTION	GENERAL CONTRAINDICATIONS, PRECAUTIONS, AND ADVERSE EFFECTS
Azoles (e.g., fluconazole, etc.) (continued)		
• Treatment and prophylaxis treatment for recurrent vulvovaginal candidiasis infections • Osteomyelitis, bone and joint infection caused by *Candida* • Infective endocarditis caused by *Candida* • Infected pacemaker, ICD, or VAD caused by *Candida* • Treatment of meningitis due to *Histoplasma capsulatum* in HIV-infected patients • CNS infections due to *Coccidioides*, cryptococcus, or *Candida* • Organ transplant recipients • Candida prophylaxis in bone marrow transplant or high-risk cancer patients • Pyelonephritis caused by *Candida* • UTI caused by *Candida* • Intra-abdominal infections caused by *Candida* • Pneumonia caused by *Candida* • Thrush		
Carbapenems (ertapenem, meropenem, etc.)		
Indications for both ertapenem and meropenem: • Bacterial encephalitis or meningitis • Intra-abdominal infections • Complicated skin and skin structure infections • Empiric treatment of febrile neutropenia • Bacteremia or sepsis • Pneumonia (CAP or nosocomial) Additional indications for ertapenem: • Complicated UTI and pyelonephritis • Acute pelvic infection • Surgical prophylaxis	• Inhibit cell wall synthesis by binding to penicillin-binding proteins inside bacterial cell wall, resulting in cell death to prevent organism growth	• Use caution in patients receiving carbapenem treatment who undergo concurrent hematologic testing. A positive Coombs test has been reported in patients taking carbapenems (meropenem). • Use caution in patients with cephalosporin, penicillin, or other beta-lactam hypersensitivity, as cross sensitivity is possible. • Use caution in head injury or neurologic disease due to risk of seizure associated with carbapenem administration. • Use caution in renal failure, impairment, or dysfunction, as carbapenems are excreted by the kidneys and can result in further damage.

(continued)

TABLE A.1 Common Antibiotic and Antifungal Medications (*continued*)

GENERAL INDICATIONS	GENERAL MECHANISM OF ACTION	GENERAL CONTRAINDICATIONS, PRECAUTIONS, AND ADVERSE EFFECTS
Carbapenems (ertapenem, meropenem, etc.) (continued)		
		• Use caution when administering to patients with inflammatory bowel disease due to high likelihood of developing pseudomembranous colitis and *clostridium difficile*. • Adverse effects include nausea, headache, diarrhea, rash, vomiting, confusion, delirium, hypoglycemia, pseudomembranous colitis, neutropenia, renal failure, and seizure.
Cephalosporins, first generation (cefazolin)		
• First-generation have coverage against most gram-positive cocci as well as gram-negative bacteria, for example, *Escherichia coli, Proteus mirabilis,* and *Klebsiella pneumoniae* • Upper respiratory tract infections • Skin and skin structure infections • Biliary tract infections • UTI • Infective endocarditis • Surgical infection prophylaxis • Lower respiratory tract infections (pneumococcal pneumonia and CAP) • Bacteremia • Bone and joint infections • Mastitis • Bacterial encephalitis or meningitis	• Inhibit cell wall synthesis by binding to penicillin-binding proteins inside bacterial cell wall, resulting in cell death to prevent organism growth causing bactericidal effect	• Do not administer in viral infections or organisms with antimicrobial resistance to cephalosporins. • Use caution in allergy to penicillin, as cross reaction is possible. • Use caution in renal failure, impairment, or dysfunction. Cephalosporins are excreted by the kidneys and can result in further damage. • Adverse effects include headache, diarrhea, nausea, vomiting, maculopapular rash, fever, confusion, bleeding, seizures, azotemia, and renal failure. • Medication is contraindicated in cephalosporin-resistant organisms and viral infection.
Cephalosporins, second generation (cefuroxime)		
• Second-generation cephalosporins have coverage against *Haemophilus influenza, Moraxella catarrhalis,* and *Bacteroides* spp. • Chronic bronchitis • Skin and skin structure infections • UTI • Treatment of bone and joint infection • Pharyngitis • Gonorrhea • Lyme disease	• Inhibit bacterial cell wall synthesis by binding to specific penicillin-binding proteins within the cell wall, causing bactericidal effect	• Medication is contraindicated in penicillin allergy, viral infections, or bacteria with known drug resistance. • Use caution in renal failure/impairment, pseudomembranous colitis, and phenylketonuria. • Adverse effects include nausea, vomiting, flatulence, dyspepsia, dysuria, phlebitis, jaundice, Stevens-Johnson syndrome, and vasculitis.

(continued)

TABLE A.1 Common Antibiotic and Antifungal Medications (*continued*)		
GENERAL INDICATIONS	**GENERAL MECHANISM OF ACTION**	**GENERAL CONTRAINDICATIONS, PRECAUTIONS, AND ADVERSE EFFECTS**
Cephalosporins, second generation (cefuroxime)(continued)		
• Acute otitis media • Bacteremia • Meningitis • Surgical infection prophylaxis • Tonsillitis • Sinusitis • Intra-abdominal infections • Lower respiratory tract infections • Pneumonia (CAP and nosocomial)		
Cephalosporins, third generation (ceftriaxone)		
• Bacteremia and sepsis • UTI • Acute bacterial otitis media • Skin and skin structure infections • Surgical incision site infections • Necrotizing infections • Intra-abdominal infections • Surgical infection prophylaxis • PID • Bone and joint infections • Lower respiratory tract infection • Pneumonia (nosocomial and CAP) • Infective endocarditis • Meningitis and vasculitis • Gonorrhea infection • Lyme disease • Congenital syphilis • Bacterial sinusitis • Third-generation cephalosporins: Less coverage against most gram-positive organisms, but increase coverage against Enterobacteriaceae, *Neisseria* spp., and *Haemophilus influenza*	• Inhibit bacterial cell wall synthesis by binding to specific penicillin-binding proteins within the cell wall, causing bactericidal effect	• Medication is contraindicated in penicillin allergy, jaundice, or hyperbilirubinemia in premature neonates, viral infection, or antimicrobial resistance. • Use caution in GI disease, as it may cause or worsen existing colitis. • Adverse effects include seizures, bronchospasm, pancreatitis, biliary obstruction, erythema multiforme, acute generalized exanthematous pustulosis, Stevens-Johnson syndrome, renal failure, thrombocytosis, elevated liver enzymes, anemia, thrombocytopenia, neutropenia, hypoprothrombinemia, jaundice, superinfection, edema, nausea, vomiting, headache, and itching.

(*continued*)

TABLE A.1 Common Antibiotic and Antifungal Medications (*continued*)

GENERAL INDICATIONS	GENERAL MECHANISM OF ACTION	GENERAL CONTRAINDICATIONS, PRECAUTIONS, AND ADVERSE EFFECTS
Cephalosporin, fourth generation (cefepime)		
• Monotherapy for febrile neutropenia • Complicated UTI and pyelonephritis • Intra-abdominal infections • Severe skin and skin structure infections • Pneumonia (CAP and nosocomial) • Bacterial meningitis • Infective endocarditis • Sepsis • Fourth-generation cephalosporins: Similar coverage as third-generation cephalosporins but with additional coverage against gram-negative bacteria with antimicrobial resistance (e.g., beta-lactamase)	• Inhibit bacterial cell wall synthesis by binding to specific penicillin-binding proteins within the cell wall, causing bactericidal effect	• Medication is contraindicated in penicillin allergy and antimicrobial resistance. • Use caution in colitis, GI disturbances, and renal failure. Cefepime may worsen colitis, other GI issues, and kidney function. • Adverse effects include seizure, anaphylactic shock, Stevens-Johnson syndrome, toxic epidermal necrolysis, erythema multiforme, agranulocytosis, pancytopenia, aplastic anemia, elevated liver enzymes, hypophosphatemia, hypoprothrombinemia, bleeding, colitis, vaginitis, pseudomembranous colitis, hypercalcemia, superinfection, confusion hallucination, rash, vomiting, diarrhea, itching, nausea, headache, and fever.
Cephalosporins, fifth generation (ceftaroline and fosamil)		
• Acute bacterial skin and skin structure infections • CAP • Sepsis • Coverage against methicillin-resistant staphylococci and penicillin-resistant pneumococci	• Inhibit bacterial cell wall synthesis by binding to specific penicillin-binding proteins within the cell wall, causing bactericidal effect	• Medication is contraindicated in viral infection and antimicrobial resistance. • Use caution in patients with colitis, GI disturbances, or renal impairments/failure. • Adverse effects include hyperkalemia or hypokalemia, bradycardia, seizure, renal failure, agranulocytosis, anaphylaxis, elevated liver enzymes, constipation, hepatitis, hyperglycemia, thrombocytopenia, pseudomembranous colitis, encephalopathy, diarrhea, rash, vomiting, abdominal pain, headache, and dizziness.

(*continued*)

TABLE A.1 Common Antibiotic and Antifungal Medications (*continued*)

GENERAL INDICATIONS	GENERAL MECHANISM OF ACTION	GENERAL CONTRAINDICATIONS, PRECAUTIONS, AND ADVERSE EFFECTS
Fluoroquinolones (e.g., ciprofloxacin, delafloxacin, levofloxacin, and moxifloxacin)		

GENERAL INDICATIONS	GENERAL MECHANISM OF ACTION	GENERAL CONTRAINDICATIONS, PRECAUTIONS, AND ADVERSE EFFECTS
• UTI, cystitis, and pyelonephritis • Lower respiratory tract infections, pneumonia (CAP and nosocomial) • Chronic bronchitis exacerbations • Skin and skin structure infections • Animal bite wounds • Enteric infections • Mild to moderate acute sinusitis • Acute prostatitis • Febrile neutropenia • Bacterial conjunctivitis • Ophthalmic infections related to corneal ulcers • Acute otitis externa • Bone and joint infections • Meningococcal infection/prophylaxis • Intra-abdominal infections • Peritoneal dialysis infections • Dental infections • Surgical infection prophylaxis • Pulmonary infections in cystic fibrosis • Infective endocarditis • Sepsis • Traveler's diarrhea • Broad spectrum antibiotics useful against gram-negative rods (*E. coli, Klebsiella* spp., *Proteus* spp., *Pseudomonas* spp., *Pseudomonas aeruginosa, Providencia* spp., and *Serratia marcescens. Streptococcus pneumoniae*); also effective against *H. influenzae, M. catarahalis, Legionella* spp., *Mycoplasma* spp., *Chlamydia pneumoniae*) • Effective against gram-positive organisms including *Staphylococcus aureus*, methacillin-resistant *S. aureus* • Effective against anaerobic bacteria, *Mycobacteria, Bacillus anthracis, Francisella tularensis*, and typhoid	• Inhibit DNA synthesis, causing bactericidal effect	• Use caution in patients with cardiac disease or cardiac dysrhythmias, CNS disorders, patients with history of myasthenia gravis, diabetes mellitus, renal impairments, and hepatic dysfunction. • Adverse effects include hepatotoxicity, phototoxicity, tendon rupture, neurotoxicity, hepatic dysfunction, hyper- or hypoglycemia, exacerbation of myasthenia gravis symptoms, worsening colitis or GI dysfunction, nausea, vomiting, or rash. • Discontinue immediately with any sign of tendon inflammation or tendon pain. These symptoms often present before tendon rupture.

(*continued*)

TABLE A.1 Common Antibiotic and Antifungal Medications (*continued*)

GENERAL INDICATIONS	GENERAL MECHANISM OF ACTION	GENERAL CONTRAINDICATIONS, PRECAUTIONS, AND ADVERSE EFFECTS
Glycopeptides (vancomycin)		
• Infective endocarditis • Pseudomembranous colitis due to *Clostridium difficile* infection • Enterocolitis • Sepsis and bacteremia • Serious gram-positive infections • Mastitis • Gram-positive lower respiratory infections (CAP and nosocomial pneumonia) • Pleural empyema • Surgical infection prophylaxis • Meningitis and other CNS infections • Bone and joint infections • Septic arthritis • Prosthetic joint infections • Febrile neutropenia • Intra-abdominal infections • Peritoneal dialysis-related peritonitis • Used to treat and prevent various bacterial infections caused by gram-positive bacteria, including MRSA • Effective for streptococci, enterococci, and MSSA infections	• Bind to parts of bacterial cell wall, preventing synthesis	• Medication is contraindicated in viral infection and vancomycin-resistant organisms. • Use caution in renal disease, hearing impairment, and HF. • Adverse effects include rash, itching, nausea, abdominal pain, fever, diarrhea, and Stevens-Johnson syndrome.
Lincosamides (clindamycin)		
• Bacteremia • Lower respiratory tract infections, including CAP and nosocomial pneumonia • Intra-abdominal infections • Skin and skin structure infections • Animal bites • Diabetic foot ulcer • Gynecologic infections • Bacterial vaginosis • Acne • Mastitis • Bone and joint infections • Bacterial sinusitis • Acute otitis media • Surgical infection prophylaxis	• Bind to RNA of bacteria to inhibit protein synthesis	• Medication is contraindicated in patients with a history of enteritis, ulcerative colitis, and pseudomembranous colitis. • Use caution in patients with diarrhea or hepatic disease. • Adverse effects include toxic epidermal necrolysis, Stevens-Johnson syndrome, erythema multiforme, exfoliative dermatitis, proteinuria, oliguria, superinfection, fungal overgrowth, pseudomembranous colitis, edema, leukopenia, thrombocytopenia, elevated hepatic enzyme, fever, fatigue, dizziness, vomiting, nausea, headache, and itching.

(continued)

TABLE A.1 Common Antibiotic and Antifungal Medications (*continued*)

GENERAL INDICATIONS	GENERAL MECHANISM OF ACTION	GENERAL CONTRAINDICATIONS, PRECAUTIONS, AND ADVERSE EFFECTS
Macrolides (azithromycin)		
• Mild to moderate bacterial exacerbations of chronic bronchitis in patients with COPD • Acute otitis media • Bacterial conjunctivitis • CAP • Skin and skin structure infections • PID • Gonorrhea • *Mycobacterium* infection • Acute bacterial sinusitis • Bacterial endocarditis prophylaxis	• Inhibit protein synthesis in bacterial cells, causing bacteriostatic effect • Bactericidal in high concentrations	• Medication is contraindicated in patients with a history of jaundice or hepatic dysfunction prior to macrolide use, viral infection, and drug-resistant bacteria. • Use caution in renal impairment, cardiovascular disease, colitis, or GI disease, and in patients with a history of myasthenia gravis. • Adverse effects include photosensitivity, dysrhythmia and QT prolongation, renal failure, hyperkalemia, bronchospasm, seizures, elevated liver enzymes, hyperbilirubinemia, constipation, jaundice, superinfection, anemia, dermatitis, and hypo- or hyperglycemia.
Oxazolidinones (linezolid)		
• Lower respiratory tract infections • CAP and nosocomial pneumonia • Skin and skin structure infections • Sepsis and bacteremia caused by vancomycin-resistant enterococcus • MRSA bacteremia • MRSA-associated bone and joint infection • Septic arthritis • Prosthetic joint infections • Meningitis and other CNS infections • Febrile neutropenia • Intra-abdominal infections • Peritonitis	• Inhibit bacterial protein synthesis by preventing translation and protein production, thus preventing bacterial growth	• Medication is contraindicated in concurrent use of metrizamide or iohexol during procedures requiring radiographic contrast administration. • Use caution in uncontrolled hypertension, concurrent use with MAOIs, diarrhea, pseudomembranous colitis, history of seizures, and diabetes (may cause hypoglycemia). • Adverse effects include myelosuppression, short-term decreased fertility in males, hypoglycemia, pancytopenia, optic neuritis, seizures, anaphylaxis, angioedema, anemia, thrombocytopenia, elevated hepatic enzymes, hypertension, hypoglycemia, pseudomembranous colitis, diarrhea, vomiting, abdominal pain, rash, itching, and tooth discoloration.

(continued)

TABLE A.1 Common Antibiotic and Antifungal Medications (*continued*)

GENERAL INDICATIONS	GENERAL MECHANISM OF ACTION	GENERAL CONTRAINDICATIONS, PRECAUTIONS, AND ADVERSE EFFECTS
Penicillins (ampicillin)		
• Severe infections including bacteremia • Infective endocarditis • Respiratory tract infections • Skin and skin structure infections • Genitourinary infections • UTI • GI infection	• Inhibit cell wall synthesis to produce a bactericidal effect, preventing organism growth	• Medication is contraindicated in penicillin-resistant organisms. • Use caution in renal impairments, cephalosporin and carbapenem hypersensitivity, colitis and other GI disturbances, and mononucleosis. • Adverse effects include antibiotic-associated colitis, anaphylaxis, exfoliative dermatitis, seizures, rash, nausea, vomiting, leukopenia, thrombocytopenia, platelet dysfunction, anemia, elevated hepatic enzymes, pseudomembranous colitis, superinfection, or diarrhea.
Tetracyclines (doxycycline)		
• Necrotizing ulcerative gingivitis • Treatment when penicillins are contraindicated • Uncomplicated gonorrhea • Chlamydia • Psittacosis • Respiratory tract infections • Skin and skin structure infection • Severe acne • Rocky Mountain spotted fever • Cholera	• Bind to ribosomes of susceptible bacteria and inhibit protein synthesis • Bacteriostatic, bactericidal in high concentrations	• There are no direct contraindications. • Use caution in renal impairment/failure, hepatic disease, colitis, and GI disease. • Adverse effects include photosensitivity, exfoliative dermatitis, enterocolitis, hepatic failure, pericarditis, anaphylaxis, hemolytic anemia, azotemia, blurred vision, dysphagia, erythema, thrombocytopenia, neutropenia, nail discoloration, headache, vomiting, diarrhea, nausea, rash, and tooth discoloration.

Note: All agents are contraindicated in the presence of hypersensitivity to the medication or one of its components.

AST/ALT, aspartate aminotransferase/alanine aminotransferase; CAP, community acquired pneumonia; CNS, central nervous system; COPD, chronic obstructive pulmonary disease; GI, gastrointestinal; HF, heart failure; ICD, implantable cardioverter-defibrillator; MAOIs, monoamine oxidase inhibitors; MRSA, methicillin-resistant *Staphylococcus aureus*; MSSA, methicillin-susceptible *Staphylococcus aureus*; PID, pelvic inflammatory disease; TMP-SMX, trimethoprim/sulfamethoxazole; TTP, thrombotic thrombocytopenic purpura; UTI, urinary tract infection; VAD, ventricular assist device.

RESOURCES

Hooper, D., Calderwood, S., & Bogorodskaya, M. (n.d.). Fluroquinolones. *UpToDate*. https://www.uptodate.com/contents/fluoroquinolones

Prescribers' Digital Reference. (n.d.-a). *Amikacin sulfate* [Drug information]. PDR Search. https://www.pdr.net/drug-summary/Amikacin-Sulfate-amikacin-sulfate-676

Prescribers' Digital Reference. (n.d.-b). *Ampicillin* [Drug information]. PDR Search. https://www.pdr.net/drug-summary/Ampicillin-for-Injection-ampicillin-677

Prescribers' Digital Reference. (n.d.-c). *Azithromycin* [Drug information]. PDR Search. https://www.pdr.net/drug-summary/Azithromycin-azithromycin-24249

Prescribers' Digital Reference. (n.d.-d). *Bactrim* [Drug information]. PDR Search. https://www.pdr.net/drug-summary/Bactrim-Bactrim-DS-sulfamethoxazole-trimethoprim-686

Prescribers' Digital Reference. (n.d.-e). *Cefazolin* [Drug information]. PDR Search. https://www.pdr.net/drug-summary/Cefazolin-Sodium-cefazolin-sodium-1193

Prescribers' Digital Reference. (n.d.-f). *Cefepime (Maxipime)* [Drug information]. PDR Search. https://www.pdr.net/drug-summary/Maxipime-cefepime-hydrochloride-3215.5755

Prescribers' Digital Reference. (n.d.-g). *Ceftriaxone* [Drug information]. PDR Search. https://www.pdr.net/drug-summary/Ceftriaxone-ceftriaxone-1723

Prescribers' Digital Reference. (n.d.-h). *Cefuroxime* [Drug information]. PDR Search. https://www.pdr.net/drug-summary/Zinacef-cefuroxime-242

Prescribers' Digital Reference. (n.d.-i). *Ciprofloxacin* [Drug information]. PDR Search. https://www.pdr.net/drug-summary/Ciprofloxacin-Injection-ciprofloxacin-3255

Prescribers' Digital Reference. (n.d.-j). *Clindamycin* [Drug information]. PDR Search. https://www.pdr.net/drug-summary/Cleocin-Phosphate-Injection-clindamycin-1865

Prescribers' Digital Reference. (n.d.-k). *Doxycycline* [Drug information]. PDR Search. https://www.pdr.net/drug-summary/Doxycycline-doxycycline-24308

Prescribers' Digital Reference. (n.d.-l). *Ertapenem* [Drug information]. PDR Search. https://www.pdr.net/drug-summary/Invanz-ertapenem-359

Prescribers' Digital Reference. (n.d.-m). *Fluconazole* [Drug information]. PDR Search. https://www.pdr.net/drug-summary/Diflucan-fluconazole-1847

Prescribers' Digital Reference. (n.d.-n). *Gentamicin sulfate* [Drug information]. PDR Search. https://www.pdr.net/drug-summary/Gentamicin-Injection-40-mg-mL-gentamicin-sulfate-3299

Prescribers' Digital Reference. (n.d.-o). *Merrem* [Drug information]. PDR Search. https://www.pdr.net/drug-summary/Merrem-meropenem-2055

Prescribers' Digital Reference. (n.d.-p). *Neomycin* [Drug information]. PDR Search. https://www.pdr.net/drug-summary/Neomycin-Sulfate-neomycin-sulfate-819

Prescribers' Digital Reference. (n.d.-q). *Pentamidine* [Drug information]. PDR Search. https://www.pdr.net/drug-summary/NebuPent-pentamidine-isethionate-1408

Prescribers' Digital Reference. (n.d.-r). *Streptomycin* [Drug information]. PDR Search. https://www.pdr.net/drug-summary/Streptomycin-streptomycin-1600

Prescribers' Digital Reference. (n.d.-s). *Teflaro (ceftaroline fosamil)* [Drug information]. PDR Search. https://www.pdr.net/drug-summary/Teflaro-ceftaroline-fosamil-158

Prescribers' Digital Reference. (n.d.-t). *Tobramycin* [Drug information]. PDR Search. https://www.pdr.net/drug-summary/Tobramycin-tobramycin-916

Prescribers' Digital Reference. (n.d.-u). *Vancomycin* [Drug information]. PDR Search. https://www.pdr.net/drug-summary/Vancocin-vancomycin-hydrochloride-802

Prescribers' Digital Reference. (n.d.-v). *Zyvox (Linezolid)* [Drug information]. PDR Search. https://www.pdr.net/drug-summary/Zyvox-linezolid-2341

TABLE A.2 Common Pain and Sedation Medications

GENERAL INDICATIONS	GENERAL MECHANISM OF ACTION	GENERAL CONTRAINDICATIONS, PRECAUTIONS, AND ADVERSE EFFECTS
Analgesics with antipyretic activity: Acetaminophen		
• Fever • Mild pain or temporary relief of headache, myalgia, back pain, musculoskeletal pain, dental pain, dysmenorrhea, arthralgia and minor aches, and pains with the common cold or flu • Moderate to severe pain with adjunctive opioid analgesics • Osteoarthritis pain • Acute migraine	• Increase pain threshold by inhibiting prostaglandin synthesis through the COX pathway	• Medication is contraindicated in severe hepatic impairment or severe active hepatic disease. • Use caution in renal disease or patients with G6PD. • Adverse effects include elevated hepatic enzymes, rash, jaundice, hypoprothrombinemia, neutropenia, angioedema, hemolytic anemia, and rhabdomyolysis.
Barbiturates (phenobarbital)		
• Status epilepticus • Maintenance of all types of seizures • Short-term treatment of insomnia • Procedural sedation • Relief of preoperative anxiety • Sedation maintenance • Relieves anxiety, tension, and apprehension	• Nonselective CNS depressant with sedative hypnotic actions	• Medication is contraindicated in pulmonary disease in which obstruction or dyspnea is present, hepatic disease or hepatic encephalopathy, pregnancy, and porphyria. • Use caution in acute pain, as paradoxical reactions can occur. • Use caution during rapid IV administration, as this can cause bronchospasm. • Do not abruptly discontinue medication, as withdrawal can occur. • Adverse effects include suicidal ideation, megaloblastic anemia, bradycardia, depression, tolerance, impaired cognition, respiratory depression, confusion, elevated liver enzymes, hepatitis, jaundice, neutropenia, dependence, emotional lability, rash, nausea, vomiting, fatigue, decreased libido, and ptosis.

(continued)

TABLE A.2 Common Pain and Sedation Medications (*continued*)

GENERAL INDICATIONS	GENERAL MECHANISM OF ACTION	GENERAL CONTRAINDICATIONS, PRECAUTIONS, AND ADVERSE EFFECTS
Gabapentinoids (gabapentin)		
• Adjunct treatment of partial seizures • Neuropathic pain • Moderate to severe restless leg syndrome • ALS • Tremor • Nystagmus • Spasticity due to MS • Pruritis • Fibromyalgia • Dysautonomia following severe TBI • Alcohol dependence	• Exact mechanism of action with GABA receptors unknown • Show a high affinity for binding sites throughout the brain correspondent to the presence of the voltage-gated calcium channels, especially alpha-2-delta-1, which seems to inhibit release of excitatory neurotransmitters in presynaptic area which participate in epileptogenesis	• There are no contraindications to use. • Use caution in renal failure and pulmonary disease. Gabapentin is excreted in the kidneys; dose adjustments may be required for patients in renal failure or with renal impairments. • Do not abruptly discontinue, as withdrawal symptoms can occur. • Adverse effects include hyperglycemia, tolerance, depression, confusion and memory impairments, dehydration, jaundice, respiratory depression, dizziness, headache, fatigue, nausea and vomiting, tremor, decreased libido, back pain, emotional lability, skin irritation, diarrhea, and irritability.
General anesthetics: Etomidate		
• General anesthesia induction • Sedation during RSI • Procedural sedation	• Increase GABA transmission by increasing the number of GABA receptors available through displacement of natural binding of GABA inhibitors	• There are no true contraindications. • Avoid use, if possible, with sepsis or septic shock. • Use caution in geriatric patients, as it can cause cardiac depression. • Use caution in hepatic disease, as etomidate is metabolized in the liver. • Adverse effects include apnea, laryngospasm, bradycardia, dysrhythmia, anaphylaxis, respiratory depression, hypoventilation, hypo/hypertension, sinus tachycardia, nausea, and vomiting.
General anesthetics: Ketamine		
• General anesthesia induction/maintenance • Preanesthetic sedation • Treatment of refractory bronchospasm in status asthmaticus • Treatment-resistant depression in adults • Moderate to severe pain • Induction agent during RSI • ICU sedation	• Interrupt pathways in the brain prior to producing somesthetic sensory blockade and selectively depress the thalamo-neocortical system	• Medication is contraindicated in which additional blood pressure increase would be hazardous, including hypertension, hypertensive crisis, stroke, head trauma, intercranial mass, or intracranial bleeding. • Use caution in glaucoma or patients with increased ICP, alcoholism, substance abuse, and thyrotoxicosis. • Adverse effects include bradycardia, diabetes insipidus, dysrhythmia, laryngospasm, apnea, ocular hypertension, increased ICP, hallucinations, delirium, hypertension, respiratory depression, confusion, withdrawal, psychosis, dysphoria, urinary incontinence, nightmares, nausea, vomiting, anxiety, and insomnia.

(*continued*)

TABLE A.2 Common Pain and Sedation Medications (*continued*)

GENERAL INDICATIONS	GENERAL MECHANISM OF ACTION	GENERAL CONTRAINDICATIONS, PRECAUTIONS, AND ADVERSE EFFECTS
General anesthetics: Propofol		
• General anesthesia • ICU sedation • Conscious sedation • Refractory status epilepticus • Refractory migraine • Postoperative nausea and vomiting prophylaxis • Agitation associated with alcohol withdrawal	• Inhibit NMDA receptors through channel gating modulation with agonistic activity at the GABA receptor	• Propofol is contraindicated when general anesthesia or sedation is contraindicated. • Use caution in cardiac disease, sepsis, and hypovolemia, as these patients will be more susceptible to propofol-induced hypotension. • Use caution in pancreatitis and hyperlipidemia; due to high lipid content, propofol can exacerbate or worsen these conditions. • Adverse effects include bradycardia, dysrhythmia, laryngospasm, bronchospasm, hyperkalemia, ileus, hypotension, edema, hypoventilation, euphoria, wheezing, elevated hepatic enzymes, respiratory depression, hypertriglyceridemia, hepatomegaly, and drowsiness.
Opioids: Fentanyl		
• Control of moderate to severe pain • Intraoperative or procedural management of severe pain • Postoperative pain management • Management of chronic severe pain in opioid-tolerant patients requiring around the clock long-term opioid treatment • Management of severe breakthrough cancer pain in opioid tolerant patients • Short-term management of acute postoperative pain • Adjunctive management of general anesthesia maintenance • Major surgery	• Bind to pain receptors in the body to decrease pain pathways and alleviate pain	• Transdermal fentanyl patches are contraindicated in patients with known or suspected paralytic ileus or GI obstruction. • Nonparenteral fentanyl is contraindicated in status asthmaticus or severe respiratory depression. • Do not stop taking medication abruptly, as it may cause withdrawal symptoms. • Use caution in patients with history of alcoholism or substance abuse, as there is a high risk for psychologic dependence. • Use with caution in patients with respiratory disorders, as it may cause respiratory depression. • Use caution in head trauma and neurologic disorder, as it may increase drowsiness and decrease respirations. • Adverse effects include GI obstruction, bradycardia, laryngospasm, respiratory depression, pneumothorax, apnea, chest wall rigidity, ileus, dysrhythmia, constipation, hypokalemia, hypoventilation, dyspnea, confusion, hallucinations, dysphoria, blurred vision, psychologic and physiologic dependance, withdrawal, rash, vomiting, abnormal dreams, drowsiness, fatigue, paranoia, anxiety, agitation, emotional lability, and nausea.

(continued)

TABLE A.2 Common Pain and Sedation Medications (*continued*)

GENERAL INDICATIONS	GENERAL MECHANISM OF ACTION	GENERAL CONTRAINDICATIONS, PRECAUTIONS, AND ADVERSE EFFECTS
Opioids: Fentanyl (continued)		
• Analgesia/sedation in mechanically ventilated patients • Sedation and analgesia prior to RSI • Management of dyspnea in patients with end-stage cancer or lung disease • Procedural sedation		
Opioids: Hydrocodone		
• Treatment of chronic severe pain requiring around the clock long-term opioid treatment • Treatment of refractory restless leg syndrome	• Agonistic activity at the mu receptors resulting in changes in the perception of pain at the spinal cord and into the CNS	• Medication is contraindicated in patients with significant respiratory depression, acute or severe asthma, known or suspected GI obstruction, or paralytic ileus. • Use caution in substance abuse, depression, geriatric populations, CNS depression and/or head trauma, increased ICP, psychosis, opioid naïve patients, seizures, cardiac disease, adrenal insufficiency, hypothyroidism, or myxedema. • Long-term use may increase risk of infertility. • Adverse reactions include GI obstructions, seizures, apnea, SIADH, respiratory arrest, constipation, depression, dyspnea, confusion, withdrawal if abruptly discontinued, respiratory depression, hypoxia, hypotension, psychologic and physiologic dependence, infertility, nausea, tremor, anxiety, dizziness, and drowsiness.
Opioids: Hydromorphone		
• Relief of moderate to severe pain • Management of chronic severe pain in opioid-tolerant patients requiring around the clock long-term opioid treatment • Analgesia and/or sedation in mechanically ventilated patients	• Acts at the mu receptor causing changes in perception to pain at the spinal cord and into the CNS	• Medication is contraindicated in patients with respiratory depression, status asthmaticus (immediate release tablets), paralytic ileus (extended-release tablets), and sulfite hypersensitivity. • Use caution in substance abuse, opioid naïve patients, head trauma or CNS depression, cardiac disease, geriatric populations, adrenal insufficiency, hypothyroidism, and myxedema.

(*continued*)

TABLE A.2 Common Pain and Sedation Medications (*continued*)

GENERAL INDICATIONS	GENERAL MECHANISM OF ACTION	GENERAL CONTRAINDICATIONS, PRECAUTIONS, AND ADVERSE EFFECTS
Opioids: Hydromorphone (continued)		
		• Adverse reactions include bronchospasm, GI obstruction, bradycardia, anaphylaxis, laryngospasm, apnea, respiratory arrest, ileus, constipation, depression, dysphoria, hallucinations, confusion, euphoria, withdrawal if abruptly discontinued, urinary retention, nausea, drowsiness, vomiting, fatigue, dizziness, diarrhea, anxiety, tremor, paranoia, and lethargy.
Opioids: Morphine		
• Acute and chronic moderate to severe pain • Management of chronic severe pain in patients who require daily around the clock long-term opioid treatment • Dyspnea in patients with end-stage cancer or pulmonary disease • Procedural sedation • Painful diabetic neuropathy • Refractory restless leg syndrome	• Act at the mu receptor, causing changes in perception to pain at the spinal cord and into the CNS	• Medication is contraindicated in significant respiratory depression in unmonitored settings, acute or severe bronchial asthma (oral solutions), respiratory depression or hypoxia, upper airway obstruction, acute alcoholism, delirium tremens (rectal route), known or suspected GI obstruction or paralytic ileus, hypovolemia, circulatory shock, cardiac dysrhythmia or HF secondary to chronic lung disease, and concurrent use with MAOI therapy. • Use caution in substance abuse, alcoholism, opioid naïve patients, CNS depression, head trauma, seizures or increased ICP, cardiac disease, adrenal insufficiency, hypothyroidism, and myxedema. • Do not abruptly discontinue, as withdrawal symptoms can occur. • Adverse effects include ileus, bradycardia, dysrhythmia, increased ICP, bronchospasm, GI obstruction, laryngospasm, depression, confusion, hypoxia, edema, euphoria, delirium, dysphagia, hallucinations, psychosis, physiologic dependence, adrenocortical insufficiency, drowsiness, diarrhea, constipation, headache, fever, nausea, restlessness, and vomiting.

(continued)

TABLE A.2 Common Pain and Sedation Medications (*continued*)

GENERAL INDICATIONS	GENERAL MECHANISM OF ACTION	GENERAL CONTRAINDICATIONS, PRECAUTIONS, AND ADVERSE EFFECTS
Opioids: Oxycodone		
• Treatment of severe pain • Management of chronic severe pain in patients requiring daily around the clock long-term opioid management • Painful diabetic neuropathy • Restless leg syndrome	• Mu receptor agonist that changes pain perceptions at the spinal cord and into the CNS	• Medication is contraindicated in patients with significant respiratory depression, patients with hypercarbia, GI obstruction, and paralytic ileus. • Use caution in opioid naïve patients, with abrupt discontinuation, CNS depression, head trauma, psychosis and increased ICP, cardiovascular disease, seizures, adrenal insufficiency, hypothyroidism, and myxedema. • Adverse effects include laryngospasm, seizure, ileus, bradycardia, GI obstruction, constipation, euphoria, dysphoria, confusion, blurred vision, dysuria, dyspnea, hypotension, hallucinations, nausea, drowsiness, vomiting, diarrhea, abdominal pain, or fatigue.
Opioids: Tramadol		
• Moderate to moderately severe acute pain • Moderate chronic pain or moderately severe chronic pain in patients requiring continuous around the clock treatment for an extended period of time • Adjunctive treatment of osteoarthritis • Diabetic neuropathy • Postherpetic neuralgia • Postoperative shivering	• Agonistic activity at the central opiate receptor	• There are no direct contraindications. • Use caution in polysorbate 80 hypersensitivity, CNS depression, head trauma, seizure and increased ICP, severe pulmonary disease, biliary disease, GI obstruction or GI disease, substance abuse, renal or hepatic impairments, geriatric population, adrenal insufficiency, hypothyroidism, and myxedema. • Adverse effects include hepatic failure, pancreatitis, bradycardia, seizures, pulmonary edema, dysrhythmia, bronchospasm, constipation, hallucinations, hypertension, hypertonia, dyspnea, urinary retention, peripheral edema, blurred vision, withdrawal with abrupt discontinuation, hepatitis, amnesia, confusion, nausea, dizziness, headache, vomiting, drowsiness, agitation, and pruritus.
Sedatives: Benzodiazepines (midazolam)		
• Procedural sedation • Amnesia induction • Control of preoperative anxiety • General anesthesia induction and maintenance • Seizures	• Act on the hypothalamic, thalamic, and limbic regions to produce CNS depression	• Medication is contraindicated in sleep apnea or severe respiratory insufficiency/failure that is not mechanically ventilated, acute closed angle glaucoma. • Use caution in geriatric populations; psychiatric conditions including bipolar disorder; depression; mania; psychosis, or suicidal ideation; CNS depression; hepatic disease; substance use/abuse; and dementia.

(continued)

TABLE A.2 Common Pain and Sedation Medications (*continued*)

GENERAL INDICATIONS	GENERAL MECHANISM OF ACTION	GENERAL CONTRAINDICATIONS, PRECAUTIONS, AND ADVERSE EFFECTS
Sedatives: Benzodiazepines (midazolam) (continued)		
• Sedation maintenance in mechanically ventilated patients • Relief of agitation and/or anxiety • Treatment of status epilepticus refractory to standard therapy • Sedation during RSI • Treatment of alcohol withdrawal including delirium tremens		• Adverse effects include coma, seizure, apnea, pneumothorax, dysrhythmia, bradycardia, delirium, confusion, hypotension, hallucinations, memory impairment, constipation, respiratory depression, tolerance, psychologic dependance, withdrawal if abruptly discontinued, drowsiness, dizziness, weakness, headache, and tremor.
Sedatives: Dexmedetomidine		
• Sedation induction and maintenance of mechanically ventilated ICU patients • Procedural sedation of nonintubated patients undergoing surgical procedure • Preanesthetic sedation	• Centrally act as agonist to alpha2-adrenoceptors, resulting in sedation and analgesia without significant ventilatory effects	• There are no direct contraindications. • Use caution in patients with hypovolemia, diabetes, bradycardia, hypotension, uncontrolled hypertension, hepatic disease, and renal failure. • Adverse effects include hypotension and bradycardia (may require decreased dose or discontinuation), dysrhythmia, hyperkalemia, renal failure, apnea, respiratory depression, hypoxia, hypovolemia, anemia, nausea, anxiety, fever, vomiting, diaphoresis, dizziness, headache, and diarrhea.

ALS, amyotrophic lateral sclerosis; CNS, central nervous system; GABA, gamma-aminobutyric acid; GI, gastrointestinal; HF, heart failure; ICP, intracranial pressure; IV, intravenous; MAOIs, monoamine oxidase inhibitors; MS, multiple sclerosis; NMDA, N-methyl-d-aspartate; RSI, rapid sequence intubation; SIADH, syndrome of inappropriate antidiuretic hormone; TBI, traumatic brain injury.

RESOURCES

Prescribers' Digital Reference. (n.d.-a). *Acetaminophen* [Drug information]. PDR Search. https://www.pdr.net/drug-summary/Ofirmev-acetaminophen-1346

Prescribers' Digital Reference. (n.d.-b). *Amidate (etomidate)* [Drug information]. PDR Search. https://www.pdr.net/drug-summary/Amidate-etomidate-675

Prescribers' Digital Reference. (n.d.-c). *Ativan* [Drug information]. PDR Search. https://www.pdr.net/drug-summary/Ativan-Injection-lorazepam-996

Prescribers' Digital Reference. (n.d.-d). *Ativan* [Drug information]. PDR Search. https://www.pdr.net/drug-summary/Precedex-dexmedetomidine-hydrochloride-1271

Prescribers' Digital Reference. (n.d.-e). *Dilaudid* [Drug information]. PDR Search. https://www.pdr.net/drug-summary/Dilaudid-Injection-and-HP-Injection-hydromorphone-hydrochloride-490

Prescribers' Digital Reference. (n.d.-f). *Diprovan* [Drug information]. PDR Search. https://www.pdr.net/drug-summary/Diprivan-propofol-1719

Prescribers' Digital Reference. (n.d.-g). *Fentanyl* [Drug information]. PDR Search. https://www.pdr.net/drug-summary/Fentanyl-Citrate-fentanyl-citrate-2474

Prescribers' Digital Reference. (n.d.-h). *Ketamine* [Drug information]. PDR Search. https://www.pdr.net/drug-summary/Ketalar-ketamine-hydrochloride-1999#10

Prescribers' Digital Reference. (n.d.-i). *Morphine* [Drug information]. PDR Search. https://www.pdr.net/drug-summary/Morphine-Sulfate-Tablets-morphine-sulfate-1520

Prescribers' Digital Reference. (n.d.-j). *Neurontin* [Drug information]. PDR Search. https://www.pdr.net/drug-summary/Neurontin-gabapentin-2477.4218

Prescribers' Digital Reference. (n.d.-k). *Oxycodone* [Drug information]. PDR Search. https://www.pdr.net/drug-summary/Oxycodone-HCl-oxycodone-hydrochloride-24333

Prescribers' Digital Reference. (n.d.-l). *Phenobarbital* [Drug information]. PDR Search. https://www.pdr.net/drug-summary/Phenobarbital-Elixir-phenobarbital-2669#10

Prescribers' Digital Reference. (n.d.-m). *Zohydro-ER (hydrocodone)* [Drug information]. PDR Search. https://www.pdr.net/drug-summary/Zohydro-ER-hydrocodone-bitartrate-3389

TABLE A.3 Common Intravenous Fluids

GENERAL INDICATIONS	GENERAL MECHANISM OF ACTION	GENERAL CONTRAINDICATIONS, PRECAUTIONS, AND ADVERSE EFFECTS
D5NS		
• Parenteral (IV) treatment for hypoglycemia and hyperkalemia • Nutritional and parenteral nutrition	• Replace and supplement glucose, supplies energy to cells	• Medication is contraindicated in hyperglycemia and severe dehydration. Dextrose solutions can worsen the patient's hyperosmolar state. • Use caution in hypernatremia, hyperchloremia, metabolic acidosis, infection, diabetes, hepatic disease, in HF with fluid overload, and electrolyte imbalance. • Adverse effects include hyperglycemia.
D5W		
• Parenteral (IV) treatment for hypoglycemia and hyperkalemia • Nutritional and parenteral nutrition • Oral glucose tolerance test	• Replace and supplement glucose • Supply energy to cells	• Medication is contraindicated in hyperglycemia and severe dehydration. Dextrose solutions can worsen the patient's hyperosmolar state. • Use caution in infection, diabetes, hepatic disease, HF with fluid overload, and electrolyte imbalance. • Adverse effects include hyperglycemia.

(continued)

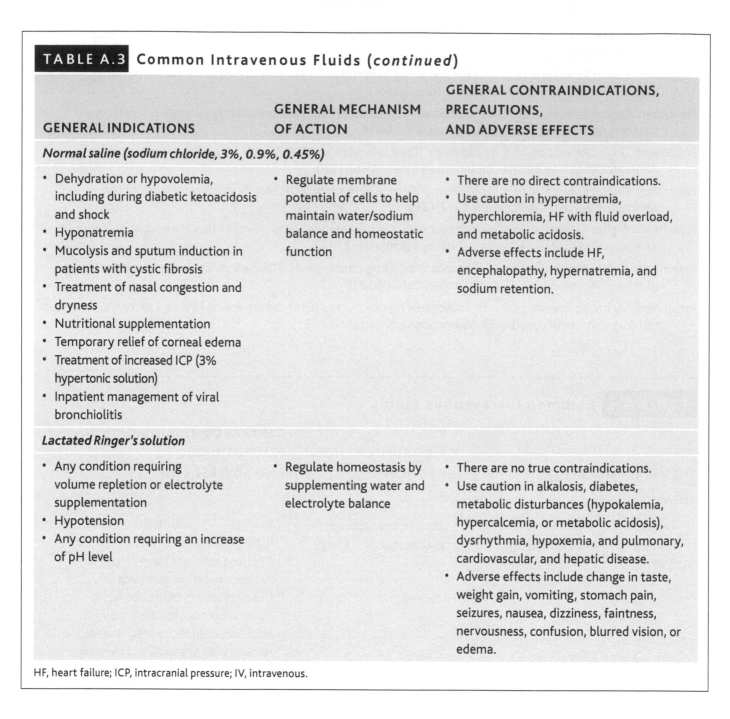

TABLE A.3 Common Intravenous Fluids (*continued*)

GENERAL INDICATIONS	GENERAL MECHANISM OF ACTION	GENERAL CONTRAINDICATIONS, PRECAUTIONS, AND ADVERSE EFFECTS
Normal saline (sodium chloride, 3%, 0.9%, 0.45%)		
• Dehydration or hypovolemia, including during diabetic ketoacidosis and shock • Hyponatremia • Mucolysis and sputum induction in patients with cystic fibrosis • Treatment of nasal congestion and dryness • Nutritional supplementation • Temporary relief of corneal edema • Treatment of increased ICP (3% hypertonic solution) • Inpatient management of viral bronchiolitis	• Regulate membrane potential of cells to help maintain water/sodium balance and homeostatic function	• There are no direct contraindications. • Use caution in hypernatremia, hyperchloremia, HF with fluid overload, and metabolic acidosis. • Adverse effects include HF, encephalopathy, hypernatremia, and sodium retention.
Lactated Ringer's solution		
• Any condition requiring volume repletion or electrolyte supplementation • Hypotension • Any condition requiring an increase of pH level	• Regulate homeostasis by supplementing water and electrolyte balance	• There are no true contraindications. • Use caution in alkalosis, diabetes, metabolic disturbances (hypokalemia, hypercalcemia, or metabolic acidosis), dysrhythmia, hypoxemia, and pulmonary, cardiovascular, and hepatic disease. • Adverse effects include change in taste, weight gain, vomiting, stomach pain, seizures, nausea, dizziness, faintness, nervousness, confusion, blurred vision, or edema.

HF, heart failure; ICP, intracranial pressure; IV, intravenous.

RESOURCES

Mayo Foundation for Medical Education and Research. (2021, February 1). *Lactated Ringer's (INTRAVENOUS route) side effects*. https://www.mayoclinic.org/drugs-supplements/lactated-ringers-intravenous-route/side-effects/drg-20489612?p=1

Prescribers' Digital Reference. (n.d.-a). *Dextrose monohydrate* [Drug information]. PDR Search. https://www.pdr.net/drug-summary/5--Dextrose-dextrose-monohydrate-24283

Prescribers' Digital Reference. (n.d.-b). *Sodium chloride* [Drug information]. PDR Search. https://www.pdr.net/drug-summary/Sodium-Chloride-sodium-chloride-24245

TABLE A.4 Common Steroid Medications

GENERAL INDICATIONS	GENERAL MECHANISM OF ACTION	GENERAL CONTRAINDICATIONS, PRECAUTIONS, AND ADVERSE EFFECTS
Corticosteroids (prednisone, dexamethasone, methylprednisolone)		
• Maintenance therapy of primary or secondary adrenocortical insufficiency • Congenital adrenal hyperplasia • Kidney transplant rejection prophylaxis • Chronic graft versus host disease • Acute lymphocytic leukemia • Chronic lymphocytic leukemia • Short-term treatment of hypercalcemia secondary disease • Inflammatory bowel disease • Crohn's disease • Ulcerative colitis • Rheumatic conditions • Systemic autoimmune conditions • Hemolytic anemia • Asthma exacerbation • Thrombocytopenia or ITP • Myasthenia gravis • Psoriatic arthritis • Proteinuria in nephrotic syndrome • Severe erythema multiforme or Stevens-Johnson syndrome • Treatment of ACE-inhibitor-induced angioedema • Allergic disorders including anaphylaxis • ARDS • Pneumonia • Hodgkin lymphoma • Multiple myeloma • Duchenne muscular dystrophy • Carpal tunnel syndrome • Autoimmune hepatitis • Primary amyloidosis • Exacerbation of COPD • Idiopathic or viral pericarditis • Interstitial nephritis • Bell's palsy • Transplant rejection • Guillain-Barré syndrome	• Inhibit steps in the inflammatory pathway to prevent systemic infection and inflammation of the lungs and to reduce mucus production	• Patients receiving corticosteroids for an extended time or in high doses are at increased risk of immunosuppression, making them more prone to infection. • Avoid in patients with Cushing's syndrome. • Use caution in untreated infection, diabetes, glaucoma, immunosuppression, and liver disease. • Adverse effects include growth inhibition, osteoporosis, osteopenia, impaired wound healing, immunosuppression, candidiasis, fluid retention, hypernatremia, euphoria, hallucinations, hyperglycemia, nausea, weight gain, fluid retention, emotional lability, headache, hoarseness, diaphoresis, and bronchospasm. • Medication may reduce glucose tolerance, causing hyperglycemia in diabetic patients.

ACE, angiotensin-converting enzyme; ARDS, acute respiratory distress syndrome; COPD, chronic obstructive pulmonary disease; ITP, immune thrombocytopenic purpura.

RESOURCES

Prescribers' Digital Reference. (n.d.). *Prednisone* [Drug information]. PDR Search. https://www.pdr.net/drug
-summary/Prednisone-Prednisone-Intensol-prednisone-2575

INDEX

Page entries that appear in italics refer to content in the practice test and practice test answer chapters.